Smart Devices for Medical 4.0 Technologies

The aim of this book is to identify some of the challenges that need to be addressed to accelerate the deployment and adoption of smart health technologies for ubiquitous healthcare access especially in wearable devices. These wearable devices may include pacemakers, defibrillators, RFID devices, assistive devices for the visually impaired, magnifiers, and talking assistants. It also explores how Internet of Things (IoT) and big data technologies can be combined with these wearable devices to provide better healthcare solutions.

Features:

- Focuses on real-time implementation of deep and machine learning techniques as well as novel algorithms for smart healthcare.
- Explores innovative challenges and solutions to complex problems in assistive devices with Medical 4.0 technologies.
- Presents an overview of challenges in the design of medical wearable devices.
- Discusses different techniques on VLSI for medical devices.
- Includes a case study on an AI-tuned cardiac pacemaker.

This book is aimed at graduate students and researchers in biomedical, electrical, computer engineering, and medical technologies.

Advances in Smart Healthcare Technologies

Editors: Chinmay Chakraborty and Joel J. P. C. Rodrigues

This book series focus on recent advances and different research areas in smart health-care technologies including Internet of Medical Things (IoMedT), e-Health, personalized medicine, sensing, Big Data, telemedicine, etc. under the healthcare informatics umbrella. Overall focus is on bringing together the latest industrial and academic progress, research, and development efforts within the rapidly maturing health informatics ecosystem. It aims to offer valuable perceptions to researchers and engineers on how to design and develop novel healthcare systems and how to improve patient's information delivery care remotely. The potential for making faster advances in many scientific disciplines and improving the profitability and success of different enterprises is to be investigated.

Blockchain Technology in Healthcare Applications
Social, Economic and Technological Implications
Bharat Bhushan, Nitin Rakesh, Yousef Farhaoui, Parma Nand Astya and Bhuvan Unhelkar

Digital Health Transformation with Blockchain and Artificial Intelligence
Chinmay Chakraborty

Smart and Secure Internet of Healthcare Things
Nitin Gupta, Jagdeep Singh, Chinmay Chakraborty, Mamoun Alazab and Dinh-Thuan Do

Practical Artificial Intelligence for Internet of Medical Things
Emerging Trends, Issues, and Challenges
Edited by Ben Othman Soufiene, Chinmay Chakraborty, and Faris A. Almalki

Intelligent Internet of Things for Smart Healthcare Systems
Edited by Durgesh Srivastava, Neha Sharma, Deepak Sinwar, Jabar H. Yousif, and Hari Prabhat Gupta

Future Health Scenarios
AI and Digital Technologies in Global Healthcare Systems
Edited by Maria Jose Sousa, Francisco Guilherme Nunes, Generosa do Nascimento and Chinmay Chakraborty

Machine Learning and Deep Learning Techniques for Medical Image Recognition
Edited by Ben Othman Soufiene and Chinmay Chakraborty

Artificial Intelligence Technology in Healthcare
Security and Privacy Issues
Edited by Neha Sharma, Durgesh Srivastava and Deepak Sinwar

Federated Deep Learning for Healthcare
A Practical Guide with Challenges and Opportunities
Edited by Amandeep Kaur, Chetna Kaushal, Md. Mehedi Hassan and Si Thu Aung

Smart Devices for Medical 4.0 Technologies
Edited by Manisha Guduri, Chinmay Chakraborty and Martin Margala

For more information about this series, please visit: www.routledge.com/Advances-in-Smart-Healthcare-Technologies/book-series/CRCASHT

Smart Devices for Medical 4.0 Technologies

Edited by
Manisha Guduri, Chinmay Chakraborty, and
Martin Margala

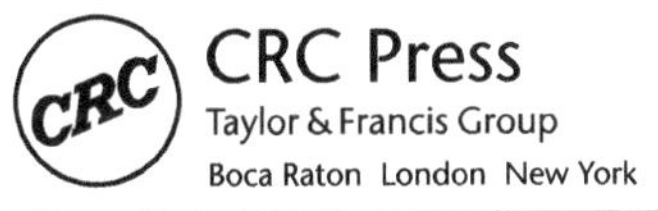

CRC Press
Taylor & Francis Group
Boca Raton London New York

CRC Press is an imprint of the
Taylor & Francis Group, an **informa** business

First edition published 2025
by CRC Press
2385 NW Executive Center Drive, Suite 320, Boca Raton FL 33431

and by CRC Press
4 Park Square, Milton Park, Abingdon, Oxon, OX14 4RN

CRC Press is an imprint of Taylor & Francis Group, LLC

ISBN: 978-1-032-60962-1 (hbk)
ISBN: 978-1-032-99342-3 (pbk)
ISBN: 978-1-003-60361-0 (ebk)

DOI: 10.1201/9781003603610

Typeset in Times
by KnowledgeWorks Global Ltd.

Contents

Preface

Enhancing the quality of healthcare and improving ease of access to health records while maintaining reasonable costs is challenging for health-care organizations globally. The problem is further exacerbated by the rapidly increasing world population, especially the rate of increase of senior people (65 years old and older). According to the World Health Organization (WHO, 2024), the number of senior people will increase to about 1.5 billion by 2050. An aging population implies an increase in chronic diseases that require frequent visits to health-care providers, as well as increased hospitalization needs. The rise in the number of patients requiring constant care significantly increases medical treatment costs. For example, in the USA, the cost of health care was about 17.9% of the gross domestic product in 2017 (CMS, 2019) and is expected to hit 19.4% in 2027 (HealthAffairs, 2019). Over the past few decades, Information and Communication Technologies (ICT) have been widely adopted in the health-care environment to make health-care access and delivery easier and most cost-effective. The use of ICT has led to the development of electronic health record (EHR) systems. EHRs contain complete patient health history (current medications, immunizations, laboratory results, current diagnosis, and so on) and can be easily shared among various providers. They have shown to enhance patient-provider interaction. This book mainly focuses on technological challenges and solutions in smart devices and assistive devices for healthcare. Wearable technology in healthcare includes electronic devices that consumers can wear, like Fitbits and smartwatches, and are designed to collect the data of users' personal health and exercise. Growing demand for wearables has generated a booming market, and now insurers and companies are seeing how supplying wearable health technology to their consumers and employees is beneficial. Wearable fitness technology has weaved itself into society so that FitBits and smartwatches are seen as mainstream; and the future of wearable devices shows no sign of slowing down. Piloted by the increasing demand of consumers to monitor their own health and keep track of their own vital signs, use of wearable technology has more than tripled in the last four years. According to research from Insider Intelligence, more than 80% of consumers are willing to wear fitness technology. Wearable ECG monitors are on the cutting edge of consumer electronics, and what sets these monitors apart from some smartwatches, is their ability to measure electrocardiograms, or ECGs. Biosensors are up-and-coming wearable medical devices that are radically different from wrist trackers and smartwatches. The Philips' wearable biosensor is a self-adhesive patch that allows patients to move around while collecting data on their movement, heart rate, respiratory rate, and temperature.

The book presents the new paradigm of open innovation used by the most prolific research teams around the world. The latest developments in the field of smart devices for Medical 4.0 technologies, healthcare monitoring, Artificial Intelligence approached for smart healthcare, IoT Based Smart Devices in Healthcare Monitoring Systems, Smart Paralysis Revolution, etc., are given. Overall, this book will be a reference for researchers, practitioners, and engineers. Therefore we need to establish intelligent digital healthcare systems using various emerging technologies like Blockchain and Artificial Intelligence (AI).

BOOK ORGANIZATION

The book consists of ten chapters in the field of smart healthcare systems. A summary of each chapter is presented below:

Chapter 1 Secured Smart Devices for Medical 4.0 Technologies: Threats and Approaches

This chapter offers a thorough assessment of security threats and approaches in securing smart devices used in Medical 4.0 technologies.

Chapter 2 Low-Cost Versatile Remote Healthcare Monitoring of Bedridden Patients

In this chapter, the objective is to integrate low-cost and software components for sensor data acquisition and storage into a functional system to monitor the physiological parameters of bedridden patients.

Chapter 3 Transfer Learning and Domain-Specific Adoption Algorithms for Image Classification

In this chapter, a unique transfer learning framework is presented with domain adoption algorithm.

Chapter 4 Artificial Intelligence and Internet of Things Mechanism for Smart Healthcare 4.0

This chapter focuses on the challenges in implementing various new technologies such as AI, IoT, and BD and provides the feasible solution. This chapter is helpful for the medical practitioner and Healthcare 4.0 industries.

Chapter 5 Significance of Quality Attributes of IoT-Based Smart Devices in Healthcare Monitoring Systems: Leading Towards Success or Failure

This chapter highlights the importance and challenges associated with critical quality attributes of existing healthcare monitoring IoT-based systems.

Chapter 6 Smart Paralysis Revolution: BCI Virtual Keyboards Unleashed in Healthcare

This work introduces a groundbreaking and transformative virtual keyboard that harnesses the principles of brain-computer interface (BCI) technology, offering a revolutionary solution for individuals grappling with paralytic diseases.

Chapter 7 Hardware Enhanced Secure Data Forwarding Protocol for Optimized Throughput in Wireless Body Area Networks

This chapter investigates wireless body area networks (WBANs) enhanced secure data forwarding protocol that attempts to boost network performance while maintaining security and dependability.

Chapter 8 HealthCoin: Solidity-Backed Blockchain Ventures in Smart Healthcare Technologies

This chapter introduces a novel approach to record management, utilizing a time-stamped structure coupled with a private mapping, allowing individuals to store and retrieve their health records efficiently.

Chapter 9 AI-Driven Smart Healthcare System for Monitoring Drought and Analyzing Climate Change Impacts in Healthcare for Medical 4.0

The healthcare-centric system showcases the feasibility of leveraging satellite imaging for drought analysis and climate change observations, providing valuable insights into crucial environmental issues.

Chapter 10 Fortifying Healthcare Cybersecurity: A Sturdiness-Based Approach to Threat Modeling and Risk Analysis

This research contributes to the field of healthcare cybersecurity by providing a novel framework that addresses the challenges of threat modeling and risk analysis in a decentralized and efficient manner.

Manisha Guduri
Chinmay Chakraborty
Martin Margala

REFERENCES

1. WHO, 2024. https://www.who.int/news-room/fact-sheets/detail/ageing-and-health
2. CMS, 2019. https://www.cms.gov/newsroom/press-releases/cms-office-actuary-releases-2018-2027-projections-national-health-expenditures

About the Editors

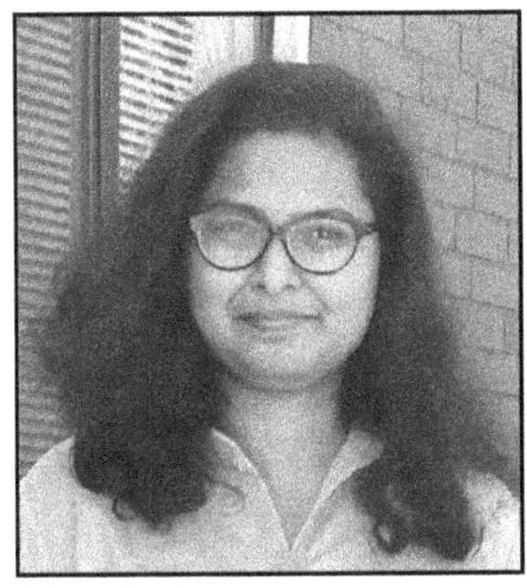

Manisha Guduri, PhD, is full-time teaching faculty at the University of Louisiana at Lafayette, USA. She is the author/coauthor of more than 65 research papers in reputed journals, book chapters, and international conferences. Her research interests include Artificial Intelligence, Biomedical Applications and VLSI/CAD design. She is currently working on VLSI and AI in the biomedical field. She has published five patents, two of which are under FER. She has received one patent grant and is a reviewer for *IEEE TVLSI, Microelectronics Journal, IET Digital Circuits, IEEE Journal of Biomedical and Health Informatics,* and other journals. She has one ongoing funded project from the Department of Science and Technology.

She is a senior member of IEEE, USA. She is also currently member of various IEEE Societies such as IEEE Young Professionals, IEEE Women in Engineering, Circuits and Systems, Computer Society and the Sensor Council. She is appointed as IEEE WiE CASS representative for 2023 and 2024. She was executive committee member in Women in Engineering Affinity Group IEEE Hyderabad Section 2022. She is IEEE WiE DL Program Coordinator and 2024 IEEE Computer Society Lafayette Section Vice Chair. She has delivered more than 35 talks at international conferences, technical programs and various other platforms. She has helped to organize ten international conferences across different roles.

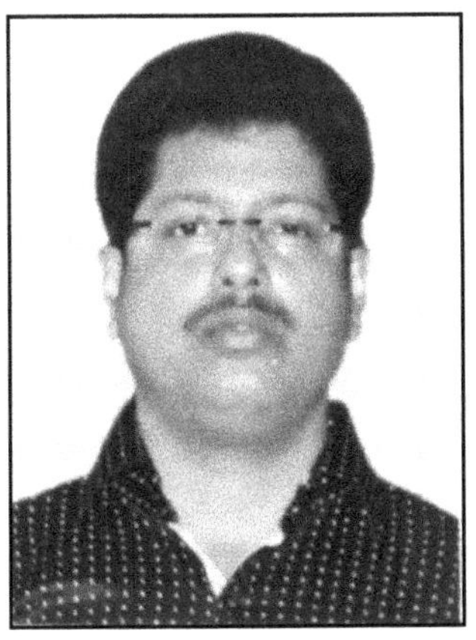

Chinmay Chakraborty, PhD, SMIEEE, MACM, is an Associate Professor at Birla Institute of Technology, Mesra, India. He completed a Post-Doctoral fellowship at the Federal University of Piauí, Brazil. He worked as a Senior Lecturer at the ICFAI University, Tripura, India. He worked as a Research Consultant in the Coal India project at Industrial Engineering and Management, IIT Kharagpur. He worked as a Project Coordinator of the Telecommunication Convergence Switch project under the Indo-US joint initiative. He also worked as a Network Engineer in System Administration at MISPL, India. His main research interests include the Internet of Medical Things (IoMT), AI/ML, Communication and Computing, Telemedicine, m-Health/e-health, and Medical Imaging. Dr. Chakraborty has widely published 200+ articles in peer reviewed international journals, conferences, book chapters, 25+ books, 4+ patents, and 20+ special issues in the field (Google h-index

35/i10-index 88, Scopus h-index 26, ISI-WoS h-index 22). He is an Editorial Board Member for several journals and conferences. Dr. Chakraborty has co-edited several books on IoMT, Healthcare Technology, and Sensor Data Analytics. He has served as a Publicity Chair member at renowned international conferences, including IEEE Healthcom, IEEE SP-DLT. He is a member of ACM and a senior member of IEEE.

He received a Best Session Runner-up Award, Young Research Excellence Award, Global Peer Review Award, Young Faculty Award, Outstanding Researcher Award, and Outstanding Paper in the 2022 Emerald Literati Awards and secured rank #1 from amongst 500 authors at BIT Mesra in Scival-Elsevier published by Scopus.com in 2023. He was selected as one of the top 2% of scientists in the world in the fields of Artificial Intelligence and Image Processing Stanford University, USA, 2021, 2022. He was the speaker for AICTE, DST-sponsored FDP, and CEP short-term course.

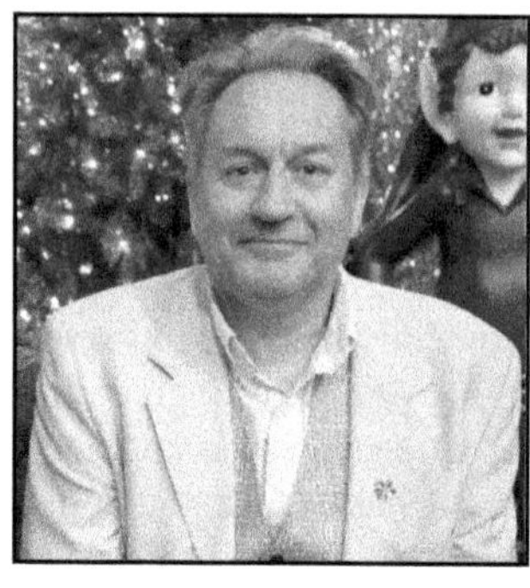

Martin Margala, PhD, joined the School of Computing and Informatics as Professor and Director in August 2021. Before joining UL Lafayette, from September 2011 to July 2021, Dr. Margala was Professor and Chair of the Electrical and Computer Engineering Department at the University of Massachusetts Lowell and a Co-Director of the Center for Smart Cyber-Physical Systems (SCyPS). He received his PhD degree in Electrical and Computer Engineering from the University of Alberta, Canada (#61 in Global Ranking in North America region; #13 in Global subject-specific ranking Electrical and Electronic Engineering in North America region US News) in the spring of 1998. He is a senior member of ACM, IEEE, and SPIE with more than 50 journal and 200 peer-reviewed conference publications in the areas of Design for Testability for Energy Efficient Architectures and Systems, High-Performance Reliable Low-Power Architectures and Reconfigurable Secure Architectures and Systems. Dr. Margala has directed 22 PhD students and 19 MS students, many of whom now hold leading positions in academia and industry. He has served on numerous program committees of international conferences and on workgroups (such as the International Technology Roadmap for Semiconductors) that have a great impact on the future direction of academia and industry.

Contributors

Sruthi Akinapally
Vallurupalli Nageswara Rao Vignana
    Jyothi Institute of Engineering &
    Technology, Hyderabad, India

Sainath Akula
Vallurupalli Nageswara Rao Vignana
    Jyothi Institute of Engineering &
    Technology, Hyderabad, India

Rajanikanth Aluvalu
Chaitanya Bharati Institute of
    Technology, Hyderabad, India

Pravallika Ambati
Vallurupalli Nageswara Rao Vignana
    Jyothi Institute of Engineering &
    Technology, Hyderabad, India

Fahim Arif
National University of Sciences and
    Technology (NUST), Islamabad,
    Pakistan

Ashima
Swami Vivekanand Subharti
    University, Meerut, India

Suneetha Bandeela
Department of Computer Science
    and Engineering, Koneru
    Lakshmaiah Education Foundation,
    Vaddeswaram, Guntur, India

José Hugo Barrón-Zambrano
Digital Systems Group, Electronics
    Department, Instituto Nacional de
    Astrofísica Óptica y Electrónica,
    Luis Enrique Erro\#1, Tonantzintla,
    Puebla, Mexico

Anil Kumar Chevella
Vallurupalli Nageswara Rao Vignana
    Jyothi Institute of Engineering &
    Technology, Hyderabad, India

Alan Díaz-Manriquez
Facultad de Ingeniería y Ciencias,
    Universidad Autonoma de
    Tamaulipas, Victoria,
    Mexico

Juan Carlos Elizondo-Leal
Facultad de Ingeniería y Ciencias,
    Universidad Autonoma de
    Tamaulipas, Victoria,
    Mexico

Ali El-Moursy
Department of Computer Engineering,
    College of Computing and
    Informatics, University of Sharjah,
    Sharjah, United Arab Emirates

Manisha Guduri
University of Louisiana at Lafayette,
    Louisiana, LA, USA

Yahir Hernández-Mier
Intelligent Systems Department,
    Polytechnic University of Victoria,
    Victoria, Mexico

Ganesh Jaina
Vallurupalli Nageswara Rao Vignana
    Jyothi College of Engineering and
    Technology, Hyderabad, India

Nimala K.
Department of Networking and
  Communications, School of
  Computing, College of Engineering
  and Technology, SRM Institute of
  Science and Technology,
  Tamil Nadu, India

Harika Kandukuri
Vallurupalli Nageswara Rao Vignana
  Jyothi College of Engineering and
  Technology, Hyderabad, India

Mahnoor Khan
National University of Sciences and
  Technology (NUST), Islamabad,
  Pakistan

Rohit Khethavath
Vallurupalli Nageswara Rao Vignana
  Jyothi College of Engineering and
  Technology, Hyderabad, India

Amit Kishor
Swami Vivekanand Subharti University,
  Meerut, India

Allada Harish Kumar
Department of Electronical
  Instrumental Engineering, V R
  Siddhartha Engineering College,
  Vijayawada, India

Tapeshwar Mandotra
Vallurupalli Nageswara Rao Vignana
  Jyothi Institute of Engineering &
  Technology, Hyderabad, India

Martin Margala
University of Louisiana at Lafayette,
  Louisiana, LA, USA

Aleena Nadeem
National University of Sciences and
  Technology (NUST), Islamabad,
  Pakistan

Marco Aurelio Nuño-Maganda
Intelligent Systems Department,
  Polytechnic University of Victoria,
  Victoria, Mexico

Sonu Kumar Pandit
Department of Computer Science
  and Engineering, Koneru
  Lakshmaiah Education Foundation,
  Vaddeswaram, Guntur, India

Suresh K. Peddoju
Cullen College of Engineering,
  University of Houston, Texas, USA

Said Polanco-Martagón
Intelligent Systems Department,
  Polytechnic University of Victoria,
  Victoria, Mexico

Mukesh Prasad
School of Computer Science, University
  of Technology, Sydney, Australia

Mallellu Sai Prashanth
Vardhaman College of Engineering,
  Hyderabad, India

Nareshkumar R.
Department of Networking and
  Communications, School of
  Computing, College of Engineering
  and Technology, SRM Institute of
  Science and Technology,
  Tamil Nadu, India

Sravanth Kumar Ramakuri
Anurag University, Department
  of AI, Telangana, India

A. Roshini
Department of Computer Science
  and Engineering, Koneru
  Lakshmaiah Education Foundation,
  Vaddeswaram, Guntur, India

Shaik Roshini
Department of Computer Science
and Engineering, Koneru
Lakshmaiah Education Foundation,
Vaddeswaram, Guntur, India

Saddaf Rubab
Department of Computer Engineering,
College of Computing and
Informatics, University of Sharjah,
Sharjah, United Arab Emirates

Pranavi S.
Florida International University,
Florida, USA

Mithileysh Sathiyanarayanan
University of London, London,
United Kingdom

Seetha Srujana
Salesforce India Pvt Limited,
Hyderabad, India

Uma Maheswari V.
Chaitanya Bharati Institute of
Technology, Hyderabad, India

V. Sagar Reddy
Vallurupalli Nageswara Rao Vignana
Jyothi Institute of Engineering &
Technology, Hyderabad, India

1 Secured Smart Devices for Medical 4.0 Technologies
Threats and Approaches

Suresh K. Peddoju and Pranavi S.

1.1 INTRODUCTION

The concept of Internet of Things (IoT) is initially coined by Kevin Ashton in the year 1999 [1]. According to him, it's a technological system which connects real world physical objects through the internet with a computing capacity. Over several years it has different evolutions and has been adopted in a wide variety of application domains such as healthcare, retail, home, defense, automobile, waste management, traffic controlling, and others. Most attracted area for IoT is healthcare and related area due to its potential applicability in different medical applications like health monitoring, disease identification, elderly care, childcare, fitness programs, and many more [2]. Another important application is the availability of treatment and medication at home and lots of coordination between different healthcare providers. Thus, several medical devices such as diagnostic, imaging, and other devices need to be smart [3] and can be connected to each other for providing automated services. Healthcare IoT services [4–5] are useful in terms of providing quality life to humankind with reduced costs and increasing the user's experience with the assistance of advanced technologies. To provide better healthcare IoT services, there is a need for secure connectivity [6] across healthcare stakeholders like patients, clinics, and healthcare organizations.

IoT is swiftly gaining recognition in diverse sectors, spanning automation of home, agriculture, retail, automotive, cities, and other application areas, especially healthcare. There is an exponential growth in IoT usage as reported by Gartner, projecting that over 50 billion connected devices will be in operation by 2025. This surge in IoT adoption necessitates responsive services to meet the growing demands in different sectors, compelling the IT industry to embrace IoT for enhanced customer service. The healthcare sector, in particular, is experiencing a pressing need for technological advancements such as federated learning, big data (BD), cloud computing, and quantum computing to provide quick and fast healthcare services to the end users. There are various components involved in healthcare operations which generate substantial data on a daily basis. Predictive analytics emerges as a crucial tool in extracting valuable inputs from health data, facilitating the records

DOI: 10.1201/9781003603610-1

of patient's health information, and enabling immediate responses in critical health situations. Given the vast amounts of data generated in healthcare, leveraging technologies like IoT become imperative. Wearables, in particular, play a pivotal role in this landscape, offering consumers the means to monitor their health conditions. The current market boasts a variety of wearable devices designed to continuously collect data and transmit it to the cloud, where it undergoes analysis to provide actionable insights. Wearables also empower users by issuing alerts related to their health, and these notifications can extend to healthcare providers. However, the potential latency in data propagation poses a challenge to the timely delivery of patient care. In the healthcare IoT ecosystem, wearables serve as indispensable tools for health monitoring. These devices offer real-time data collection, enabling individuals to proactively manage their well-being. The data collected by wearables is transmitted to cloud platforms, where sophisticated analytics and machine learning algorithms can extract meaningful patterns and insights. This wealth of information not only benefits individuals by providing personalized health insights but also contributes to a broader understanding of population health trends. Despite the current advancements in wearables and healthcare IoT, there are challenges to address. Latency in data transmission is a critical concern, as delays in receiving and processing health data can impact the timeliness of patient care. Additionally, ensuring the security and privacy of health-related data is paramount to foster trust among users and healthcare providers. To address these challenges, continuous innovation and integration of technologies are essential. The healthcare industry must collaborate with IoT developers, AI experts, and data scientists to create a seamless and secure ecosystem. The focus should be on reducing latency through optimized communication protocols and ensuring data security through robust encryption measures. In conclusion, the intersection of IoT and healthcare holds immense potential for revolutionizing patient care and well-being. Wearables and IoT technologies offer unprecedented opportunities to monitor health in real-time, but addressing challenges related to data latency and security is crucial. By fostering collaboration and driving technological advancements, the healthcare sector can harness the full benefits of IoT, paving the way for a more responsive and patient-centric healthcare experience.

The latest advancements have enabled IoT to provide reliable connectivity between patients and physicians through telemedicine and collect data from critical care situations in a secure manner for making faster decisions. The massive usage of IoT in medical field and various vulnerabilities with IoT devices have opened the doors for attackers to hack the systems and steal valuable patient's data [7]. Hackers also spread denial of services (DoS) attacks on various IoT devices, spawn malicious activities on healthcare devices to mislead healthcare monitoring and diagnosis, cyberattacks on healthcare prescriptions, and many more [8–11]. To overcome these vulnerabilities with healthcare IoT devices, there is an acute need for strong encryption and cryptography techniques.

In the healthcare industry, federated learning is quickly becoming a game-changing idea that offers a potent remedy for pressing problems with data security and privacy. Protecting patient privacy is crucial in the IoT world of healthcare, where enormous amounts of sensitive patient data are generated, gathered, and analyzed. Traditional centralized data processing and analysis methods have frequently sparked worries about data breaches and illegal access, posing serious hazards to patients' private health data. However, federated learning presents a decentralized strategy in which data stays on local servers or edge devices and only aggregated insights are exchanged, protecting the security and privacy of patient data.

In a nutshell, federated learning in the healthcare sector signifies a significant change in how the sector views data security and privacy. Healthcare stakeholders are given the ability to maximize the potential of their data collectively while adhering to strict privacy laws since collaborative model training is made possible without disclosing raw patient data. This novel strategy safeguards patient privacy while fostering ground-breaking research and advancements that will ultimately raise the standard of healthcare and lead to better patient outcomes. We can anticipate the fusion of cutting-edge technology with strict data protection as the healthcare sector continues to implement federated learning, propelling the industry into a new era of secure, patient-centric, and data-driven healthcare innovation.

In this chapter, we highlight cutting-edge research on IoT in healthcare and recent research trends in providing secured approaches for safeguarding healthcare data. This chapter looks at the most recent research on developments in IoT for healthcare and how modern technologies are tackling problems associated with cyberattacks on data related to healthcare and smart devices in Medical 4.0 technologies. The primary goal of this chapter is to describe various contributions made by researchers in developing various techniques for identifying security vulnerabilities and solutions. It also highlights various technology developments, innovations, industrial efforts, and provides challenges, threats, and issues.

In the healthcare industry, there are many latest advancements happening and they are streamlined in the form of Medical 4.0. This framework empowers all stakeholders to design and develop insightful products for continuous monitoring which in turn increases the performance, tailored to unique configurations. The motive behind all these advancements is to develop smart facilities that operate autonomously with the help of analytics and visualizations. Rapid migration to online operations, partly due to a lack of preparedness, has become essential for sustaining momentum. In the era of connected IoT and advancements in robotics, organizations must reimagine their structures, enhance skills, and redirect investments to align with Industry 4.0 technologies.

Industry 4.0 seeks to improve conventional mechanisms in production environments and timely treatments in healthcare, bringing new methods in industrialization by incorporating latest cutting-edge technologies. Furthermore, cutting down the expenditures in these sectors especially in areas like telemedicine systems that leverage advanced technologies for efficient infection prevention and management. Latest advancements in the areas of virtual reality (VR) and augmented reality (AR) are playing an important role in preventative maintenance, asset management, and communication within the healthcare sector.

AR products are helping technicians to view the things live and virtual to assess and react to the supply chain, asset, and other application areas data. Human-machine collaboration enhances connectivity, boosts efficiency, and minimizes costs. VR headsets serve as interfaces for accessing healthcare facilities remotely, facilitating collaborative environments for distant workers, partners, and customers.

In the transition to Industry 4.0, cybersecurity becomes paramount. Establishing a cybersecurity strategy encompassing both IT and OT equipment is crucial for securing factory and field operational equipment. The intelligent asset management ushered in by Industry 4.0 brings forth a paradigm shift from reactive to proactive. All the processes are interconnected dynamically to make significant advancement. The digital revolution inherent in Industry 4.0 allows for the development of digital twins, which is a process of replicating virtual operations especially in the fields of manufacturing, supply chain, healthcare, and other fields. Manufacturers enhance their efficiency and optimize their operations by producing innovative products by analyzing IoT sensor data and other connected devices information. Digital twins offer a platform for testing modifications, identifying opportunities to reduce downtime, and boosting manufacturing process capacity.

For industrial organizations, embedded sensors generate substantial data, allowing the concerned manufacturers to perform analysis over data to study tendencies, recognize relationships, and make informed decisions. Smart factories integrate data from various business sections and their broader ecosystem to help in analyzing data to take production oriented decisions by considering all factors such as sales, personnel, and warehouse data insights.

The healthcare sector stands to benefit significantly from the adoption of Industry 4.0 principles, giving rise to what is now referred to as Healthcare Industry 4.0, or simply Health 4.0. In this paper, we will use the term Health 4.0 to denote this transformation. Unlike the industrial systems, the healthcare systems did not progress through versions 3.0, 2.0, and 1.0; hence, the 4.0 in Health 4.0 is inherited from its origin, Industry 4.0.

The use of integrated healthcare platforms with advancing virtualized, distributed, and real-time healthcare services for professionals, patients, and informal and formal caregivers is known as "Health 4.0." In order to move healthcare services away from empirical data-based models and toward precision medicine or individualized healthcare services, it seeks to promote cooperation, coherence, and convergence. This fits with the worldwide movement toward a patient-centered, decentralized healthcare system. In order to improve operations and save costs, Health 4.0 also includes the integration, sharing, and optimization of healthcare personnel, systems management, and service resources. The predicted \$18.28 trillion in global healthcare spending by 2040 makes the adoption of Industry 4.0 technology essential for improving efficacy and efficiency.

Adopting Health 4.0 has numerous benefits for the healthcare sector, including increased cost-effectiveness, flexibility, scalability, dependability, agility, and overall quality of operations and services. As the difficulties caused by COVID-19 demonstrate, these qualities can greatly support national and international responses to pandemics.

However, there are significant obstacles in the way of creating and delivering Health 4.0-compliant healthcare applications. It is necessary to properly handle problems such as increased design complexity, a plethora of architectural options, and the incorporation of strong security and privacy measures. An effective approach to address these issues is to make use of a sophisticated service-oriented middleware (SOM) architecture. The integration and utilization of cutting-edge technologies, such as cloud computing, edge/fog computing, IoT, IIoT (Industrial IoT), cyber-physical system (CPS), and BD, is demonstrated by this framework. By using this method, some of the challenges related to developing Health 4.0 apps can be reduced, current services can be improved, and new, high-value Health 4.0 applications can be more easily introduced. In order to keep up with the constantly changing environment of technology integration in the medical field, this chapter explores the advances in Medical 4.0 technologies and their profound impact on healthcare. It emphasizes the importance of embracing disruptive techniques.

Further, the remainder of the chapter is organized into three sections. A general overview and architecture of healthcare IoT is mentioned in Section 1.2. Section 1.3 provides modern study in the area of healthcare IoT security threats and approaches. Conclusion of the chapter is presented in Section 1.4.

1.2 HEALTHCARE IOT

Recent years drastic advancements and innovations have taken place with healthcare IoT. Due to these technological enhancements several stakeholders benefited in terms of cost-effective healthcare services. Figure 1.1 showcases the reliable and secured general architecture of healthcare IoT.

As shown in the diagram, there are multiple stakeholders (patient, doctors, diagnosis providers, wearable devices, other healthcare providers) participating in healthcare IoT system to generate/access the healthcare data. Multiple IoT devices are interconnected in the system to make automated services available to all the stakeholders anytime, anywhere. It is very important to have a secure environment surrounding this healthcare data and all the communications links accessed by all the healthcare stakeholders. Various researchers proposed many security approaches surrounding this healthcare system to provide reliable and secured communication channel and security provisions to healthcare data. Still there is an acute need for identifying security threats and corresponding countermeasures in order to provide

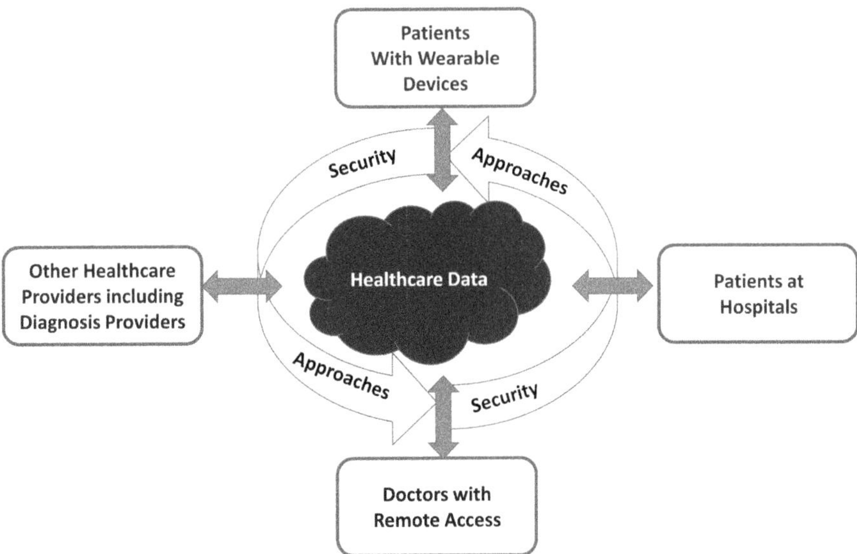

FIGURE 1.1 General healthcare IoT system architecture.

secure and safe healthcare data access. Next section will provide an extensive survey on Medical 4.0 and healthcare IoT security issues and approaches presented by different researchers in state-of-the-art research.

1.2.1 MEDICAL 4.0

The goal of Medical 4.0 is to create a plan that will enable them to change from being manufacturers to service providers. This evolution has been streamlined to better cater services to clients depending on their needs and convenience. Medical 4.0 connects patients and healthcare professionals to organization and treatment methods using contemporary technologies. These technologies are developing into a patient-centered strategy in which data will be made available to industry players so they can improve technology and healthcare delivery models. Healthcare delivery will become more specialized because of the Medical 4.0 development as shown in Figure 1.2. It aims to focus aggressively on patient orientation and individualized care using cutting-edge technologies.

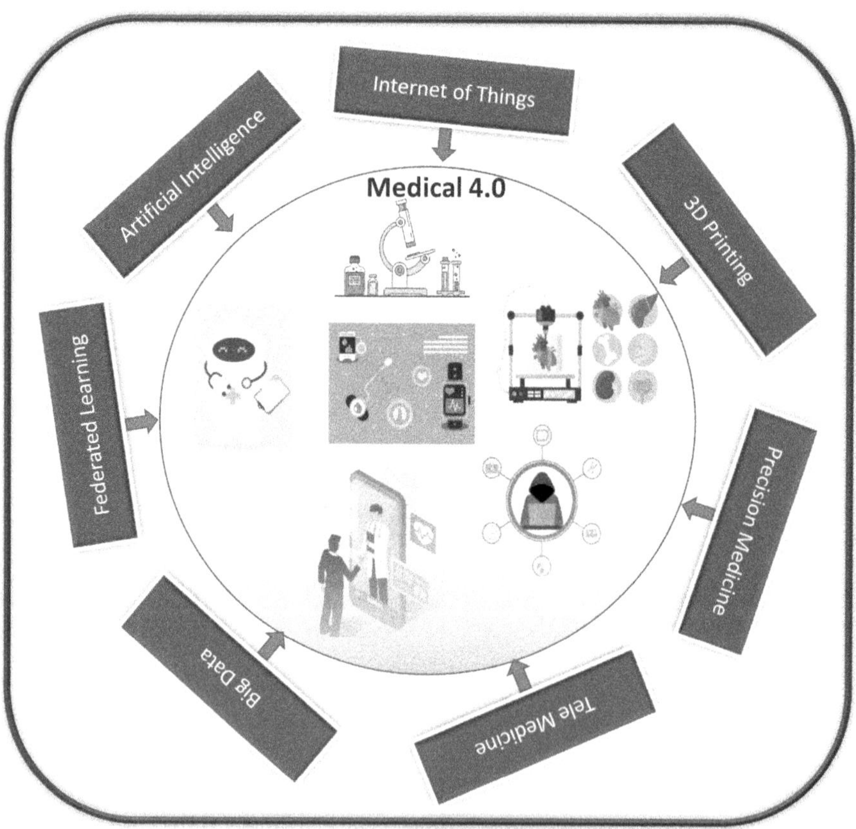

FIGURE 1.2   Medical 4.0 technologies.

With the use of software and mobile medical apps that use artificial intelligence to support doctors' clinical choices, Medical 4.0 technologies have been transforming the way that healthcare is provided. Hospitals may also utilize sensors to control their supply inventories, maximizing their use of and spending on gases, chemicals, and disposable items like masks and gloves. Healthcare workers can get confidential patient information. In addition to protecting user data, IoT devices need to be dependable in connectivity, performance, and real-time data transfer. By linking other physician networks to handle referrals and send prescriptions to pharmacies, electronic health records (EHR)-related technologies help doctors diagnose patients more accurately and quickly. Drawing influence from Industry 4.0 concepts, Health 4.0 functions as a strategic deployment and managerial framework in the healthcare industry. Personalized healthcare in near real time for patients, healthcare providers, and informal and formal caregivers is the main goal of Health 4.0, which aims to enable a progressive shift toward virtualization. The push for customized healthcare requires a greater use of cloud computing, CPSs, and an enlarged IoT, sometimes known as the internet of everything (IoE). Things like devices, services, people, and the incorporation of 5G networks are all included in the IoE.

Tools, techniques, and objects related to BD and software developed for distributed systems are virtualized using a spatial-temporal matrix in the context of the CPS paradigm. Small space-time frames can be examined in real-time within the real environment thanks to this virtualization process. As a result, this ability allows for theragnostics in precise and individualized treatment, allowing for a seamless integration of therapeutic interventions and diagnostics. This strategy promotes innovation by combining cutting-edge technologies to improve healthcare delivery without sacrificing customization and accuracy. Inspired by the ideas of Industry 4.0, Health 4.0 functions as a strategic deployment and administrative framework in the healthcare industry. Health 4.0's primary goal is to enable a progressive shift toward virtualization, allowing for near-real-time tailored healthcare for patients, healthcare providers, and informal and formal caregivers.

A lack of adequate management in conjunction with a lack of understanding of a health issue can aggravate diseases and raise mortality. It is critical that the mobile internet of things (MIoT) be used effectively in health education and illness management. By utilizing the IoT and 5G, a variety of multimedia materials pertaining to disease education can be sent to patients' mobile devices, improving their understanding of their medical issues and including both non-pharmaceutical and pharmaceutical treatment choices.

Additionally, MIoT is essential to the assessment and tracking of diseases. For example, patients can use their phones to frequently manage their tests and surveys, which make it possible for medical staff to regularly check on their patients' well-being. On the other hand, medical professionals, decision-makers, and service providers can use MIoT to dynamically evaluate circumstances and comprehend their interplay with environmental or behavioral factors. This integrated approach not only enhances patient education but also enables proactive and informed healthcare decisions.

Medical 4.0 aims to formulate a strategy for the transition from traditional manufacturing to becoming service providers. This shift involves tailoring services to clients based on their specific demands and preferences. By harnessing modern technologies, Medical 4.0 establishes connections between patients, healthcare professionals, and the organization, thereby facilitating an evolution toward a patient-centered approach. The data generated in this process is made available to industry participants to drive advancements in technology and healthcare delivery concepts.

1.2.2 MEDICAL 4.0 AND CUTTING-EDGE TECHNOLOGIES

Medical 4.0 is growing with its innovations by providing efficient and effective patient services by the way of delivering enhanced healthcare services. It uses cutting-edge technologies such as IoT, AI, and ML, deep learning, federated learning, BD, robotics, and others to process and manage data to take firm and timely decisions and provide precise medicine/treatment based on lifestyle based approaches. New innovations are evolving in this industry on daily basis to help the needs of the healthcare industry and better life of stakeholders of healthcare systems. It also provides an insightful framework for the doctors and patients to interact and provide services to all the stakeholders of the patient in a highly visualized manner even though they located in different geographical locations especially remote places.

Similarly, VR has emerged as a valuable contributor to healthcare technology during the transition to Medical 4.0. VR wearable technology headsets enable patients to virtually explore uncharted environments, providing a more engaging and less clinical experience. Beyond offering an escape, VR has demonstrated efficacy in pain management and shown improvements in chronic pain patients. Patients can access virtual therapy and self-care remedies through commercial platforms, using VR headsets to experience pain relief similar to hospital settings.

The digital healthcare sector continues to evolve with the growing advancements in the areas of AI, cloud computing, federated learning, edge computing, and robotics which produce modern and smart devices and applications. These innovations in supply chain process are ensuring prompt delivery of services and provide right time right treatment to the needy people. Medical 4.0 is playing a key role in providing access to healthcare assistance and monitoring for those who are suffering from long-term diseases especially chronic issues. Wearable devices, including heart rate, oxygen, cardiography, glucose monitoring related devices offer valuable data for extensive analysis, aiding in patient health information and to take preventive measures.

The transformative impact of Medical 4.0 extends to mobile medical applications, clinical decision support software powered by artificial intelligence, and the use of sensors in hospitals to optimize supply inventories. Patient engagement technologies and EHR contribute to better and faster patient diagnoses, streamlined referral processes, and efficient prescription transmissions to pharmacies. Safeguarding sensitive personal information and ensuring the reliability of IoT devices in terms of connectivity, performance, and real-time data transmission are critical considerations. This digital transformation not only enhances patient engagement but also allows individuals to establish a stronger connection with their health, enabling them to assess the costs of pharmaceutical items and healthcare services. For pharmaceutical firms, this presents an opportunity to engage with potential patients online during their exploration of various products.

Advancements in biology and technology have prompted a call for the simplification of doctors' procedures in treating chronic patients. Medical 4.0 technologies play a pivotal role in achieving this goal by enabling individualized therapy, swift symptom management, and real-time monitoring of patients' health. This technological revolution revolves around tracking breakthroughs that provide consistent patient data, emphasizing the importance of data-recording and data-display devices such as sensors and monitors.

As Medical 4.0 emerges as a new trend in healthcare, the sector stands to benefit from the integration of cloud computing and artificial intelligence. Cloud computing, coupled with artificial intelligence, offers several advantages, enhancing personalized purchasing experiences by recognizing trends in customers' browsing and purchasing habits. Artificial intelligence enables the automation of client interactions, with chatbots capable of engaging with multiple clients simultaneously.

Artificial intelligence's real-time assistance capabilities further extend to data mining, swiftly identifying valuable insights by extensively studying, and analyzing the data. Further, usage of AI is pretty much important in performing operational automation by facilitating cross-sector innovations in healthcare sector.

The proliferation of data in the Medical 4.0 era significantly contributes to the growth of medical research. The ability to gather and analyze massive amounts of data accelerates medical research, fostering a better understanding of patients' unique conditions through real-time monitoring and tailored information delivery during interactions with their doctors.

Medical 4.0 technologies not only monitor patients but also administer individualized care. The development of biometric devices allows for scanning between appointments to detect and treat diseases at their earliest stages. As technology progresses, increased access to high-quality healthcare at reduced costs becomes a reality. This, in turn, contributes to the overall health of the population, leading to lower healthcare expenses over time. The holistic integration of technology in healthcare holds the promise of a healthier future with improved patient care and cost-effective outcomes.

Medical 4.0 has many advantages with it but also have some challenges to it. With advancing Medical 4.0 lots a medical data generated in centralized storage locations and served to various devices connected to those centralized systems. There is vast range of chances for hackers to attack on this data and exploit it for bad purposes. These attacks may take place in network, data transmission, and data collection stages. There are several security and privacy approaches evolved in the industry and securing health data from hackers. One of them is to use cloud to store the data and provide security provisions. The subsequent section provides vast literature on security threats and approaches in healthcare IoT with respect to Medical 4.0.

1.3 STATE OF THE ART

People's quality of life is one of their top concerns, and they are searching for cutting-edge medical technologies and healthcare solutions to meet their needs [12–13]. The IoT (IoT) is now playing a critical role in delivering high-quality healthcare solutions. In the healthcare industry, technology has been rapidly advancing to meet the needs of both the patients and the healthcare workers. In fact, an exponential growth of 10 billion IoT devices has been recorded in present day since the first mention of them in 1999 [14]. IoT is the term for connecting any gadget to the internet, together with other devices in a vast network of similarly connected items, as well as individuals who gather and exchange data [15]. Society as an entity comprises of a massive amount of IoT devices, with places like healthcare facilities containing thousands of them, operating on a regular basis, and most of these IoT devices need security to protect them from harm [16]. Furthermore, IoT security is a cybersecurity technique and defense system that guards from the threat of cyberattacks that target real-world IoT devices that could be connected to a network [17].

A healthcare facility is a large entity that contains a myriad of IoT devices, many of which in turn contain subsets of multiple IoT devices. These IoT devices allow for remote monitoring of patients [18–19], enable better detection of medical conditions, and consist of wearable technology and other digital tools; however, they also pose a significant threat to security and privacy, as they are vulnerable to cyberattacks, data breaches, and unauthorized access to sensitive patient information. The number of organizations that reported attacks surged during 2021, reaching an all-time high [20]. IoT devices have no doubt revolutionized the healthcare industry, but they have also expanded the scope for attacks, and given the sensitivity surrounding healthcare, cyberattacks can be detrimental.

Considering common cyberattacks on healthcare organizations it is imperative that necessary steps are taken to mediate them. Many IoT devices are implanted in a healthcare facility, these devices regularly need maintenance. Therefore, having a thorough surveillance system, along with an access control system is a necessity to prevent physical access [21]. Facilities often overlook the need for physical security when accounting for attacks when they should be higher prioritized. Healthcare organizations house important operations, matters that deal with the well-being of others, and IoT security should be implemented every step of the way.

Wearable sensors can be used to measure vital parameters collected from patients and stream information to the required storage at remote server with the support of wireless technologies such as Bluetooth and Wi-Fi for anytime anywhere accessibility. Similar work is carried out by Sultan [18] using cloud-based systems to store gathered information.

This research endeavors to design and implement a health monitoring framework focused on identifying health risks through the application of anomaly detection techniques. The initial phase of development involves refining the framework to align with the specific requirements of the proposed solution. Subsequently, the study aims to analyze and highlight the efficacy of various machine learning models in discerning anomalous behavior within health monitoring. The anticipated outcomes of the research encompass the creation and refinement of a comprehensive framework, the selection of machine learning algorithms based on their performance, identification of optimal deployment modes on wearable devices or gateways, and an evaluation of the overall framework's performance. Currently, the research is ongoing to identify a suitable machine learning algorithm that can effectively detect anomalies in health data. The subsequent steps involve designing and developing models based on data received from wearable devices, distinguishing between normal and anomalous data.

In the upcoming stages, the developed model will be deployed either on wearable devices or IoT gateways. The health data will be scrutinized based on established health risk patterns, and anomalous data will be filtered to trigger alert messages to patients or caretakers. The proposed framework aims to contribute valuable insights into health conditions such as wound healing, diabetes, or respiratory diseases, providing immediate responses to critical health situations.

The strategic plan of ASSIST is supported by this study, which focuses on wound healing as a disease of interest. By providing real-time health emergency notifications, the suggested architecture and monitoring IoT devices present a fresh way for ASSIST to help patients with wounds and other medical issues. The findings will be compiled and presented, highlighting the potent machine learning models found for efficient anomaly detection and monitoring, once the framework has been adjusted as a workable anomaly detection solution. Real-time wound monitoring is the main emphasis of the experimental phase. Traditionally, wound supervision has involved a long series of repeated clinical trials and laboratory investigations. The suggested architecture is used to address this time lag, as seen by the experimental setup's initial findings. ASSIST's enzymatic biosensor for measuring uric acid in wound fluid, the wound monitoring sensor, is used to measure uric acid levels in a variety of lab environments throughout time. Elevations of uric acid are used as a diagnostic marker for wound healing, and their changes over time are detected by electrochemical sensors. The project is presently investigating a number of machine learning methods, such as One-Class SVM, K-means Clustering, LSTM, and Autoencoders. The work will eventually be deployed for clinical trials in hospital settings as the application is further improved through more lab tests and sensors. This all-encompassing strategy promises revolutionary consequences for patient care and monitoring as it attempts to close the gap between conventional wound monitoring and real-time, data-driven health solutions. Numerous publications discuss the vast range of applications that these kinds of frameworks offer, including data analytics, machine learning model creation, and the use of AI techniques to identify high-risk circumstances with various diseases [22–33].

According to some of the researchers, security, and privacy challenges are prevalent in healthcare IoT devices with lack of security provisions [34]. Due to this reason most of the patient's data is compromised and privacy information of patient is misused [35]. Authors in [36–37] state the reasons why these devices may be vulnerable to attacks: lack of standardization, insufficient testing, lack of necessary solutions, lack of quality skills from medical staff, and the lack of regulation. These authors further explain the different types of attacks related to IoMT: ransomware, side-channel, tag, cloning, sensor tracking, account hijacking, and brute force. In the paper [38] the author also lists the different types of attacks, directly relates it to fog based IoT systems, and breaks it down into three different categories: authentication, confidentiality, and non-repudiation. The authors propose a solution that combines cipher text and encrypted keys forwarded to the fog layer for authentication [39]. Like the previous solution, authors in [40] propose a solution for body sensor security that requires two different communication procedures: system initialization and authentication phases. This solution uses encrypted keys to secure body sensors. Authors in [41] propose a system for security of patient data exchanging devices that include five different modules or steps: handshaking, listener, cryptographic security layer, conversion, and an encryption layer. In [42], the authors propose three crucial types of algorithms that can be used to combat IoMT security problems: supervised, unsupervised, and semi-supervised algorithms. This chapter also provides a more generalized analysis and solution to the security problems present in IoMT devices. Authors in [43] formed a methodology to categorize the security of IoMT devices to determine the vulnerabilities of different devices using a survey from medical staff. A common solution to the security problems pertaining to IoMT based on these research papers are to use encrypted keys for authentication using different types of systems as seen in [44–51].

The authors in [52] recognized four crucial segments which are to be focused with regards to cybersecurity capacity over the medical field, apart from that the nine main challenges of cybersecurity, and eleven major approaches that healthcare entities have considered to address the difficulties. They did notice that cyberattacks in various forms such as ransomware attacks, phishing, distributed denial-of-service attacks (DDoS), and attacks related to malware were the most crucial ones that occurred frequently in the period of pandemic. To protect the privacy of IoT devices, the authors of [53] suggested a simple two-factor authentication system. The broad and open use of IoT devices has led authors to place more focus on device authentication because this makes those devices more susceptible to physical and cyberattacks. This method creates random physical variations within the IC's microstructure, making it unique, by using certain hash values based on single side along with unclonable functions (PUFs), which are constructed based on integrated circuits (ICs). Reduced sensor data processing framework (REDPF), which Wang et al. [54] mentioned, is a data processing system that enhances network dependability and accuracy when transferring medical information of a patient across the IoT architecture. The creators of this model, which is dependent on fog computing, applied the reduced variable neighborhood search (RVNS) method to improve transmission reliability of data and efficiency of load balancing. The newly developed framework contains a self-adaptive filter that automatically gathers faulty or missing data. Consequently, it becomes a fault-tolerant system. A cloud-based authentication of user's approach was put forth by Srinivas et al. [55] for the secure access of health data in the IoT health surveillance system. To protect interactions between an authorized individual and a device's sensor node, this technique generates a private session key. The suggested mechanism was subjected to a security study using the real-or-random (ROR) paradigm to determine how resilient it was to several well-known assaults.

Medical 4.0 brought so many smart technologies such as wearable devices, cloud, BD, and many to gather and store data. As a result, securing such data is very much obvious otherwise sensitive data can be leaked and used it for unlawful purposes. This itself showcases that Medical 4.0 systems need to be robust in order to face such security threats in EHR, networks, and directories located in different areas. In support of various approaches followed by Medical 4.0 [56] there is also a need of federated learning to build AI models to assess the data and find anomalies by comparing with baseline data. Federated learning brings robust to healthcare systems in terms of building robust clinical models [57–59] with the help of state of the art research carried out on healthcare data.

After performing vast research on healthcare IoT and its security issues, we found that there are various methods and approaches presented by different researchers are providing kind of security to the existing systems but there are many research gaps. Summary of all the research gaps is, most of the research focusing on detecting, preventing, and avoiding threats but not providing a stable and robust systems.

Identified outcomes of this study is, there is an acute need of robust and trustworthy security approaches and standardization of procedures are required to the existing healthcare IoT systems to safeguard from the attackers especially in the era of Medical 4.0. Also, innovative technology provides convenience to healthcare stakeholders, but it should retain security and privacy of Healthcare IoT systems data and resources. Especially usage of Medical 4.0 and federated learning mechanisms are playing a major role in providing fast, accurate, and secure healthcare data to the stake holders of the healthcare system.

The deliverables of this study is

- Providing a state-of-the-art literature with respect to healthcare IoT, Medical 4.0, and federated learning including role of other cutting edge technologies in healthcare systems.
- Identify research gaps related to securing smart devices in the era of Medical 4.0 and provide a study of current approaches in relation to security aspects of Healthcare industry.
- Provide approaches and insights on improving the existing systems.
- Provide future research directions and security aspects.

1.4 CONCLUSION

In this study, we summarized the most recent state-of-the-art research on healthcare IoT conducted by different researchers. We explored different security threats and issues related to IoT devices, wearable devices, communication channel, healthcare professionals, and others. The motive of this study is to present current research trends in the field of healthcare IoT and summarize different solutions or frameworks with security aspects. After performing a state of the art study, we conclude that there needs a strong security approaches and standards to safeguard the healthcare data in healthcare IoT system even after adopting new techniques and/or technologies in healthcare industry.

1.5 FUTURE SCOPE

In future, we will work in building a robust and trustworthy framework to secure smart devices used in Medical 4.0 technologies and safeguard healthcare data from advanced security threats and breaches by using modern technologies like cloud, BD, edge computing, artificial intelligence, deep learning, and federated learning.

There are lot many advancements took place in current technologies especially AI, it is being used in both good and bad purposes. Issues like deepfake, weapons automation, and privacy issues are most dangerous aspects of AI to the humankind whereas good side of AI is usage of generative AI, trustworthy AI, standardization of law, and policies with respect to AI usage in daily life of mankind. In the context of this chapter, there is a lot of scope in these areas to contribute and provide research insights toward healthcare services by making use of good impacts of cutting-edge technologies and brining world class advancements into the lives of people across the globe by overcoming security threats.

REFERENCES

1. Tan, N. L., Wang, N. 2010. Future internet: The internet of things. Proceedings of Third International Conference on Advanced Computer Theory and Engineering (ICACTE), 5, pp. 376–380.
2. Guduri, M., Chakraborty, C., Margala, M. 2023. Blockchain-based federated learning technique for privacy preservation and security of smart electronic health records. IEEE Transactions on Consumer Electronics.
3. Yamada, I., Lopez, G. 2012. Wearable sensing systems for healthcare monitoring. Proceedings of the Symposium on VLSI Technology, Honolulu, HI, USA, pp. 5–10.
4. Ahmed, S., Millat, S., Rahman, M. A. et al. 2015. Wireless health monitoring system for patients. 2015 IEEE International WIE Conference on Electrical and Computer Engineering (WIECON-ECE), Dhaka, pp. 164–167.
5. Aminian, M., Naji, H. R. 2013. A Hospital healthcare monitoring system using wireless sensor networks. Journal of Health & Medical Informatics, 4, p. 121.
6. Patel, S., Singh, N., Pandya, S. 2016. IoT based smart Hospital for secure healthcare system. International Journal on Recent and Innovation Trends in Computing and Communication, 5, 5, pp. 404–408.
7. Christodoulakis, C., Asgarian, A., Easterbrook, S. 2017. Barriers to adoption of information technology in healthcare. Proceedings of the 27th Annual International Conference on Computer Science and Software Engineering. USA: IBM Corp., pp. 66–75.
8. Park, Y. J., Lee, Kh. 2018. Constructing a secure hacking-resistant IoT U-healthcare environment. Journal of Computer Virology and Hacking Techniques, 14, pp. 99–106.
9. Pradhan, J. D., Prasad, L. V. N., Dash, T. K., et al. (2024) Cascaded PFLANN model for intelligent health informatics in detection of respiratory diseases from speech using bio-inspired computation. Journal of Artificial Intelligence and Technology. DOI: 10.37965/jait.2024.0435.
10. Moosavi, S. R., Gia, T. N., Rahmani, A.-M., et al. 2015. SEA: A secure and efficient authentication and authorization architecture for IoT-based healthcare using smart gateways. Procedia Computer Science, 52, pp. 452–459.
11. Yang, Y., Zheng, X., Guo, W., et al. 2019. Privacy-preserving smart IoT-based healthcare big data storage and self-adaptive access control system. Information Sciences, 479, pp. 567–592.
12. Chaudhary, A., Peddoju, S. K., Peddoju, S. K. 2020. Cloud based wireless infrastructure for health monitoring. Virtual and Mobile Healthcare, pp. 34–55.
13. Murthy, S., Peddoju, S. K. 2020. IoT based patient health monitoring: A comprehensive survey. Springer 5th International Conference on ICT for Sustainable Development, Goa, India, pp. 349–356.

14. Thomas, V. S., Darvesh, S., MacKnight, C., et al. 2001. Estimating the prevalence of dementia in elderly people: A comparison of the Canadian study of health and aging and national population health survey approaches. International Psychogeriatrics, 13, pp. 169–175.
15. Sanghavi, J. 2019. Review of smart healthcare systems and applications for smart cities. ICCCE, 570, pp. 325–331.
16. Ashfaq, Z., Rafay, A., Mumtaz, R., et al. 2022. A review of enabling technologies for internet of medical things (IOMT) ecosystem. Ain Shams Engineering Journal, 13, 4, pp. 101660.
17. Palo Alto Networks. 2022. What is IOT security?.
18. Sultan, N. 2014. Making use of cloud computing for healthcare provision: Opportunities and challenges. International Journal of Information Management, 34, 2, pp. 177–184.
19. Dash, S. P. 2020. The impact of IoT in healthcare: Global technological change & the roadmap to a networked architecture in India. Journal of the Indian Institute of Science, 100, pp. 773–785.
20. McKeon, J. 2021. IOT security incidents increase as healthcare leans into Connected Health. HealthIT Security.
21. Roy, D. 2022. How healthcare facilities can use IoT to bolster security. TechTarget. https://www.techtarget.com/iotagenda/post/How-healthcare-facilities-can-use-IoT-to-bolster-security
22. Kumar, P. S., and Umatejaswi, V., 2016. Diagnosing diabetes using data mining techniques. International Journal of Scientific and Research Publications, 7, 6, pp. 705–709.
23. Rishika Reddy, A, Kumar, P. S. 2016. Predictive big data analytics in healthcare. Proceedings of IEEE Second International Conference on Computational Intelligence & Communication Technology, Ghaziabad. pp. 623–626.
24. Kumar, P. S., Pranavi, S. 2017. Performance analysis of machine learning algorithms on diabetes dataset using big data analytics. Proceedings of IEEE International Conference on Infocom Technologies and Unmanned Systems, Dubai, United Arab Emirates, pp. 580–585.
25. Kumar, P. S., Kavitha, K., Sharma, S. C. 2019. Big data analytics for childhood pneumonia monitoring. IGI global edited book, pp. 1–17.
26. Peddoju, S. K., Upadhyay, H., Bansali, S. 2019. Health monitoring with low power IoT devices using anomaly detection algorithm. Proceedings of IEEE Conference FMEC-2019, Rome, Italy, pp. 278–282.
27. Abdelgawad, A., Yelamarthi, K., Khattab, A. 2016. IoT-based health monitoring system for active and assisted living. International Conference on Smart Objects and Technologies for Social Good (GOODTECHS), Venice, Italy, 195, pp. 11–20.
28. Kodali, R. K., Mahesh, K. S. 2017. Smart emergency response system. Proc. IEEE Region Conf. (TENCON), Penang, Malaysia, pp. 712–717.
29. Dar, B. K., Shah, M. A., Islam, S. U., et al. 2019. Delay-aware accident detection and response system using fog computing. IEEE Access, 7, pp. 70975–70985.
30. Wu, X., Dunne, R., Yu, Z., et al.. 2017. STREMS: A smart real-time solution toward enhancing EMS pre-hospital quality. IEEE/ACM International Conference on Connected Health: Applications, Systems and Engineering Technologies, Philadelphia, PA, pp. 365–372.
31. Bartoletti, I. 2019. AI in healthcare: Ethical and privacy challenges. Proceedings of 17th Conference on Artificial Intelligence in Medicine, Berlin, Heidelberg, Springer-Verlag, pp. 7–10.
32. Choi, J., et al. 2019. Medical information protection frameworks for smart healthcare based on IoT. Proceedings of the 9th International Conference on Web Intelligence, Mining and Semantics. New York, NY, USA, ACM. Web. 29, pp. 1–5.

33. Zhang, C., Shahriar, H. 2020. The adoption, issues, and challenges of wearable healthcare technology for the elderly. Proceedings of the 21st Annual Conference on Information Technology Education. New York, NY, USA, ACM, pp. 50–53.
34. Abbas, N., Asim, M., Tariq, N., et al. 2019. A mechanism for securing IOT-enabled applications at the fog layer. Journal of Sensor and Actuator Networks, 8, 1, pp. 16.
35. WAL-mawee, W. 2012. Privacy and security issues in IoT healthcare applications for the disabled users a survey. Master's Theses, pp. 651.
36. Kashani, M. H., Madanipour, M., Nikravan, M., et al. 2021. A systematic review of IOT in healthcare: Applications, techniques, and trends. Journal of Network and Computer Applications, 192, 103164.
37. Landaluce, H., Laura A., Asier P., et al. 2020. A review of IoT sensing applications and challenges using RFID and wireless sensor networks. Sensors, 20, 9, pp. 2495.
38. Hasan, M. K., Ghazal, T. M., Saeed, R. A., et al. 2021. A review on security threats, vulnerabilities, and counter measures of 5G enabled internet-of-medical-things. IET Communications, 16, 5, pp. 421–432.
39. Hireche, R., Mansouri, H., Pathan, A. S. K. 2022. Security and privacy management in internet of medical things (IOMT): A synthesis. Journal of Cybersecurity and Privacy, 2, 3, pp. 640–661.
40. Dwivedi, R., Mehrotra, D., Chandra, S. 2022. Potential of internet of medical things (IOMT) applications in building a smart healthcare system: A systematic review. Journal of Oral Biology and Craniofacial Research, 12, 2, pp. 302–318.
41. Alotaibi, Y. K., Federico, F. 2017. The impact of health information technology on patient safety. Saudi Medical Journal, 38, 12, pp.1173–1180. DOI: doi: 10.15537/smj. 2017.12.20631
42. Binbusayyis, A., Alaskar, H., Vaiyapuri, T. et al. 2022. An investigation and comparison of machine learning approaches for intrusion detection in IOMT network. The Journal of Supercomputing, 78, 15, pp. 17403–17422.
43. Anandarajan, M., Malik, S. 2018. Protecting the internet of medical things: A situational crime-prevention approach. Cogent Medicine, 5, 1, p. 1513349.
44. Gopalan, S., Raza, A., Almobaideen, W. 2020. IOT Security in Healthcare Using AI: A Survey. Proceedings of International Conference on Communications, Signal Processing, and their Applications (ICCSPA), Sharjah, United Arab Emirates, pp. 1–6.
45. Hameed, S. S., Hassan, W. H., Latiff, L. A., Ghabban, F. 2021. A systematic review of security and privacy issues in the internet of medical things; The role of machine learning approaches. Journal of Computer Science, 7, pp. 414.
46. Cogniteq 2022. Importance of IOMT Security: What to consider in development. https://www.cogniteq.com/blog/importance-iomt-security-what-consider-development
47. Koutras, D. Stergiopoulos, G., Dasaklis, T. et al. 2020. Security in IOMT communications: A survey. Sensors, 20, 17, pp. 4828.
48. Putta, S. R. 2018. Security and privacy of wearable internet of medical things: Stakeholders perspective. Culminating Projects in Information Assurance, pp. 69.
49. Rana, A., Chakraborty, C., Sharma, S. et al. 2022. Internet of medical things-based secure and energy-efficient framework for health care. Big Data, 10, 1, pp. 18–33.
50. Razdan, S., Sharma, S. 2021. Internet of medical things: Overview, emerging technologies, and case studies. IETE Technical Review, 39, 4, pp. 1–14.
51. Wazid, M., Das, A. K., Rodrigues, J. J. et al. 2019. IOMT malware detection approaches: Analysis and research challenges. IEEE Access, 7, pp. 182459–182476.
52. He, Y., Aliyu, A., Evans, M., Luo, C. 2021. Health care cybersecurity challenges and solutions under the climate of COVID-19: Scoping review. Journal of Medical Internet Research, 23, 4, p. e2174.
53. Gope, P., Sikdar, B. 2019. Lightweight and privacy preserving two-factor authentication scheme for IoT devices. IEEE Internet of Things, 6, 1, pp. 580–589.

54. Wang, K., Shao, Y., Xie, L., et al. Jan.–March. 2020. Adaptive and fault-tolerant data processing in healthcare IoT based on fog computing. IEEE Transactions on Network Science and Engineering, 7, 1, pp. 263–273.
55. Srinivas, J., Das, A. K., Kumar, N., et al. 2020. Cloud centric authentication for wearable healthcare monitoring system. IEEE Transactions on Dependable and Secure Computing, 17, 5, pp. 942–956.
56. Kishor., Amit, Chakraborty C. 2021. Artificial intelligence and internet of things based healthcare 4.0 monitoring system. Wireless Personal Communications, pp. 1–14.
57. Guduri, M., Chakraborty, C., Maheswari, U., et al. 2023. Blockchain-based federated learning technique for privacy preservation and security of smart electronic health records. IEEE Transactions on Consumer Electronics, pp. 1–11.
58. Ahmed, S., Hossain, M. F., Kaiser, M. S., et al. 2021. Artificial Intelligence and Machine Learning for Ensuring Security in Smart Cities. Data-Driven Mining, Learning and Analytics for Secured Smart Cities. Advanced Sciences and Technologies for Security Applications. Springer, vol. 16, pp. 1–44.
59. Gaur, R., Prakash, S., Prasad, L.N., et al. 2023. A secure and efficient scheme based on unlinkability and anonymous traceable protocol for cloud-assisted IoT environment. Journal of Circuits, Systems and Computers, 32, 18, p. 2350316.

2 Low-Cost Versatile Remote Healthcare Monitoring of Bedridden Patients

Marco Aurelio Nuño-Maganda, Yahir Hernández-Mier, Said Polanco-Martagón, José Hugo Barrón-Zambrano, Juan Carlos Elizondo-Leal, and Alan Díaz-Manriquez

2.1 INTRODUCTION

Telehealthcare focuses on distance measurement of human physiological parameters to detect disease abnormalities. Remote care must include patient monitoring outside the hospital, primarily supported by wireless sensors, embedded systems, networked systems, and mobile applications. Remote patient monitoring must enable real-time disease detection, the ability to continuously monitor patients, prevent deterioration and premature death, reduce hospitalization costs, reduce hospital admissions, and provide more accurate measurements while maintaining patients' daily activities through communications technology, emergency medical nursing, support for patients with limited mobility to improve healthcare efficiency (Malasinghe et al., 2019).

Medical advances will give patients more rapid access to medicines and treatments. Healthcare 4.0 leverages new technologies to make significant healthcare advances, from mobile to cloud computing. As life expectancy continues to increase, there is a need to develop valuable tools to improve older people's care. Medicine 4.0 envisions a highly networked healthcare system. With the Internet of Things (IoT), hospital beds can be connected to the network and use patient data. Medicine 4.0 reduces the health burden of rich countries and provides good services with comprehensive, high-quality treatment to less developed countries. Patient data is collected electronically and used through technology to better understand and diagnose them. Patient-centered paradigms replace physician-centered treatment techniques.

There are several main approaches to performing vital signals monitoring. Non-wearable devices are related to sensors or electronic devices located outside the body but in contact with some parts of it, and manual activation can be required for monitoring a specific vital sign, for example, blood pressure (BP). The sensor has a fixed location, generally connected to an embedded monitoring device, which may need to be connected to a power source, or in some cases, power is obtained from a

DOI: 10.1201/9781003603610-2

battery pack. The main advantage of this approach is its low cost. Wearable devices are related to electronic devices that a user can wear to collect health and activity data. Although these devices use last-generation sensing technologies, their main disadvantage is their high cost, and due to their high grade of miniaturization, their battery drops when utilized extensively. Finally, hybrid devices use a smartphone or a PC as a container for the obtained data, sensors attached to the monitored body parts, and wireless connectivity is required to transfer sensor measurements to the data container. The approach combines the advantage of the low cost of non-wearable devices and the connectivity of wearable devices.

Digital health can improve healthcare delivery in low- and middle-income countries even when its implementation faces several challenges (Mitchell & Kan, 2019). Wearable devices aid in several health areas, such as healthcare and biomedical monitoring systems. Widespread adoption of wearable devices requires solving some technical challenges. Calibration of personal wearable devices is a technical issue in this area (Guk et al., 2019). In Qaosar et al. (2018), the authors proposed a device for monitoring health physiological parameters and emergency medications, including information and communication modules enabling physicians and health centers to track patient health status remotely. The communication module enables the proposed device to communicate automatically with emergency services when necessary.

In Distefano et al. (2017), the authors combine the IoT paradigm and resource ecosystem with a customized cloud-oriented solution to solve several e-health scenarios, such as monitoring and early treating hospital patients. In Hoppe et al. (2019), the authors proposed a severe hypertension monitoring strategy for postpartum women through remote BP monitoring.

Wearable health devices and their integration into healthcare systems have evolved. Personal monitoring devices provide patient data and transmission. Still, integrating multiple biosensors, intelligent processing, and alerts are crucial in medical applications interacting with healthcare (Dias & Paulo Silva Cunha, 2018). Caregivers can customize wireless health data monitoring in hospitals to support patient mobility and make the patient journey through the hospital stay cost-effective (Andersen & Mihovska, 2019).

Existing systems monitor vital functions, namely BP and the force of blood circulation through vessel walls. BP (measured in mm/Hg) is the systolic/diastolic pressure ratio. The average BP value for adults is below 120/80 and above 90/60. Heart rate (HR), or pulse, is the rhythmic expansion of the arteries caused by the opening and closing of the heart's aortic valve. HR expresses the heart contractions (beats) per minute. During sleep, a slow heartbeat is expected, with a frequency of about 40–50 beats per minute considered normal. The number of breaths per minute (respiratory rate) is based on a person's chest rises and falls at rest. Respiratory or breathing rate could be affected by fever and other illnesses. The standard breathing rate is 12–20 when resting. Healthy adult body temperature ranges from 36.5 degrees Celsius to 37.2 degrees Celsius. A fever occurs when the body temperature is 1 degree or above the average temperature of 37 degrees Celsius. Oxygen saturation (SO_2), also named blood oxygen (BO), is a measurement of the concentration of oxygen dissolved or transported in a specific medium. Oxygen saturation in adults typically ranges from 94% to 99%. People with oxygen saturation below 90% may need supplemental oxygen. Electrodermal activity (EDA), or galvanic skin response, is a change in the skin's electrical resistance, a physiochemical response to emotional arousal, increasing that increases sympathetic nervous system activity.

The main contribution of this paper is a remote monitoring system focused on most of the relevant physiological parameters to adequately monitor the health of bedridden patients, which consists of an embedded system that acquires the parameters, sends them to a local smartphone through a Bluetooth connection, and local app packages and transfer the parameters over the network to a cloud platform, where a remote caregiver accesses the data graphically. This chapter proposes a configurable platform to support e-health control for bedridden patients through a real-time vital signs monitoring system. We have two types of caregivers in this system. The local caregiver located close to the patient (possibly with the responsibility of caring for other patients as well) has no medical knowledge but will only assist the patient in solving his physiological needs and checking the status of the embedded system. The other type of caregiver is the responsible caregiver, who, through the App, monitors the patient's status remotely and can communicate with the physician in charge in case of abnormal readings of physiological variables. The developed project involves monitoring patients lacking internet connectivity infrastructure, but 3G/4G/5G connectivity is a common denominator in underdeveloped countries. We propose the use of a smartphone, which is not necessarily of a recent model (those used in this project are old-generation devices); it is sufficient that it has a Bluetooth interface for obtaining data from the sensors and through the mobile application (ReViSiAApp) allows the caregiver to make a diagnosis of the hardware and send to the server in the cloud the data obtained from the sensors.

We designed this platform to require minimal human intervention after its initial setup. From the four commonly observed vital signs, the proposed platform monitors three of them: body temperature, BP, and pulse (HR), as well as three complementary physiological parameters: electrodermal activity (galvanic resistance (GR)), oxygen saturation, and electric heart signals (through an electrocardiogram (ECG)). The main components of this platform are an interface for smartphones that receives information from a microcontroller-based embedded system that interacts with sensors to monitor vital signs. These parameters are monitored and integrated into a distributed system that stores them in a web server. Finally, a caregiver application manages the patient profile and generates reports of the monitored parameters for a specific patient. This chapter is organized as follows. Section 2.2 summarizes existing systems and approaches. Section 2.3 describes the main modules using the most sensors compared with previous methods, including the hardware required, and explains in detail the software components and interfaces of the proposed applications. Section 2.4 presents and discusses the main results. Finally, Section 2.5 establishes the conclusion and addresses future work.

2.2 RELATED WORK

The system proposed in this paper monitors as many vital signs as possible. Some articles only deal with ECG or HR monitoring for heart health among the existing technologies. In Ahsanuzzaman et al. (2020), the authors report an Android prediction system to detect real-time cardiac arrhythmias by monitoring ECG signals, which uses recurrent neural networks and long short-term memory algorithms to predict arrhythmias. Some of the system's components are a Raspberry Pi 3 and Arduino UNO embedded computers, the HC-05 Bluetooth device, and an ECG sensor, among other circuit operation components. In Antonius and Dachyar (2020), the authors use IoT technology for remote cardiac monitoring of patients to reduce emergency response and outpatient processing times. In Hasan and Ismaeel (2020), they proposed an ECG monitoring system with the following hardware components: AD8382 ECG sensor, Arduino Uno, ESP8266 WiFi module, and the doctor receives the patient's EKG information through the IoT Blynk application. In Mallidi et al. (2022), the authors report on IoT (Internet of Things) devices for temperature and HR monitoring. In Villanueva-Miranda et al. (2018), the authors developed an ECG monitor whose hardware components use a three-port Arduino, allowing the NodeJS framework to exchange data with remote servers using the NodeJS framework to provide cloud-based services and features. In Wijaya et al. (2020), the authors proposed an ECG monitoring solution that employs an AD8382 ECG and an Arduino Kit coupled with an ESP8266 WiFi module that sends the caregiver's ECG data through the IoT Blynk application. An IoT Blynk app monitors the patient remotely, allowing the physician to visualize the patient's ECG signal using the facilities provided by a cloud module. In Devi and Roy (2017), the authors proposed a mobile physiological measurement platform that continuously monitors the patient's HR and oxygen level. The system records the ECG and the photoplethysmogram (PPG) to estimate the HR and oxygen saturation level. An Android app displays the physiological parameters stored in text files and shared via a wireless network. In Brezulianu et al. (2019), the authors developed a wearable sensor to monitor the heart designed to monitor the heart's mechanical in a non-invasive way through its insertion in sports clothes. In Megalingam et al. (2014), the authors proposed a system with sensors attached to the patient's body to monitor the HR, body temperature, ECG, respiration rate, tilt, and fall of bedridden patients. In critical situations, the system informs the caregiver and transfers sensor data to a smartphone with Bluetooth connectivity. In Pereira et al. (2016), the authors developed a device for home care of bedridden patients, which acquires the patient's pulse, oxygen in the blood, airflow, body temperature, ECG, blood glucose meter, galvanic skin response, and BP. Their solution allows the caregiver to access patient data remotely through a web system. Related to body electric signals in Gupta et al. (2019), the authors acquired the electroencephalogram (EEG) from epileptic patients using an IoT-enabled cloud module and a smartphone app to monitor epileptical seizures. Even when we do not include the EEG in this study, its integration into the current system in a future version is straightforward.

Other authors focus on measuring patient temperature, such in Rahimoon et al. (2020), where the authors propose a non-invasive and wearable Arduino-based body temperature sensor with integrated embedded communication platforms. In Azizulkarim et al. (2017), the authors report a patient monitoring system that continuously monitors patient's temperature and pulse rate. The device records the measurements and sends them to a PC. Other vital sign is the oxygen saturation. In Agustine et al. (2018), the authors developed a system that uses a battery powered pulse oximeter sensor coupled with a WLAN router to display cardiovascular data on an Android app.

Another vital sign is BP, which provides insight into a patient's health status. Some works have focused on remotely monitoring a patient's BP, including wearable technologies that reduce weight but require continuous charging. In Varghese et al. (2013), the authors report a remote monitoring system focused on measuring patient (BP) coupled with a wireless network-based data storage. In Lazazzera et al. (2019), the authors proposed a smartwatch with two pulse oximeters on the device's back and front sides for real-time BP estimation. In Samartkit et al. (2022), the authors developed promising fiber optic-based HR and BP sensors unavailable to the general public. So, using standard sensors that require user intervention to take measures is necessary.

Advances have been reported regarding multiple vital signs measurements using the same platform. Some were limited to locally communicating results to a computer, while others included interfaces that remotely inform the monitored signs to the doctor or caregiver. In Sangeethalakshmi et al. (2023), the authors proposed a healthcare monitoring system that measures the patient's temperature, heartbeat rate, ECG, BP, and SPO2 and provides real-time patient health feedback through a mobile app. In Zhang and Ling (2020), the authors developed other healthcare monitoring solutions that measure the patient's temperature, respiration, oxygen saturation, HR, BP, and ECG. In Abdul Rahman and Jambek (2019), the authors report a remote monitoring device which get on electrocardiography (ECG), airflow, galvanic skin response, and temperature from biomedical sensors. In Bunkum et al. (2018), the authors present a patient monitoring system for bedridden patients with a bed lift control module. A caretaker or physician monitors the patient's HR, BP, and temperature through a web interface available in this system. In Miramontes et al. (2017), the authors present a platform called PlaIMoS, a fixed measurement station that uses wearable sensors that obtain data through network infrastructure and transmit collected data to a server for later analysis through apps created for diverse mobile operating systems. The proposed app records the patient's data, and the wearable sensors can detect the patient's falls. In Prasanth et al. (2019), the authors combine Arduino hardware and LabVIEW tools to develop a system that monitors patient ECG, HR, and temperature. Through a GSM module, the system sends SMS or email alerts if the patient's parameters are outside of normal limits. In Raja et al. (2019), the authors proposed a nonstop monitoring patient's health conditions, by obtaining parameters of patient's body complemented with patient's video monitoring algorithms which allows the physician to constantly monitor the patient's condition. In Malathi et al. (2023), the authors proposed a monitor solution to acquire patient data such as BP, temperature, and HR, developed using C language to receive the sensor data. This project included an IoT data cloud in reporting the health status of patients and sending notifications related to patient's health status to caregivers and nurses while being updated on a web page for doctors to access. In Bhardwaj et al. (2022), the authors proposed an embedded solution for health monitoring of patient's BP, HR, BO level, and body temperature. The proposed solution eases the integration of real-time data acquisition with IoT technologies. In Al-Naggar et al. (2019), the authors developed a smartphone-based real-time remote monitoring system with several physiological parameters such as ECG, HR, respiratory rate, BO saturation, and temperature). The patient and doctor apps get the wearable sensors data, which were acquired and stored by an Arduino Kit, for its visualization in graphical format. In Feng et al. (2022), the authors proposed a system that combines Arduino, Android, and Bluetooth technologies to interact with a reflective photoelectric sensor to obtain HR signals, a digital BP module to obtain BP information, and a MAX30102 BO sensor to obtain BO information. An Arduino processes the data collected by the sensors and displays it in real-time on an LCD. An app obtains the sensor's measurements from the Arduino via Bluetooth.

There are some systems that monitor the patient using image sensors, either capturing photographs or short time-lapse videos. This is particularly useful when it is desired to monitor the evolution of a visible lesion. Image sensors can increase the cost of the monitoring system since they require compression algorithms, such as the one developed by Chakraborty (2021), focused on estimating the healing status of chronic wounds. These systems demand colossal storage and bandwidth, especially those allowing users to capture and send wound images to a remote medicine center. Chakraborty proposed a compression algorithm, which, aided by a clustering module, improves its performance by reducing the execution time. Other authors are concerned about improving the security of data collected in the IoT but focused on medical apps by designing specialized secure communication techniques (Rana et al., 2022). Innovative city technologies include safer healthcare systems, a concern of the academic community, where the integration of mobile and ambient sensors with private and safety edge computing techniques to obtain valuable health information (Faria et al., 2021).

2.3 PROPOSED SYSTEM

Figure 2.1 shows the main components of the proposed system. Each component is described below:

- *Remote Vital Signs Monitoring Embedded System (ReViSMoES)*. This system is enclosed in a box with the required circuits to acquire the vital signs of a bedridden patient. It also includes a wireless communication interface that reports to the ReViSiMoApp, which transfers the sensor measurements to the remote server.
- *Remote Vital Signs Acquisition Application (ReViSiAApp)*. Each sensor sends its monitoring information through Bluetooth to the smartphone that hosts the ReViSiAApp.
- *Cloud Monitoring Module (CMoM)*. This module allows the storage of the sensor measurements connected to the ReViSMoES and reports to the server through ReViSiApp. In addition, through an API, the ReViSiMoApp, the caregiver receives information on the monitored patient's vital signs.
- *Remote Vital Signals Monitoring Application (ReViSiMoApp)*. The caregiver's smartphone hosts this application, allowing the caregiver to obtain information on the monitored vital signs and to administrate the monitoring times of the parameters acquired by the ReViSiMoApp.

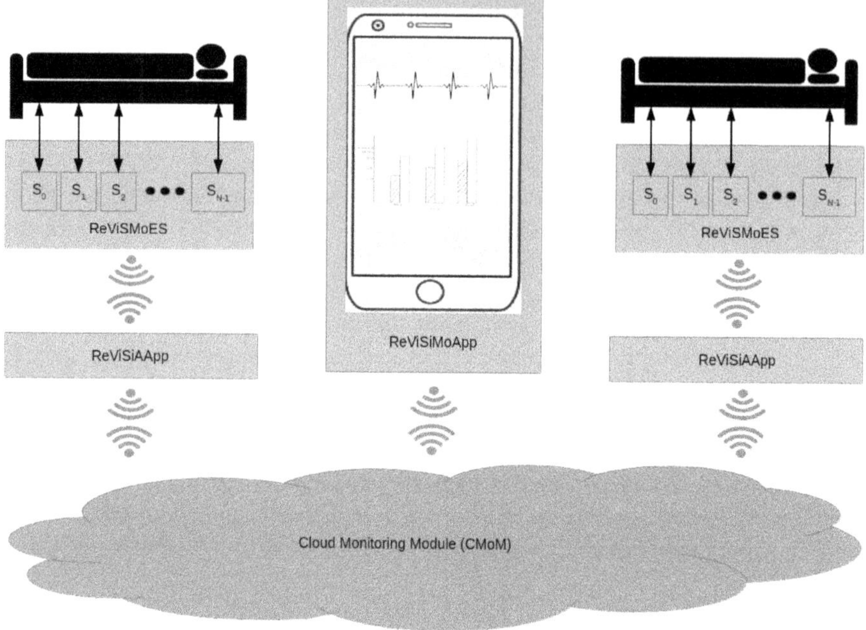

FIGURE 2.1   The proposed remote monitoring system's architecture includes the primary components such as ReViSMoES, ReViSiAApp, ReViSiMoApp, and CMoM.

2.3.1   SENSOR MONITORING PLATFORM

This part of the system includes the devices near the patient, both the ReViSMoES and the ReViSiAApp. The ReViSiAApp allows initializing of the ReViSMoES through a Bluetooth connection, performing initial system tests, configuring the remote servers, perform data transmission tests, among other functions.

2.3.1.1   Hardware Components of the ReViSMoES

The ReViSMoES includes a battery backup, which provides electrical power to the sensors and the smartphone that hosts the ReViSiAApp. This monitoring will not be interrupted when a power failure occurs. The ReViSiAApp saves the sensor measurements locally in case of Internet failure and performs the measurement transfer to the cloud app when the service is restored. The hardware parts of the ReViSMoES and their specifications are:

- *Microcontroller.* This element is the core of the ReViSMoES, since it hosts the required interface functions to obtain data of the attached sensors, and sends information to the ReViSiAApp using wireless connectivity, specifically Bluetooth serial communication.
- *HC-05 module.* This module makes possible to link the microcontroller with the smartphone that hosts the ReViSiAApp.

- *KY-001 temperature sensor module.* This module is required for measuring body temperature.
- *AD8232 ECG sensor.* This sensor measures the electrical activity of the heart. It extracts, amplifies, and filters bio-potential signals even in noisy conditions.
- *BPW34 silicon PIN photodiode.* This device is coupled with a 555 timer in order to generate the signals required to compute and report the BO levels.
- *OMRON HEM-7114 Blood pressure monitor.* This device is utilized for measuring BP levels. It was required to open the device and to monitor the generated signals in order to create the interface from ReViSMoES to start the measurement and to obtain the systolic/diastolic BP to be send to the ReViSiAApp.
- *Handmade galvanic sensor.* For building this sensor, the following components are required: (1) Two 220 Ohm resistors, (2) Velcro tape, (3) aluminium foil, and (4) regular adhesive tape. To construct the sensor, a jumper cable is connected to a piece of wrapped aluminium foil. Velcro tape is wrapped around the aluminium fold, which serves as a retainer for the fingers. A second sensor connected to the breadboard through two 220 resistors must be constructed.

In Figure 2.2, a control flow diagram of the ReViSMoES is shown. A brief description of each function is given below:

- *Device connection to smartphone.* This function performs the Bluetooth pairing between the smartphone hosting the ReViSiAApp and the ReViSMoES. If the ReViSMoES has already connected, then the connection is opened and tested.
- *Patient's profile loading.* This function transfers data between the ReViSMoES and the ReViSiAApp. Basically, the profile must contain the vital signs to be monitored and its respectively monitoring frequency (for example, daily or hourly).
- *Sensor configuration.* This function configures each sensor attached to the ReViSMoES according to the patient profile.
- *Vital signs acquisition.* This function processes each sensor measurement using the patient profile.
- *Vital signs filtering and integration.* This function processes the data obtained by each sensor and packages them into a string.
- *Vital signs transmission to smartphone.* This function sends the vital signs package using Bluetooth serial connectivity.

2.3.1.2 ReViSiAApp and Cloud Monitoring Module

The app provides a minimal interface that allows the local caregiver to diagnose any problem with Internet or Bluetooth connectivity or sensor problems. It is also possible to obtain the sensor measurements locally in case of any failure in the internet

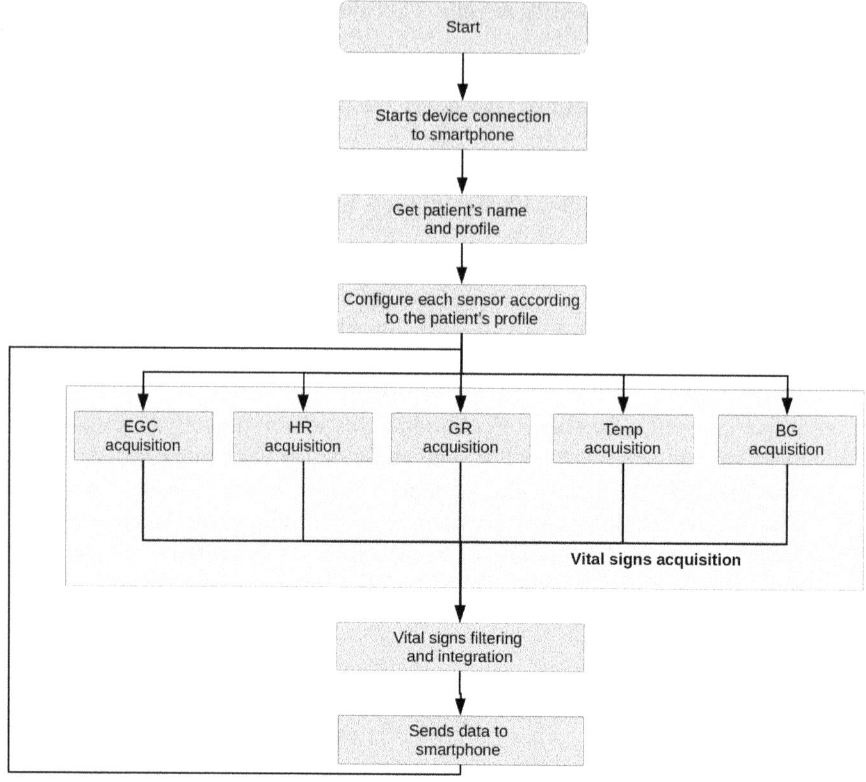

FIGURE 2.2 ReViSMoES flowchart. In the initial stage, ReViSMoES pairs with the ReViSiApp, which asks for the caregiver patient's general data. Once configured, ReViSMoES starts a continuous data acquisition cycle by the attached sensors. When the sensors acquire the data, these are stored and sent to the ReViSiApp.

connection that prevents the transmission of the sensor measurements to the cloud application.

Figure 2.3 shows a screen of the ReViSiA App. The local caregiver must configure the app before its first use to guarantee that it sends the obtained measurements to the remote server. The user interface components are:

- *Current server information label.* Initially, there is no default server, so the rest of the controls of the mobile application are disabled.
- *Manage servers button.* This button allows the user to add a default server. Only one server set is active when the manager adds other servers to backup monitoring results. This button becomes enabled when the user adds at least one server to the server's list. The *current user panel* displays the current server.
- *Request access button.* This button enables the ReViSiA App to connect to the current active remote server and to obtain the device identification.

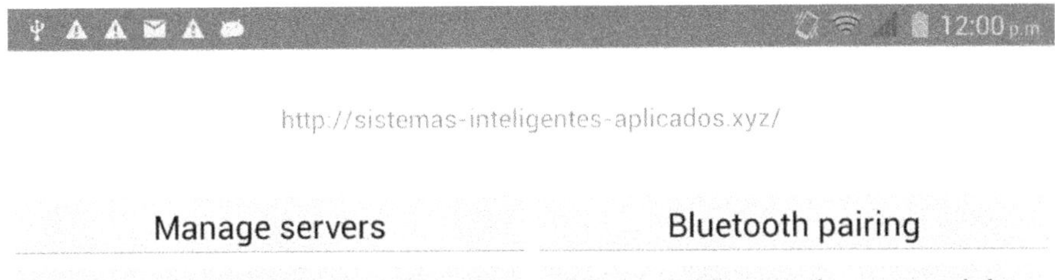

FIGURE 2.3 The main interface of the ReViSiApp includes several buttons to test each sensor individually, configure patient data, pair the device with the ReViSMoES, and verify the connection with the CMoM.

- *Bluetooth pairing/unpairing button.* This button allows the ReViSiAApp to be paired with the ReViSMoES using Bluetooth. When ReViSiAApp pairs with the ReViSMoES, the data transfer between them is ready to be performed. This button allows the ReViSiAApp to be unpaired with the ReViSMoES. When the function associated with this button finishes, the app will turn off the controls in the *vital signal test panel*, so it is required to press the *Bluetooth pairing button* to pair the ReViSiAApp with the ReViSMoES again.
- *Current user panel.* Once the user establishes the patient profile, this panel shows information such as the MAC address of the smartphone hosting the ReViSiAApp, the device identification, and the patient's name.
- *Vital signal test panel.* This panel allows the user to test each sensor attached to the ReViSMoES by sending the appropriate command by Bluetooth connectivity. Selecting one button of this panel turns off the other buttons until the specific vital sign is acquired.

The CMoM is mounted in the cloud and includes an MQTT server for receiving sensor data captured by the ReViSMoES through the ReViSiApp. It consists of the necessary APIs for reading data from the ReViSiApp, in addition to providing the management to replace the patient's profile from the ReViSMoES, store the history of the readings, and query the data based on the doctor's or caregiver's requirements.

2.3.2 REMOTE VITAL SIGNALS MONITORING APPLICATION

In Figure 2.4, a screen of the *ReViSiMoApp* app is shown. This application is designed to be used by any caregiver without medical training, for example a relative of the

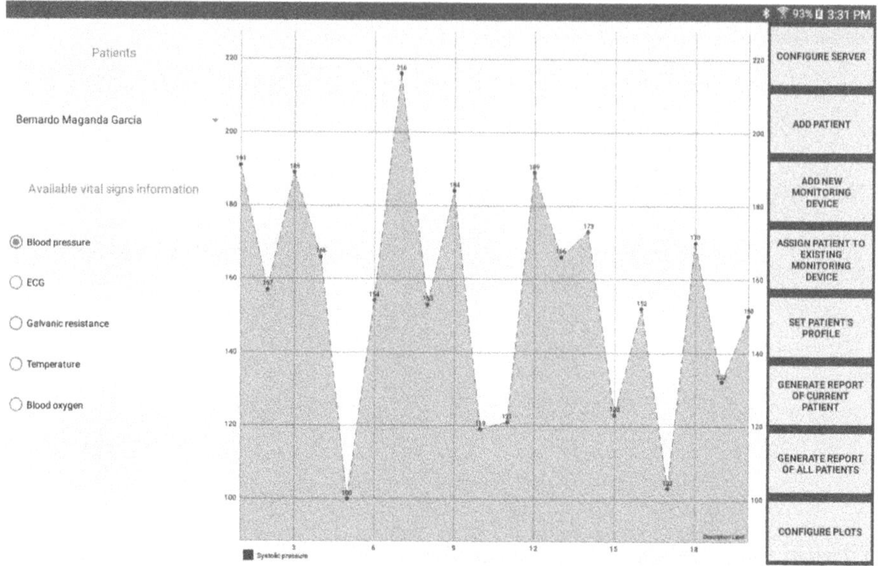

FIGURE 2.4 The main interface of the ReViSiMoApp includes several buttons where the remote caregiver chooses the patient to monitor. The caregiver could have a different setting for each patient based on each requirement. The central panel plots the selected physiological variable, and the caregiver can generate reports related to the monitored variables.

patient to be monitored. The application is divided into three panels: left panel, that allows the selection of the name of the patient, and the specific vital sign to be monitored; the center panel, that displays a graph related to the patient vital sign selected in the left panel; and the right panel with several user-configurable functions. The user interface components are described below:

- *Patient spinner.* The caregiver uses this control to select the patient's name for vital signs visualization.
- *Available vital signs Radiogroup.* This control allows the user to select the available vital signs to be monitored for the selected patients. When both, patient spinner and available vital signs groups are updated, the vital signs plot located in the center is also updated.
- *Vital signs plot.* Depending on the selection of patient and vital sign, this panel shows a bar plot to visualize the behavior of a selected vital sign in the last 24 hours. The configuration of this panel can be changed by selecting the *Configure plots button* in the right panel of the UI.
- *Configure server button.* This button allows the user to add and set a default server. In the case that the manager adds other servers to backup monitoring results, each server can be added to the application, but only one is marked as active.
- *Add patient button.* This button allows the user to add patients, so the vital signs of multiple patients can be managed by the same ReViSiMoApp.

- *Add new monitoring device button.* This button allows to add new monitoring device. The user must input the mac address and the device identifier of the smartphone that hosts the ReViSiAApp, and from this moment, this device is ready to be used.
- *Assign patient to existing monitoring device button.* This button allows the user to assign a specific ReViSMoES to a previously created patient register. One ReViSMoES can be only assigned to one patient, so if a patient is marked as the current user, this setting can be changed by the caregiver in this function.
- *Patient profile setting.* This button allows the user to configure the monitoring frequency for each vital signal for the target patient. A relevant issue is that each vital sign can have a different monitoring frequency, so it is possible to monitor HR every 30 minutes. Still, the system can monitor the same patient's temperature every 2 hours. Remotely, the caregiver must define the timing of the measurements, establishing a minimum periodicity of 1 minute and a maximum separation of 90 minutes. Once the user sets the time interval, it is possible to make changes based on the evolution of the patient.
- *Generate report for the current patient.* This button allows the user to generate a report for the current patient by asking the date range and the desired vital sign, and the user select the location where the report will be generated as a PDF file.
- *Generate report of all patients.* This button allows the user to generate a global PDF report for all the patients monitored by the system, by date range.
- *Configure plots.* This button allows the user to configure titles, legends, X and Y ranges, resolution, colors and other fancy effects in the visualized plot located in the center panel.

2.4 IMPLEMENTATION AND RESULTS

2.4.1 PRELIMINARY PROTOTYPE

We tested the circuits using protoboards and wires to implement a prototype. In the first phase, we programmed a requests API and circuits to obtain BP for the sphygmomanometer using a Bluetooth serial interface. An initial version of the app performs the BP measurement using the BT serial interface, waits until the sphygmomanometer obtains the BP measurement, and displays the BP in the ReViSiAApp. Later, we added the interface elements for the local APP and the necessary circuitry to monitor the rest of the vital signs. Figure 2.5(a) shows the ReViSiAApp obtaining data from the prototype (in a wooden box). Figure 2.5(b) shows the operation of the sphygmomanometer remotely operated by the ReViSiAApp. At a later stage, we designed a printed circuit board to reduce the size of the circuit, assembled on a plastic box with the necessary holes for sensors attached to the patient's body.

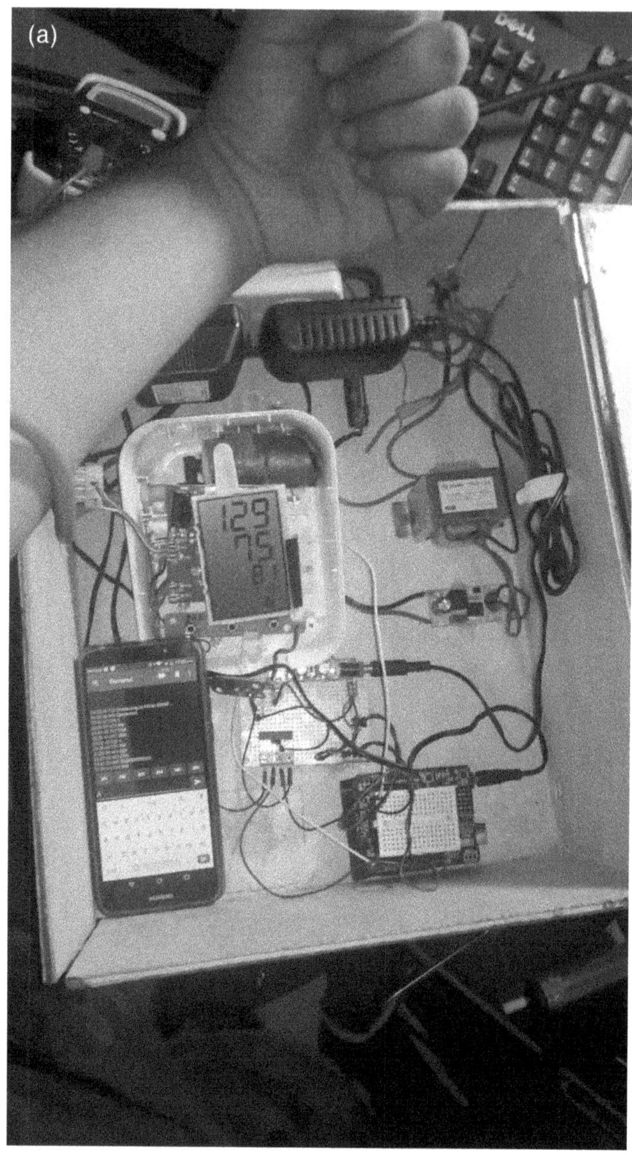

FIGURE 2.5 We validated the remote monitoring system by integrating the ReViSMoES, ReViSiAApp, ReViSiMoAp, and ReViSiMoAp. (a) We used an initial version of the ReViSMoES to perform a Bluetooth connectivity test with the ReViSiApp and to verify the data sensor acquisition reliability. *(Continued)*

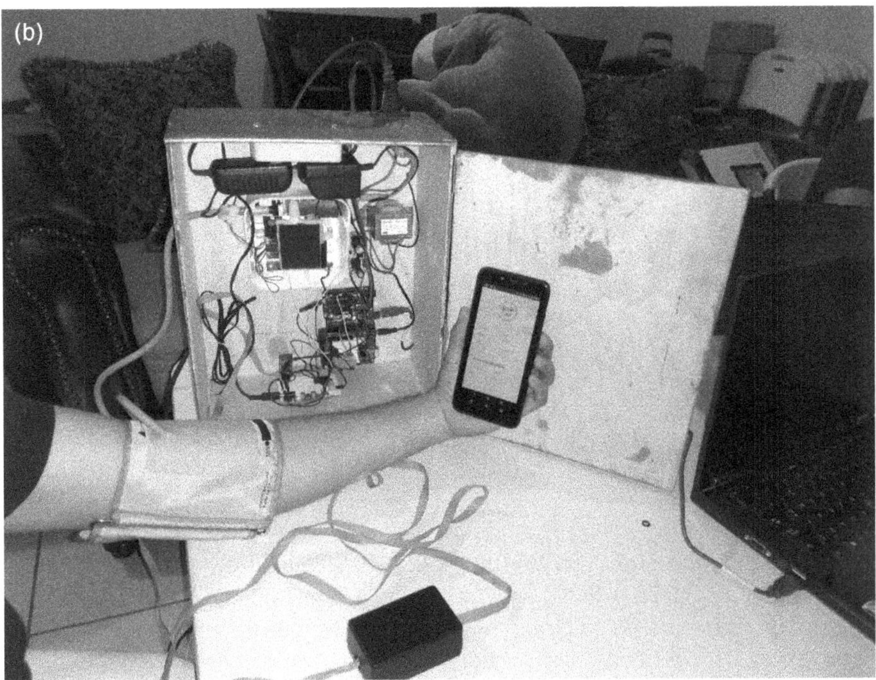

FIGURE 2.5 *(Continued)* (b) We test the ReViSiMoApp to perform a BP measurement remotely with the ReViSiApp connected and properly configured. We repeated the same test with the other sensors attached to the ReViSMoES.

2.4.2 Deployment of ReViSiAApp and ReViSiMoApp

We tested four remote monitoring prototypes simultaneously through the same platform. We used smartphones with different Android versions to test the proposed system. When we tried the ReViSiApp application, the most recent Android version was 13, while the oldest version of the device on which we tested the app was 2.3.4, as reported in Table 2.1.

Although we assume that the smartphone hosting the ReViSiAApp must have a power supply, we perform tests to estimate the maximum monitoring autonomy in the event of a power failure. We suggest that smartphones hosting the ReViSiAApp cannot be of the last generation. However, they may be functional devices already in disuse due to their memory limitations and the number of applications allowed. We cannot perform this test on one device (the oldest one) used for the ReViSiAApp deployment since it must have a power supply for continuous operation. To compare the battery performance of the app, we included in the table a modern smartphone with much more computational and memory capabilities.

We defined three policies to evaluate battery consumption and data transmission, which establishes the interval between the measurements. These intervals were 1, 5, and 20 minutes. In the first policy, the device continuously sends the acquired measurements, which involves intensive use of the battery, since to achieve this objective, each sensor carries out its respective measure in a shorter

TABLE 2.1

Devices Used to Test the Proposed Mobile Apps for Remote Monitoring.

Device	Processor	Cores	RAM	Android Version	Deployed App
Polaroid PMID706GK	Cortex-A7 (1.0 GHz)	2	512 MB	4.2.2	ReViSiAApp
LG E510F	ARM1136EJ-S (800Mhz)	1	512 MB	2.3.4	ReViSiAApp
ZUUM P50	Cortex-A7 (1.3 GHz)	4	1 GB	4.2.2	ReViSiAApp
LG G3 Stylus	Cortex-A7 (1.3 GHz)	4	1 GB	5.0.2	ReViSiAApp
Motorola E5 Play	Cortex-A53 (1.4 GHz)	4	1 GB	8.1.0	ReViSiAApp
Motorola Edge 20	Cortex-A78 (2.4 GHz)	8	8 GB	12.0.0	ReViSiAApp
Samsung Galaxy Note 10.1	Krait 400 (2.3 GHz)	4	3 GB	5.1.1	ReViSiMoApp

time than the one established by the policy. In a second test, the time interval increases to 5 minutes (which involves making a larger shipment in a much longer time). Still, it is possible to define how many measurements will be made in that interval (by default, the system sets to three measures, but it is possible to define as many measurements as long as the minimum time). In the third test, the sending time was increased to 20 minutes, reducing the number of sendings but increasing the amount of data significantly depending on the number of measurements in said time interval.

For the ReViSiAApp, we considered two energy consumption comparison profiles:

- High data demand, which implies reducing the time interval between data requests and the request to the sensors, specifically designed for caregivers who require real-time information. We determine the minimum separation time between readings of one minute, based on the sphygmomanometer's speed, which requires that time to inflate the inflatable cuff.
- Low data demand, which implies taking readings with a high interval (specifically, four measurements per hour, or a 15-minute interval between them).

Figure 2.6 shows the previously described profiles' energy consumption results (i.e., battery lifetime). We measured the battery consumption for each configuration and plotted it in Figure 2.6(a) and (b). We can note that all the smartphones maintain the system in operation for at least four hours; the older ones who power fall faster than the newest ones.

2.4.3 Heart Rate Monitoring Comparison Results

We evaluated several mobile applications, including most commercial apps and fitness bands, to compare the HR accuracy of the sensor embedded in the proposed system. Most reviewed apps focus on sports and do not provide a long-term

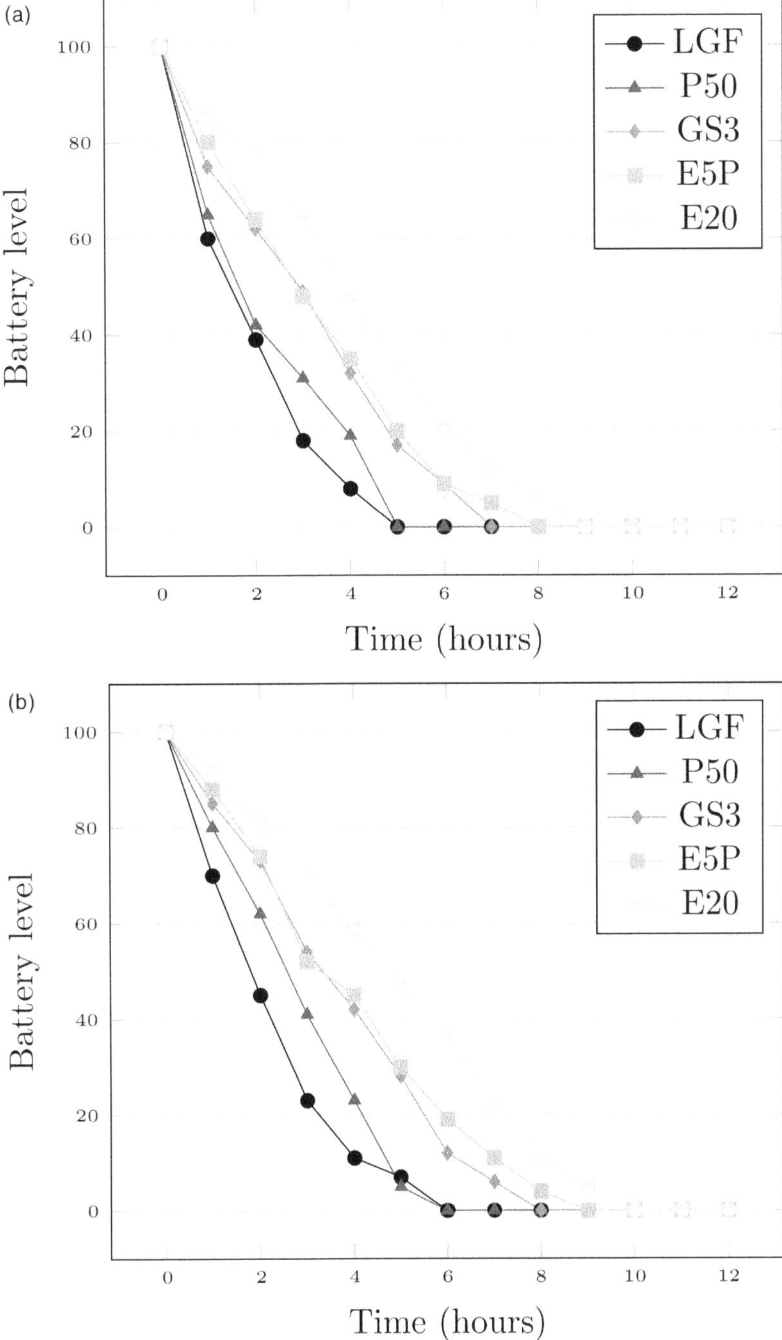

FIGURE 2.6 Power consumption of the variants of the ReViSiAAp in the tested smart-phones (LGF corresponds to the LG E510F smartphone located in the second row of Table 2.1, P50 to the third one, and so on). (a) Energy consumption over time for configuration A. (b) Energy consumption over time for configuration B.

TABLE 2.2

Comparison between Proposed App against Best Rated HR Applications

Application Name	Rating	HR Range
Health Care Monitor (iCare, 2019)	4.5	68–75
Single pulsometer (Pulsometer, 2019)	4.4	66–72
Pulse Heart Rate Monitor (Monitor, 2019)	4.3	68–76
Runtastic Heart Rate: Pulse (Runtastic, 2019)	4.3	68–76
Cardiograph (Cardiograph, 2019)	3.8	69–72
SmartBand2 (Sony, 2019)	3.4	68–75
Proposed Application	-	69–75
AVERAGE HR		68–74

functionality analysis when designing remote health monitoring systems. Six top-rated Android apps were considered and compared with the proposed system for remote vital signs monitoring. Table 2.2 shows data of the tested applications (app name, rating, and HR range). We take HRs from test subjects resting for two minutes for monitoring purposes.

As shown in Table 2.2, the HR ranges obtained by the applications are close to the application, as expected, since the sensor used for HR is of commercial type. The advantage of using the interface with the retail device is that the BP, which the applications cannot obtain, can be obtained simultaneously.

2.4.4 COMPARISON WITH EXISTING SYSTEMS

Table 2.3 summarizes related systems for vital sign monitoring. Many reviewed systems focus exclusively on cardiac symptoms reported to the physician. In this chapter, in addition to including cardiac symptoms, we include BO, HR, BP, temperature (T) and GR, and ECG (columns in Table 2.3). We also included in this comparison some devices of the wearable type, even when, in the first instance, they involve higher costs, in addition to adding discomfort, requiring multiple charging individually, and being more fragile compared to their non-wearable counterparts. Labels related to the type of technology used are wearable Device (W) and monitoring type (MT). In the last column, LM means *Local monitoring*, since the proposed platform reports results to a computer connected to the device/sensor using a wired connection. RM means *Remote monitoring*, seeing that the proposed system reports results using wireless Internet/cloud storage connectivity. These results will be available for later monitoring from a caregiver of a physician.

From the reviewer articles, we found that most focus on a single physiological parameter, while others focus on only a few, whereas we cover all those listed in the table. Some research focuses on having a local solution, where the physiological parameters are acquired but not transmitted to the cloud or other devices over a WiFi network. Other research works concentrate on predicting specifically detected diseases based on the selected physiological parameter.

TABLE 2.3

Comparison of the Proposed System Versus Existing Vital Sign Monitoring Systems

Work	Monitored Sign						Technology	
	ECG	BO	HR	BP	T	GR	WD	MT
(Chakraborty, 2021)	NO	NO	YES	YES	YES	NO	NO	RM
(Bhardwaj et al., 2022)	NO	YES	YES	YES	YES	NO	NO	RM
(Al-Naggar et al., 2019)	YES	YES	YES	NO	YES	NO	NO	RM
(Feng et al., 2022)	NO	YES	YES	YES	NO	NO	NO	LM
(Megalingam et al., 2014)	YES	NO	YES	NO	YES	NO	NO	LM
(Pereira et al., 2016)	NO	YES	NO	NO	YES	YES	NO	LM
(Bunkum et al., 2018)	NO	NO	YES	YES	YES	NO	NO	RM
(Miramontes et al., 2017)	NO	YES	YES	NO	YES	YES	NO	RM
(Devi & Roy, 2017)	YES	YES	NO	NO	NO	NO	NO	RM
(Brezulianu et al., 2019)	YES	YES	YES	NO	NO	NO	YES	RM
(Lazazzera et al., 2019)	NO	NO	NO	YES	NO	NO	YES	RM
(Wijaya et al., 2020)	NO	NO	YES	NO	YES	NO	NO	RM
(Prasanth et al., 2019)	YES	NO	YES	NO	YES	NO	NO	RM
(Agustine et al., 2018)	NO	YES	YES	NO	NO	NO	NO	RM
(Raja et al., 2019)	NO	NO	YES	NO	YES	NO	NO	RM
(Villanueva-Miranda et al., 2018)	YES	NO	YES	NO	NO	NO	NO	RM
(Abdul Rahman & Jambek, 2019)	YES	NO	NO	NO	YES	YES	NO	RM
(Sangeethalakshmi et al., 2023)	YES	YES	YES	YES	YES	NO	NO	RM
(Zhang & Ling, 2020)	YES	YES	YES	YES	YES	NO	NO	RM
Proposed Platform	YES	YES	YES	YES	YES	YES	YES	RM

2.4.5 Discussion

The initial prototype acquires sensor signals and sends them to the ReViSiAApp, which concentrates the data and sends it to the cloud. A remote caregiver application can obtain sensor data and display it in a graphical format. We built several prototypes of the embedded system, each linked to the local application to test sensor data acquisition. The local application allows the configuration of the capture interval as requested by the remote caretaker. The tests confirm the correct operation of the prototypes when linked to the local caregiver application regardless of the Android operating system version.

We concentrated only on the RH parameters to compare the embedded system with existing monitoring systems. For this, we implemented a comparison concerning existing applications. We showed that the embedded system has similar accuracy ranges to such applications, highlighting the advantage that the applications require on a smartphone. In contrast, in the embedded system, the HR acquisition is performed by the same sensor that obtains the BP.

To estimate the autonomy of the local application, we carried out battery autonomy tests by deploying the application on different devices. The first profile has high data demand, where constant sending of sensor readings is required, while in the second profile, the time-space between sensor captures is long. We installed the local monitoring application on each smartphone using each profile. We monitored the battery discharge time for each smartphone, shown its evolution in Figure 2.6. The comparison indicates that devices allow up to 8 hours of battery life using the high data demand profile, while for the low data demand profile, some smartphones achieve autonomy of up to 10 hours.

2.5   CONCLUSION AND FUTURE WORK

From the work developed, we emphasize the following deliverables:

- A ReViSMoES, which has a microcontroller receiving information from the vital signs sensors and a Bluetooth interface that sends data to a ReViSiAApp.
- A ReViSiAApp, which is a mobile app hosted on a smartphone that manages the remote connectivity with a CMoM, where the lectures obtained from the ReViSMoES are stored.
- CMoM, which stores the sensor measurements connected to the ReViSMoES and reports to the server through ReViSiApp. In addition, through an API, the ReViSiMoApp, the caregiver receives information on the monitored patient's physiological parameters.
- ReViSiMoApp, which is a mobile app hosted on a smartphone used by a caregiver located in a far location. The app obtains reports from one or more patients in order to give feedback to the clinician.

In this chapter, a system to Remote Monitoring of Vital Signs (ReMoViS) is proposed. The proposed system is integrated by three main components: the ReViSMoES composed of a microcontroller receiving information from the vital signs sensors and a Bluetooth interface that sends data to a ReViSiAApp, hosted on a smartphone; the ReViSiAApp manages the remote connectivity with a cloud server, where the lectures obtained from the ReViSMoES are stored; finally, the Remote Vital Signals Monitoring Application (ReViSiMoApp) is used by a caregiver located in a far location, obtaining reports from one or more patients in order to give feedback to the clinician. This caregiver does not necessary has medical background, but he/she informs the physician about eventual problems in order to take the appropriate actions to preserve the patient integrity. Results show that the obtained measurements are comparable to those of commercial devices. Battery consumption tests show that the GR configuration consumes the most of the stored energy. The developed system allows the caregiver to remotely access data from the sensor measurements when he has no mobility problems. In that case, the patient places the sensors (including the BP inflatable cuff and the ECG electrodes); in this way, the system should report physiological parameters as programmed by the caregiver. If the patient has no mobility, an assistant is needed to place the sensors and check the sensors' status and the embedded system's battery. The approach proposed in this paper allows the exchange of sensors without changing the system architecture simply by updating or adding the sensor to the driver base. One substantial improvement would be the inclusion of artificial intelligence to detect measurement anomalies since, at this stage, the system only reports raw data without any analysis. Adding this would reduce the bandwidth needed to transmit all the sensor readings attached to the system.

Future work is related to enhancing the system using artificial intelligence algorithms capable of predicting changes in physiological parameters and informing physicians and caregivers in advance. Another possible improvement is incorporating mechanical assistants to place or change the sensors so that monitoring is not interrupted in patients with limited mobility. The developers must evaluate this addition since these mechanical components increase the cost of the system. Another concern of the system is the security of the data interchange among the modules. In an improved version of the system, it is desirable to add cryptographic algorithms to prevent the data from being visible and manipulated in a malicious way, which was left aside in this version to reduce both the computational cost of the operations executed by the application and the bandwidth required to transmit the data between its components.

ACKNOWLEDGMENTS

The first author thanks José Eduardo Guerra Hernández, Daniel Humberto Villatoro-Carranco, Juan Eduardo Rivera López, and Victor Gloria Vázquez for their contributions to the design, implementation, testing, and validation of the circuits and software routines incorporated in this project.

REFERENCES

Abdul Rahman, N. A., & Jambek, A. (2019). Biomedical health monitoring system design and analysis. *Indonesian Journal of Electrical Engineering and Computer Science, 13,* 1056–1064. https://doi.org/10.11591/ijeecs.v13.i3.pp1056-1064

Agustine, L., Muljono, I., Angka, P. R., Gunadhi, A., Lestariningsih, D., & Weliamto, W. A. (2018). Heart rate monitoring device for arrhythmia using pulse oximeter sensor based on android. *2018 International Conference on Computer Engineering, Network and Intelligent Multimedia (CENIM),* 106–111. https://doi.org/10.1109/CENIM.2018.8711120

Ahsanuzzaman, S., Ahmed, T., & Rahman, M. A. (2020). Low cost, portable ECG monitoring and alarming system based on deep learning. *2020 IEEE Region 10 Symposium (TENSYMP),* 316–319.

Al-Naggar, N. Q., Al-Hammadi, H. M., Al-Fusail, A. M., & Al-Shaebi, Z. A. (2019). Design of a remote real-time monitoring system for multiple physiological parameters based on smartphone. *Journal of Healthcare Engineering, 2019,* 5674673.

Andersen, A. B., & Mihovska, A. (2019). Wireless smart monitoring of patient health data in a hospital setup. In V. Poulkov (Ed.), *Future access enablers for ubiquitous and intelligent infrastructures* (pp. 37–48). Springer International Publishing.

Antonius, N., & Dachyar, M. (2020). The internet of things (IoT) design for cardiac remote patient monitoring using business process re-engineering. *2020 3rd International Conference on Applied Engineering (ICAE)*, 1–7.

Azizulkarim, A., Abdul Jamil, M. M., & Ambar, R. (2017). Design and development of patient monitoring system. *IOP Conference Series: Materials Science and Engineering, 226*, 012094. https://doi.org/10.1088/1757-899X/226/1/012094

Bhardwaj, V., Joshi, R., & Gaur, A. M. (2022). IoT-based smart health monitoring system for Covid-19. *SN Computer Science, 3*(2), 137. https://doi.org/10.1007/s42979-022-01015-1

Brezulianu, A., Geman, O., Zbancioc, M. D., Hagan, M., Aghion, C., Hemanth, D. J., & Son, L. H. (2019). IoT based heart activity monitoring using inductive sensors. *Sensors, 19*(15). https://doi.org/10.3390/s19153284

Bunkum, M., Reanaree, P., Wanluk, N., & Visitsattapongse, S. (2018). Prototype modeling of bed for bedridden patients. *2018 11th Biomedical Engineering International Conference (BMEiCON)*, 1–4. https://doi.org/10.1109/BMEiCON.2018.8609992

Cardiograph. (2019). Cardiograph, (version dependent on device).

Chakraborty, C. (2021). Performance analysis of compression techniques for chronic wound image trans- mission under smartphone-enabled tele-wound network. In Information Resources Management Association (Ed.), *Research anthology on telemedicine efficacy, adoption, and impact on healthcare delivery* (pp. 345–364). IGI Global.

Devi, S., & Roy, S. (2017). Physiological measurement platform using wireless network with android appli- cation. *Informatics in Medicine Unlocked, 7,* 1–13. https://doi.org/10.1016/j.imu.2017.02.001

Dias, D., & Paulo Silva Cunha, J. (2018). Wearable health devices—Vital sign monitoring, systems and technologies. *Sensors, 18*(8). https://doi.org/10.3390/s18082414

Distefano, S., Bruneo, D., Longo, F., Merlino, G., & Puliafito, A. (2017). Hospitalized patient monitoring and early treatment using IoT and Cloud. *BioNanoScience, 7*(2), 382–385. https://doi.org/10.1007/s12668-016-0335-5

Faria, T. H., Shamim Kaiser, M., Hossian, C. A., Mahmud, M., Al Mamun, S., & Chakraborty, C. (2021). Smart city technologies for next generation healthcare. In C. Chakraborty, J. C.-W. Lin, & M. Alazab (Eds.), *Data-driven mining, learning and analytics for secured smart cities: Trends and advances* (pp. 253–274). Springer International Publishing. https://doi.org/10.1007/978-3-030-72139-812

Feng, C., Sun, Y., Wu, X., Jiang, F., Tao, L., & Zheng, J. (2022). Health monitoring system based on wireless personal area network. In Y. Lu & C. Cheng (Eds.), *International conference on computer application and information security (ICCAIS 2021)* (p. 122600X). SPIE. https://doi.org/10.1117/12.2637410

Guk, K., Han, G., Lim, J., Jeong, K., Kang, T., Lim, E.-K., & Jung, J. (2019). Evolution of wearable devices with real-time disease monitoring for personalized healthcare. *Nanomaterials, 9*(6). https://doi.org/10.3390/nano9060813

Gupta, A. K., Chakraborty, C., & Gupta, B. (2019). Sensing and monitoring of epileptical seizure under IoT platform. In B. Gupta (Ed.), *Smart medical data sensing and IoT systems design in healthcare* (pp. 201–223). IGI Global.

Hasan, D., & Ismaeel, A. (2020). Designing ECG monitoring healthcare system based on internet of things Blynk application. *Journal of Applied Science and Technology Trends, 1*(3), 106–111.

Hoppe, K. K., Williams, M., Thomas, N., Zella, J. B., Drewry, A., Kim, K., Havighurst, T., & Johnson, H. M. (2019). Telehealth with remote blood pressure monitoring for postpartum hypertension: A prospective single-cohort feasibility study. *Pregnancy Hypertension, 15,* 171–176. https://doi.org/10.1016/j.preghy.2018.12.007

iCare. (2019). Icare monitor de la salud (bp), (version 3.6.0).

Lazazzera, R., Belhaj, Y., & Carrault, G. (2019). A new wearable device for blood pressure estimation using photoplethysmogram. *Sensors, 19*(11). https://doi.org/10.3390/s19112557

Malasinghe, L. P., Ramzan, N., & Dahal, K. (2019). Remote patient monitoring: A comprehensive study. *Journal of Ambient Intelligence and Humanized Computing, 10*(1), 57–76. https://doi.org/10.1007/s12652-017-0598-x

Malathi, M., Muniappan, A., Misra, P. K., Rajagopal, B. R., & Borah, P. (2023). A smart healthcare monitoring system for patients using IoT and cloud computing. *AIP Conference Proceedings, 2603*(1), 030012. https://doi.org/10.1063/5.0126275

Mallidi, R. K., Sharma, M., & Mallidi, S. P. (2022). Health care monitoring application using IoT devices. *2022 4th International Conference on Advances in Computing, Communication Control and Networking (ICAC3N)*, 2413–2417. https://doi.org/10.1109/ICAC3N56670.2022.10074172

Megalingam, R. K., Pocklassery, G., Jayakrishnan, V., Mourya, G., & Thulasi, A. A. (2014). Smartphone based continuous monitoring system for home-bound elders and patients. *2014 International Con-ference on Communication and Signal Processing*, 1173–1177. https://doi.org/10.1109/ICCSP.2014.6950039

Miramontes, R., Aquino, R., Flores, A., Rodrıguez, G., Anguiano, R., Rıos, A., & Edwards, A. (2017). Plaimos: A remote mobile healthcare platform to monitor cardiovascular and respiratory variables. *Sensors, 17* (1). https://doi.org/10.3390/s17010176

Mitchell, M., & Kan, L. (2019). Digital technology and the future of health systems [PMID: 30908111]. *Health Systems & Reform, 5*(2), 113–120. https://doi.org/10.1080/23288604.2019.1583040

Monitor, H. (2019). Pulse heart rate monitor (version dependent on device).

Pereira, F., Carvalho, V., Soares, F., Machado, J., Bezerra, K., Silva, R., & Matos, D. (2016). Development of a medical care terminal for efficient monitoring of bedridden subjects. *Journal of Engineering, 2016*, 1–9. https://doi.org/10.1155/2016/3591059

Prasanth, K. S., Teja, P. S., Kalyan, S., Devi, R. S., Rajesh, P., Amirtharajan, R., & Praveenkumar, P. (2019). Labview based alert system for elderly bedridden cardiovascular pa- tients. *2019 International Conference on Computer Communication and Informatics (ICCCI)*, 1–6. https://doi.org/10.1109/ICCCI.2019.8821987

Pulsometer. (2019). Single pulsometer, (version 3.0.0).

Qaosar, M., Ahmed, S., Li, C., & Morimoto, Y. (2018). Hybrid sensing and wearable smart device for health monitoring and medication: Opportunities and challenges. *AAAI Spring Symposium Series.*

Rahimoon, A. A., Abdullah, M. N., & Taib, I. (2020). Design of a contactless body temperature measurement system using Arduino. *Indonesian Journal of Electrical Engineering and Computer Science, 19*(3), 1251–1258.

Raja, B., Firdous, A., Ishak, A., & Anand, M. (2019). Design and implementation of health care video monitoring system based on RTOS. *Indian Journal of Public Health Research & Development, 10*, 1260. https://doi.org/10.5958/0976-5506.2019.00885.4

Rana, A., Chakraborty, C., Sharma, S., Dhawan, S., Pani, S. K., & Ashraf, I. (2022). Internet of medical things-based secure and energy-efficient framework for health care [PMID: 34958234]. *Big Data, 10*(1), 18–33. https://doi.org/10.1089/big.2021.0202

Runtastic. (2019). Runtastic heart rate (version dependent on device).

Samartkit, P., Pullteap, S., & Bernal, O. (2022). A non-invasive heart rate and blood pressure monitoring system using piezoelectric and photoplethysmographic sensors. *Measurement, 196*, 111211. https://doi.org/https://doi.org/10.1016/j.measurement.2022.111211

Sangeethalakshmi, K., Preethi, U., Pavithra, S., et al. (2023). Patient health monitoring system using IoT. *Materials Today: Proceedings, 80*, 2228–2231.

Sony. (2019). Smartband-swr12, (version 4.4).

Varghese, T., Varghese, T., & Bhatele, M. (2013). Remote blood pressure monitoring using a wireless sensor network. In V. Kumar & M. Bhatele (Eds.), *Proceedings of all India Seminar on Biomedical Engineering 2012 (AISOBE 2012)* (pp. 153–158). Springer India.

Villanueva-Miranda, I., Nazeran, H., & Martinek, R. (2018). Cardiaqloud: A remote ECG monitoring system using Cloud services for ehealth and mhealth applications. *2018 IEEE 20th International Conference on e-Health Networking, Applications and Services (Healthcom)*, 1–6. https://doi.org/10.1109/HealthCom.2018.8531164

Wijaya, N. H., Fauzi, F. A., Helmy, E. T., Nguyen, P. T., & Atmoko, R. A. (2020). The design of heart rate detector and body temperature measurement device using ATMega16. *Journal of Robotics and Control (JRC)*, *1*(2), 40–43.

Zhang, K., & Ling, W. (2020). Health monitoring of human multiple physiological parameters based on wireless remote medical system. *IEEE Access*, *8*, 71146–71159.

3 Transfer Learning and Domain-Specific Adoption Algorithms for Image Classification

R. Nareshkumar and K. Nimala

3.1 INTRODUCTION

The capacity to apply learned skills in new contexts is innate to the human species. What we take away as information from learning about one task may be used directly to solve similar problems in other activities. The more closely linked the activities are, the simpler for us to transfer or cross-apply our prior learning. The idea of transfer learning (TL) mentions transcending the isolated learning paradigm and using information gained for one activity to tackle problems associated with other tasks.

Intelligent machine learning (ML) technologies [1] are growing at an exponential rate in this current era of independence to make real-life applications more manageable. Some examples of these innovations are regression, classification [2], and clustering.

TL is an up-and-coming approach in ML that allows us to solve a new problem by using the information we gained from solving an older problem. This helps resolve the problem of a shortage of labeled data. The most recent publications emphasize deep domain adaptation (DA) in specific, which is a subfield of TL [3]. It is an emerging strategy in ML that enables us to solve a new issue by using the knowledge we obtained from solving an earlier problem. This helps us to make better use of our previous experiences in the field. This contributes to the solution of insufficiently labeled data [4]. Deep DA in specific, a branch of TL, has received the highest amount of attention in recent papers.

Effectively representing TL, DA combines source and target data for learning despite differences in distribution. Figure 3.2 shows our discourse adaptable framework and DA technique.

Since just a little quantity of labeled train data is available, semi-supervised learning approaches are used. This means that a significant amount of unlabeled train data is combined with a small amount of labeled data to construct the learning classifier.

TL was introduced into computational models of DL so that the information gained from solving one issue could be used to the solution of a related but distinct problem. This was done so that DL models could overcome the inherent limits of their design.

DOI: 10.1201/9781003603610-3

The primary objective of this research is to apply the skills learned while working through one set of challenges to another related set. In addition to this, the suggested model includes the extraction of the characteristics.

The residual portions of this chapter are organized as shown below. In the next section, "related work and Specific works of Transfer Learning," we provide an overview and detailed definitions. In Section 3.3, we will provide a summary of the most important deep DA strategies. In Sections 3.4, 3.5, and 3.6, we discuss how deep DA should be carried out. Section 3.7 also includes an explanation of the more recent applications that are built on deep DA approaches. In the conclusion, we bring our study to a close and discuss potential future trends in Section 3.8.

3.2   RELATED WORK

TL enables training in the target domain using skills acquired in the source domain. Figure 3.1 depicts many various kinds of TL. Earlier solutions use standard mathematical systems such as instance weighting [5] and feature plotting. Deep transfer networks have proven more successful in locating domain-invariant components than these more traditional methods.

While making a picture, one may use a few different approaches. The radiofrequency signal capacity in an MRI, the sound intensity for ultrasounds, and the radiation uptake in X-ray imaging are some of the metrics that fall under this category.

A single measurement determines the location of each image point in a digital picture. Still, in multi-channel images, the location of each image point is determined by using many measurements. When we employ these models in clinical practice, the model may fail owing to unseen data, simply data not included during the model's training. Classic neural networks must consider yet another issue. Because of this, the ability of these algorithms to generalize to previously encountered clinical data is still a significant limitation.

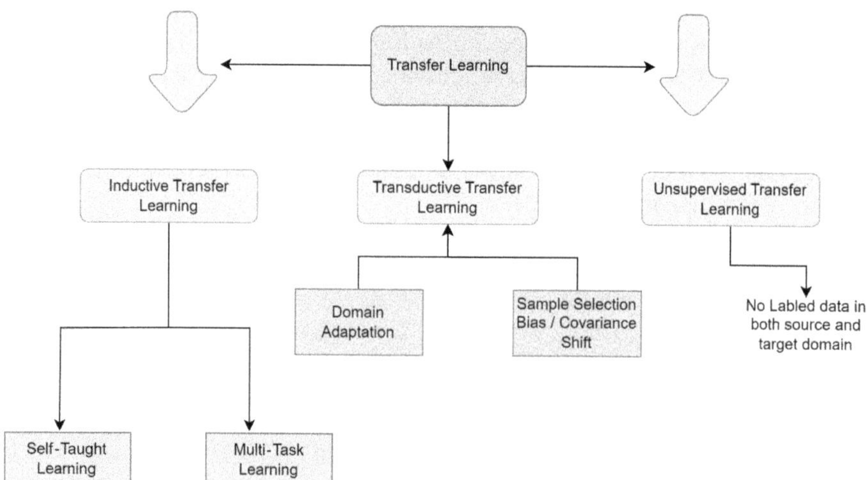

FIGURE 3.1   Different types of TL.

"Semantic segmentation" refers to adding semantic labels to each pixel in a picture. This activity is necessary for various programs, including human–machine interaction, robotics, and autonomous driving. There have been many applications of networks in downstream processes, and semantic segmentation is not a unique instance.

Before attempting automated lung image categorization utilizing statistical machine-learning techniques, a support vector machine (SVM) classifier was used to collect three statistical variables from lung texture to discriminate between malignant and benign lung nodules. Component detection is a downstream operation that recognizes an item's category and its relative location in an image. An object detection system may feed images to improve accuracy. This problem is of the utmost importance in computer vision applications like robots, autonomous driving, and scene text identification. The research conducted by Pan and Yang [6] is a groundbreaking endeavor that classifies TL and investigates the explorations that have been produced since 2010. The examination conducted by Weiss et al. provides an introduction to both homogeneous and heterogeneous TL approaches and a summary of each. TL methods have additionally been created based on recent rank minimization methodologies [7]. However, these methods apply to situations that are not structurally very distinct from face verification, and prior techniques are not used here because of this. Even though our approach is not explicitly derived from a rank minimization viewpoint, as was alluded to earlier, it may be regarded as a specific minimization problem that involves numerous concave penalties on matrix singular values that are coupled in a new way. This is because our algorithm takes into account a rank minimization perspective.

Medical professionals may visualize and monitor the disease activity using various scanning techniques, eliminating the need for intrusive treatments. Each medical imaging modality has a distinct purpose and function, enabling it to generate digital pictures containing varied amounts of information. By fine-tuning previously trained relationships, TL hopes to tackle both issues. This may be performed technically by reusing a network that has already been completely trained with a given dataset for a specific purpose. The term "reusing" refers to adapting some parts of the network to the requirements of the freshly created domain.

Classification, segmentation, and localization are just some medical imaging tasks that benefit from learning on their own with context distortion. Scan plane identification in fetal 2-D ultrasound pictures was utilized to test the method's efficacy in classification, and the results showed an enhancement in categorization in some instances.

In particular, our approach comprises two stages. Phase one involves constructing a robust classifier using TL in preparation for phase two, which consists in filtering vast quantities of photos from the Internet. Phase two incorporates pictures from the web and the previously learnt classifier to expand the training set. The severe overfitting will be mitigated, and classification accuracy will increase with this two-stage approach. Bayesian Optimization for Anything (BOA) will make it easier to tune hyper-parameters. These advantages are what make our approach superior.

Classifying an input picture into one of many predefined classes is a rapidly developing field of study. Deep learning-based picture identification, image retrieval, and other algorithms have found widespread use in various domains, from categorizing human cardiac electrocardiograms to classifying lung cancer to assessing happiness.

In this study [8], a proper definition of negative transfer is proposed, and then three significant characteristics of that concept are examined. As a result of this analysis, an innovative method for avoiding negative transfer has been developed. This method involves filtering away source data unrelated to the problem at hand. The technique, which is based on adversarial networks, is highly general and may be utilized for a wide variety of TL techniques. Influenced by the compatibility requirement announced by semi-supervised presumably roughly accurate (PAC) theory [9], propose a novel hypothesis for SsHeDA from a unique viewpoint compared to earlier DA theories. This theory is driven by the alignment constraint introduced by PAC theory. Since many researchers, particularly those in medical imaging, lack access to a large annotated dataset for training, TL is often used as an alternative.

In the field of nanoscience, where millions of pictures are often the result of characterization methods like scanning electron microscopy, image recognition programs have the potential to be a handy tool.

The long-term management of the data that is created by scientific research, particularly nanoscience, is one of the most significant issues that must be overcome. This approach has recently been guided by a clear set of principles that have been released recently. These principles state that data should be findable, accessible, interoperable, and reusable. Taking such an approach lends credence to the theory that the availability of data will confirm results, encourage the reuse of those findings, and foster the formation of new partnerships.

Classical ML techniques focus on one task at a time and depend heavily on vast volumes of training data. TL is an approach that seeks to overcome this barrier by creating techniques that can transfer the information gained from doing one job to performing another.

Because ML can handle substantially more enormous data volumes while simultaneously lowering intra-operator and inter-operator variability, the concept of supplementing and, in some circumstances, increasing human medical image analysis with ML has been losing ground in recent years. In the past, computers could only solve issues governed by rules by running algorithms that were explicitly designed for them. This method needs to be revised for modeling and carrying out all the procedures necessary to arrive at a diagnosis based on examining medical images.

Within sentiment analysis, supervised learning strategies are pretty effective in terms of their performance. A supervised sentiment classifier, on the other hand, often has abysmal performance when it is transplanted to another domain. This is a situation sometimes referred to as a domain transfer. In this research, we aim to approach this challenge by making the most use of both the old-domain data and the unlabeled new-domain data. Specifically, we focus on the old-domain data since it contains more information.

3.2.1 Roles of Smart Devices for Medical

In the context of the healthcare sector, the term "Industry 4.0" refers to the integration of intelligent and digital technologies intended to revolutionize the healthcare business. Smart devices play an essential role in making this shift possible.

Wearable technology such as fitness trackers and smartwatches can monitor various health factors, including the user's heart rate, sleep habits, and level of physical activity. They provide data in real-time, which may then be sent to healthcare practitioners for remote monitoring.

Implants with embedded sensors can monitor a patient's status and wirelessly communicate data to the personnel who offer medical treatment. For instance, intelligent pacemakers can transmit data about heart operations to cardiologists.

The Internet of Things (IoT) is used to link a variety of medical equipment. For example, intelligent inhalers may monitor how often medicine is used and relay that information to the healthcare doctors who prescribe it.

Patients suffering from chronic diseases may now undergo constant monitoring from the convenience of their own homes thanks to these technologies. They may incorporate monitors for blood pressure, glucose levels, and other parameters.

Intelligent diagnostic tools often use artificial intelligence to perform evaluations in a prompt and precise manner. Some examples include dermatological cameras driven by AI to diagnose skin conditions.

Tools for video conferencing and technology that facilitates remote examinations make it possible for medical professionals to give treatment and diagnose patients virtually. These may include digital stethoscopes, otoscopes, and even more specialized diagnostic equipment.

3.3 TRANSFER LEARNING

TL is when knowledge from one field is utilized to enhance a learner's performance in another field that is connected to the first one. We may get an understanding of why TL is feasible by drawing on experiences in the real world that could be more technical. Take, for instance, the case of two persons who are interested in picking up the piano as a new skill. The first individual has little background in performing music, whereas the second is an accomplished guitarist with a wide range of musical expertise. A person who already has a substantial musical history will have a more accessible time learning to play the piano because they will be able to use the musical information and skills that they have acquired in the past to master the piano [6]. One individual can take information gained from one activity and successfully apply it to acquiring knowledge about another task linked to the first.

Consider, as an application of ML, the problem of predicting the tone of customer evaluations, where there is a large amount of labeled data in the form of testimonials about digital cameras. Although they are not identical, assessment of digital cameras and cuisine nonetheless have many commonalities. Textual and linguistic similarities include using the same language and sharing opinions about a bought item. Target learners may benefit from TL because of the correlation between these two areas.

Compared to more conventional ML approaches, deep learning needs enormous training data. Therefore, the demand for a large volume of labeled data poses a significant obstacle in resolving specific essential domain-specific tasks. This is especially true in the case of applications for the medical domain, in which the production of large-scale, high-quality annotated medical datasets is a complicated and costly process. Further, the conventional DL model needs a great deal of computational power, such as that provided by a GPU-enabled server, despite academics working very hard to perfect it.

The weight transfer learning (WTL) method is an extension of the standard TL methodology and may be thought of as a generalization of that method. The WTL strategy involves applying a previously trained network to a new problem or set of parameters without making any adjustments to the network weights during the operation. This can be accomplished through the use of traditional TL techniques such as the reuse of a 2D network on a diverse classification task or its combination into a network planned to discourse a different problem (as is the scenario for segmentation structures with pre-trained encoders), or even its addition into a higher dimensional system. Classical TL techniques include these and many more.

TL is an excellent method for improving the outcome of medical image processing tasks by using pre-trained CNN models. This has been shown in several studies. CNNs have shown great accuracy and resilience in recognizing and categorizing various medical diseases based on medical imagery. Overall, these results highlight the critical role that TL and CNNs play in increasing medical imaging diagnosis, and they suggest that more studies in this field can substantially enhance patient outcomes.

3.4 DOMAIN ADAPTATION STRATEGIES

In recent years, there has been an increase in techniques for solving the issue of visual DA, which is also widely referred to as the problem of visual data set bias. Previous simple strategies for DA comprise reweighting the training data to the extent that they may more closely resemble those in the test distribution and discovering a transformation on a lower dimensional surface that moves the source and target subspaces of it closer together. Dealing with the changes above is the focus of the subfields of ML known as DA and TL. In the following, we will introduce these topics by focusing on the question: when and how may a classifier generalize from a source domain to a target domain? We will briefly introduce risk reduction and how TL and domain adaptability build upon this framework [10].

Approaches that use DA or TL are required to circumvent the problems that arise due to the assumptions made while utilizing supervised learning. When training the classifiers, DAs use labeled data from the source domain and unlabeled data from the target domain. This ensures that the classifiers maintain good classification capabilities when applied to data from the target domain [11].

The classification of crops presents several issues that are peculiar to the field. For example, agricultural data might have a lot of variation because of variances in topography, topology, weather, soil qualities, crop health, noise caused by the presence of other classes like cloud cover- or built-up area, and the time when the picture was acquired [12].

Training and testing data have always been taken from the same feature space in traditional ML algorithms. However, recent developments in deep neural networks have made it feasible to reuse architectures trained to extract features from training data belonging to one domain to accomplish the same thing with training data belonging to another domain.

3.4.1 Inductive Transfer Learning

Inductive TL takes as input information from a source domain D_s and a learning task T_s, as well as input knowledge from a target domain D_T and a learning task T_T, and attempts to enhance the target domain's learning of a predictive function $f_T()$ from the source domain D_s and the learning task T_s, where $T_s \neq T_T$.

To solve the issues associated with inductive TL, Dai et al. [13] suggested an adaptation of the AdaBoost boosting technique called TrAdaBoost. Supervised feature creation strategies in the inductive TL environment are analogous to individuals used in multitask learning. The core concept is to master a depiction with fewer dimensions that can be used for various similar jobs. The newly acquired representation may decrease each task's classification or regression model error.

Using an optimization problem described below, we may learn common features in an inductive TL paradigm.

$$arg\ min_{A,U} \sum_{t \in T,S} \sum_{i=1}^{n_t} L(yt_i,(a_t,U^T xt_i)) + \gamma \parallel A \parallel_{2,1}^{2} \tag{3.1}$$

$$s\ .t\ U \in O^d$$

S and T stand for the actions taken in the "source" and "target" domains, respectively, in this formula.

Models for similar tasks are often assumed to have similar parameters or previous distributions of hyperparameters. This is why maximum parameter-transfer techniques to the inductive TL scenario make this assumption. Most of the methods discussed here are optimized for multitask learning environments; examples include a regularization context and a hierarchical Bayesian framework.

3.4.2 Transductive Transfer Learning

Arnold et al. [14] initially used the phrase transductive TL, specifying that the source and target responsibilities must be identical even if the domains are free to vary. In addition to these situations, they demand that all unlabeled data in the target domain be easily accessible during training. However, this requirement may be loosened, and in our description of the transductive TL approach, we ask that some of the unlabeled target information be observed during training time to acquire the marginal probability for the target information. The most fundamental approach is to reconstruct the samples using an auto-encoder structure consisting of an encoder network and a decoder system. TL is valuable for getting an extensive network up and running with many different pictures and classes. MRI and CT are typically used as the primary datasets for these challenges because of their breadth and depth. TL then swaps the fully connected layer of a pre-trained system with a brand new fully connected layer by utilizing a substantial dataset as a guide. Last, only a subset of the larger target dataset is used for training.

3.4.3 INSTANCE-BASED TRANSFER LEARNING

In his study, Chattopadhyay [15] suggests two approaches, which rely on many labeled source domains. The central concept is to apply several classifiers from the source domain to the target domain to assign labels. A classifier is initially constructed independently for each source domain to achieve this.

3.5 PROPOSED TRANSFER LEARNING MODEL FOR CLASSIFICATION

In the next part, we will present our suggested categorization structure for TL. Figure 3.1 comprehensively represents the learning model through a flow diagram. The following sections will go through each of these procedures in further detail.

DA aims to facilitate the communication of info between the appropriate organizations or tasks and the data sources or targets [16]. One of the most challenging problems that DA must solve is how to minimize the inequality among the distributions of the source domain and the target domain while preserving the essential qualities of both domains. Therefore, in the current version of the TL model [17], we suggest a bordering probability spreading based on the distance measure of DA.

The distance between the source and the target domains is adapted by the suggested distance measure, which presents both domains.

Let us assume that $Pr_M^{(s)}$ and $Pr_M^{(t)}$ are two discrete variables marginal distribution probability for individually characteristic of the source $x^{(s)}$ and target $x^{(t)}$ domains that have been supplied. The formula for determining $Pr_M^{(s)}$ and $Pr_M^{(t)}$ may be found in Equation 3.2, and the results can be written down as follows:

$$Pr_M^{(s)} = \frac{\sum\limits_{j=1}^{m} xij^{(s)}}{\sum\limits_{i=1}^{n_s}\sum\limits_{j=1}^{m} xij^{(s)}}, \; Pr_M^{(t)} = \frac{\sum\limits_{j=1}^{m} xij^{(t)}}{\sum\limits_{i=1}^{n_t}\sum\limits_{j=1}^{m} xij^{(t)}} \tag{3.2}$$

Now, let's say that the value of d_{ij} represents the alteration among the marginal distribution probabilities of respectively basis feature and all of the target domain features. To put it another way, the distance metric, d_{ij}, may be computed as follows:

$$d_{ij} = \left| Pr_M^{(s)} - Pr_M^{(t)} \right| \tag{3.3}$$

The gap between the two probabilities, on the other hand, is not quite zero. As a result, we decided to employ a pivot value or constant (u) to determine the transformation in distribution between the two domains.

After training all the elements and variables in the learnt autoencoder, we create the classification responsible for labeling the target domain [18]. The following is how four distinct classifiers are constructed.

When training the autoencoder, utilize the source domain and the target domain directly rather than the provided DA technique. The label may be predicted by

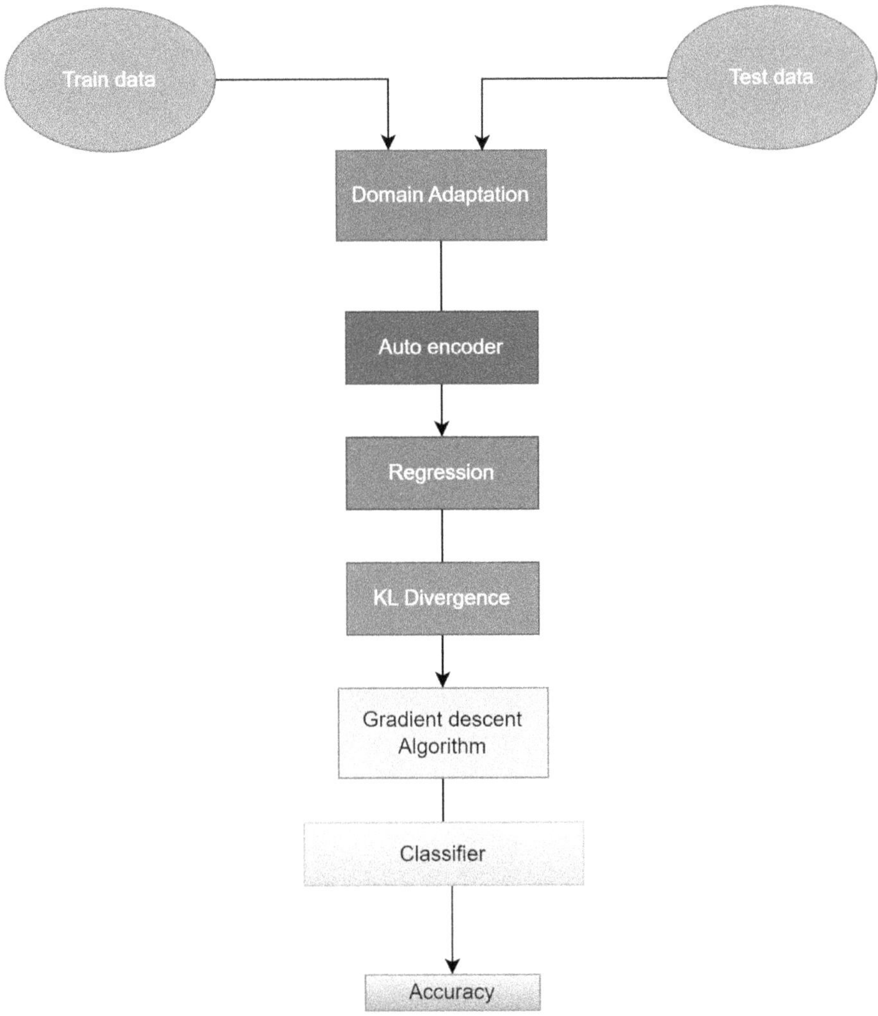

FIGURE 3.2 Architecture of domain adaptation.

taking the probability with the highest possible value. This classification method [19] is known as TL with adaptive-1 (Figure 3.2).

3.6 EXPERIMENTAL RESULTS

The effectiveness of the suggested TL adaptive concepts in correctly categorizing actual datasets, particularly the source domain and target domain (MRI vs. CT) dataset, is evaluated using a planned execution of these structures. Many subsections make up this section. The first paragraph provides an informative summary of the specifics of the datasets and the pre-processing done using the TL framework [20]. The second paragraph discusses the results that were investigated and discusses the accuracy measurements produced from the typical TL classification methods. In the last part of this section, we conducted comprehensive research to show the superiority of the new learning method [21] over alternative forms of TL [22] and classic ML approaches.

3.6.1 DATASET

The information is separated into two groups: data from the source domain and data from the destination domain. The MRIs of a brain tumor serve as the source domain data, while brain CT scans that include IPH serve as the target domain data. To prevent data leaking, the different slices obtained from a single patient are not included in the training set or the test set simultaneously. Figure 3.3 depicts the difference between the source and target domains (MRI vs. CT).

3.6.2 RESULTS AND DISCUSSION

This technique operates based on the following principle: the TL approach allows data, model, and structural knowledge acquired in one domain to be transferred to CNN training recognized in another discipline.

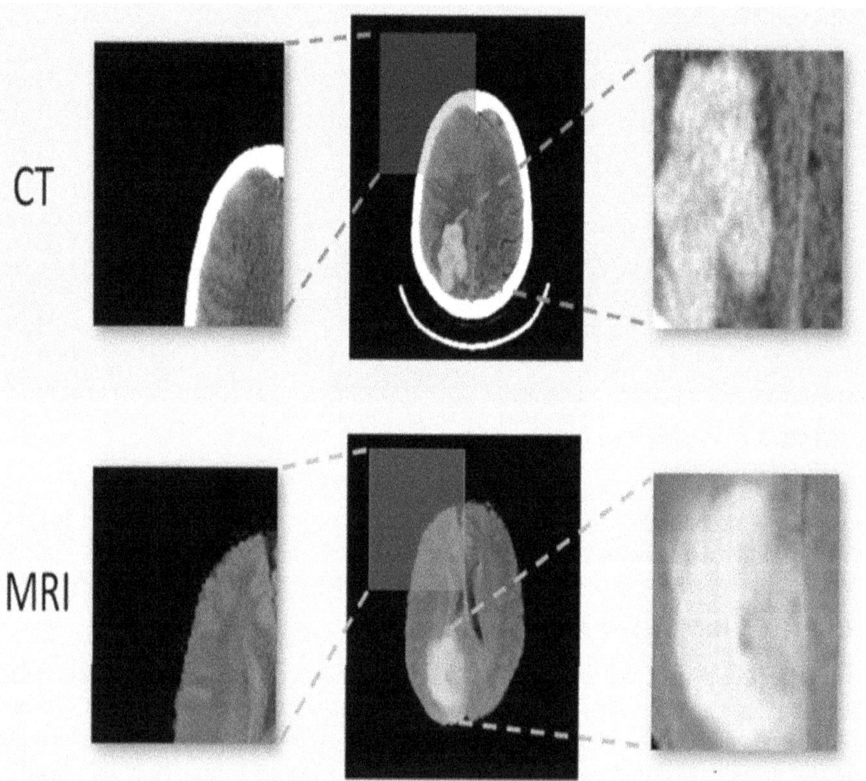

FIGURE 3.3   The difference between the source domain and target domain (MRI vs. CT).

In the final analysis, we have shown that the suggested adaptive-1 technique performs much better than all of the other algorithms that were evaluated for their ability to classify images using the source domain and target domain (MRI vs. CT). In summary, the prototypical maintained a much larger and broader margin of accuracy improvement of adaptive -2 on both datasets.

During the training phase, data augmentation techniques were also utilized to prevent neural networks from learning unnecessary characteristics and drastically enhance their general efficiency. This was accomplished by adding new data to existing data. The enhancement strategies used in this study include random horizontal flipping and random rotation in the negative fifty degrees to the positive fifty degrees range. The input picture undergoes a seemingly random transformation; the transformation established each time the training is carried out. This will result in a boost in the variety of the initial data and an improvement in the reliability of the trained model.

Collecting vast volumes of data in real-world scenarios is a complex and tedious operation, so acquiring additional data is not a viable alternative. However, increasing the quantity of data that is being used is one strategy that may be used to prevent overfitting. Increasing the overall size of the dataset that is being used for training is one of the most effective ways to cut down on overfitting.

It describes a type of training in which some neurons are purposefully and deliberately ignored. An approach that has dropout applied to it cannot depend on any particular feature and must instead learn resilient characteristics. It has been shown that utilizing this strategy significantly reduces overfitting in various problems. Furthermore, this notion was extended by applying it to a convolutional neural network using a technique known as spatial dropout. Instead of removing individual neurons, this method eliminates whole feature maps.

To provide correct predictions, a supervised learning system, whether for classification or regression issues, must first acquire the necessary knowledge from training data. However, the issue of overfitting comes anytime we attempt to train a problematic model with an inadequate amount of data for training [23]. This problem develops whenever we try to prepare a complicated model with an insufficient amount of data. The agreement, locating, and avoiding the problem of overfitting is essential for deep learning since it is the field's most significant challenge. Researchers have outlined various approaches to combating this issue, including data augmentation, weight decay, TL, batch normalization, dropout, etc.

Train and test sets have been separated from the dataset. Seventy percent of each of the two different kinds of photos are utilized for the training dataset, whereas only 30% are used for the testing dataset. The model is trained with the training dataset's help, while the TL models' accuracy [24] is tested with the help of the test set. The network parameters must be modified continuously for the deep learning system to respond appropriately to the shifting environment. This will make it more difficult to train the model and achieve convergence. This not only makes the task of training the model more complex but also makes the task of optimizing the model more challenging.

Standardization of the initial input data may ensure the reliability of that data in neural networks; however, standardization does not ensure the quality of the data fed into the hidden layer. The relatively little shifts in shallow parameters are magnified

TABLE 3.1

Comparison Results of the Source and Target MRT and CT Dataset

Methods	MRI	CT
LR	80.5	77.5
SVM	84.2	71.3
NN	80.1	66.2
ELM	85.2	72.8
Adaptive 1	90.5	93.5
Adaptive 2	92.1	93.9

by multi-layer linear transformation and activation function and the source situation adjustments at each successive system layer.

Adam is an optimization technique that is used in algorithms for deep learning that substitute random gradient descent. Adam can be utilized to repeatedly update the weights of neural networks depending on training data, and it is intended to improve accuracy. The Adam [25] method is useful for resolving issues when there are either a considerable number of factors or a high number of data points since the diagonal distribution of the gradient is invariant in this approach. The Adam method determines each parameter's adaptive parameter learning rate by computing the gradient's first- and second-moment estimations.

In the situational solution comparisons, the outcomes that are reported in Table 3.1 indicate a performance record of one victory, one defeat, and one tie. It should be noted that these findings were gathered directly from the publications that were polled. However, this information gives some fascinating insight into the comparative performances of the solutions, even though it is impossible to make accurate conclusions from it because of the reasons that were just outlined.

The demonstration is run on a computer with Windows 10 and a 64-bit operating system version. Additionally, the machine has a GPU card installed. To load the algorithm, the picture information set is first segmented into a training set and then a testing set. The primary objective of this project is to develop the most effective model possible for categorizing several types of brain tumors. It is possible to do this by finding the optimal configuration for the hyperparameters, which will allow the model to have an expanded capacity for recognition. During this stage of training, we started by training just the DDB that were put on top of the mathematical models that had already been pre-trained. The pre-trained models' neural bases were entirely frozen before training, ensuring that the weights of these layers remained constant throughout the process.

In conclusion, Figure 3.4 displays the accuracy outcomes achieved from the proposed Adaptive-1 and Adaptive-2 techniques, which have average standards of 90.4% and 92.2% for the MRI&CT dataset, respectively.

Improving the performance of CNN models requires hyper-parameter optimization (HPO) to fine-tune the models' hyper-parameters to resemble the underlying

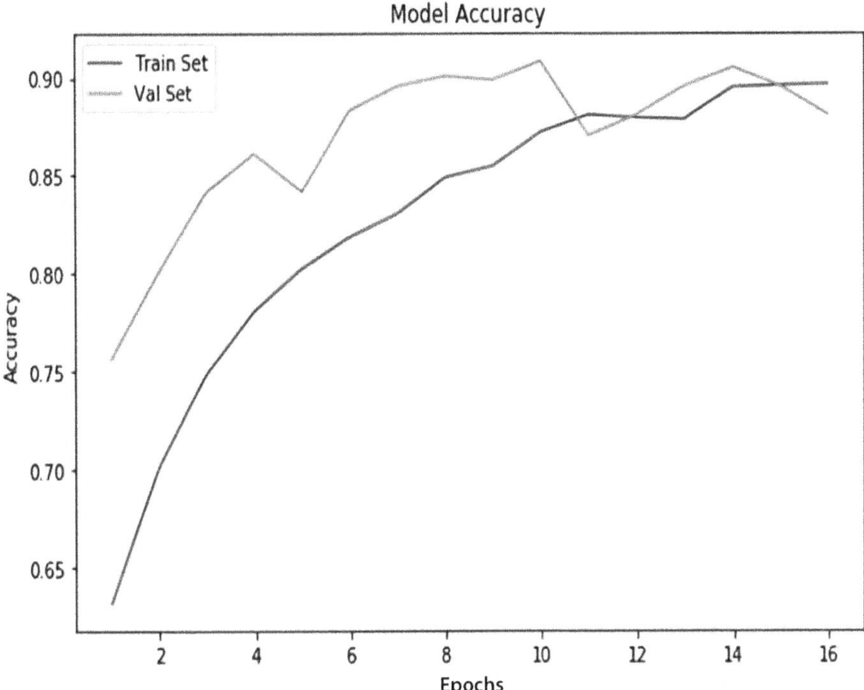

FIGURE 3.4 Accuracy results with proposed model.

models and the chosen datasets more closely. Optimizing the hyper-parameter and selecting the best possible settings for its variables is essential to get the most out of a simulation. Two categories may be used to classify these hyper-parameters: extreme parameters of either the model training or model-design operations.

The first step in designing a model is figuring out how to configure the representation's hyper-parameters. Below are the six model-design hyper-parameters that are part of the TL framework and have been recommended for optimization.

3.6.3 Evaluation Indicators

The effectiveness of the recommended model's structure in terms of system categorization is evaluated using several indicators. When assessing the classification method we had constructed, we used the metrics of accuracy, precision, recall, and specificity to determine this particular aspect of the system.

The assessment of the model's efficacy was referred to as its accuracy, while an evaluation of how well it was categorized was referred to as its precision, and a rating of how efficiently negative samples were recognized was referred to as its recall. When attempting to quantify the appropriate classification of different ship classes, specificity was the measure that was utilized. TL establishes the path for correctly anticipating potential data after accumulating past information concerning the source and target information and feature space arrangement.

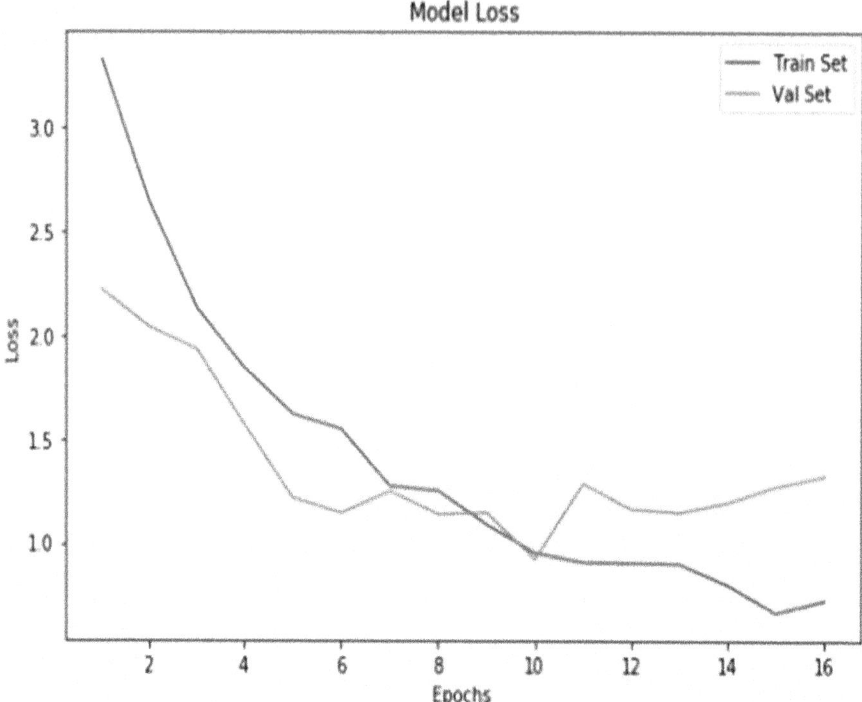

FIGURE 3.5　Loss results with proposed model.

Figure 3.5 displays the loss results data for the MRI and CT datasets. It is crystal easy to see that the suggested Adaptive 1 and Adaptive 2 deliver superior average accuracy compared to any of the well-known ML techniques we have considered for comparison.

Figure 3.6 provides the accuracy averages for the 20 classification issues found in the MRI and CT datasets. This allows for a comparative analysis of the various machine-learning methods discussed.

3.7　APPLICATIONS

In recent years, practical applications of TL strategies have been made in various real-world contexts. Raina et al. [26] and Dai et al. [27] proposed using TL strategies to study text data from other domains. Blitzer et al. [28] suggested using SCL to resolve issues with Adaptive 1 NLP.

The works reviewed for this chapter show that TL has been used in various situations that take place in the real world. Many different application examples apply to natural language processing. Image and video idea categorization are two other areas where TL has found broad application. Classification of WiFi hotspots, muscular weariness, medicine effectiveness, human activity, software defects, and irregular heartbeats are only some of the applications that have been addressed in previous articles.

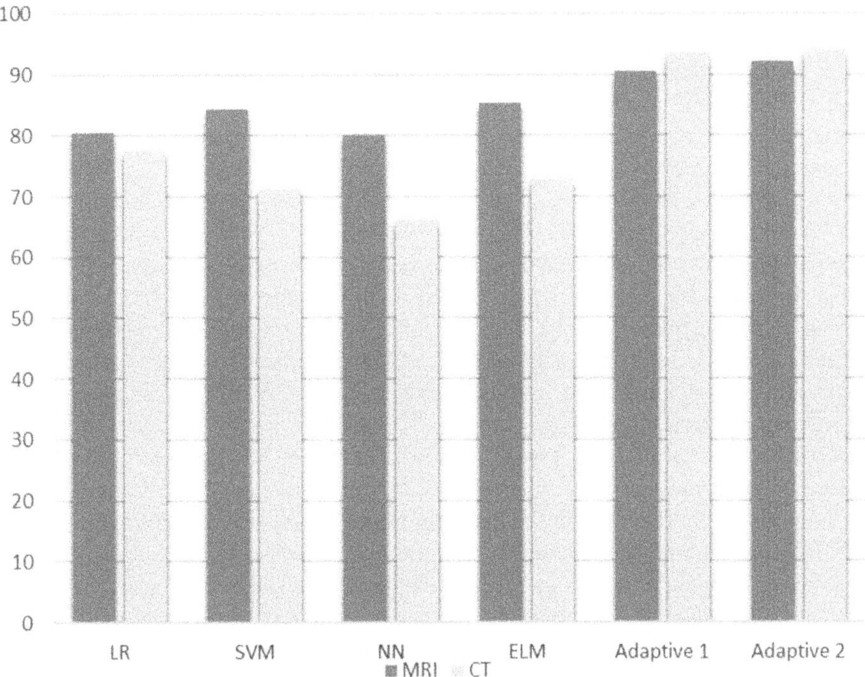

FIGURE 3.6   Comparison of the different types of TL with proposed method.

Many of the proposed solutions are generic, which means that they are easily adaptable to applications that are different from those that were actually carried out and evaluated in the articles.

The application-specific resolutions often include fields such as natural language processing [29] and image processing [30, 31] in some capacity.

TL strategies are continuously being used across a wide variety of real-world requests; in about instances, the applications in question are relatively unrecognized. The head position organization application aims to locate a learner who has been educated with previously collected labeled head poses so that they can anticipate a new head position. The categorization of people's head poses is used for a diversity of determinations, including gauging the attention of drivers, examining social behavior, and tracking how people interact with robots. Compared to the anticipated target, head positions obtained from the source exercise data will take distinct head tilt choices and angle ranges.

Learning strategies based on semi-supervision are used since only a limited amount of labeled data on trains is currently accessible. This indicates that a considerable quantity of unlabeled train data is used in conjunction with a limited amount of labeled data to create the learning classifier.

The classification of people's head positions is used for several applications, including determining whether or not drivers are paying attention, researching social behavior, and monitoring how people interact with robots. The head locations that were collected from the source training data would, when compared to the predicted target, have unique head tilt ranges and angles.

A kind of machine learning known as TL [32] occurs when an existing model that was developed for one purpose is applied to another task and utilized as the foundation for a new model. Due to the large amount of computational and temporal resources required to develop neural network models on these topics, it is common practice to start with pre-trained models when performing computer vision and natural language processing tasks. This approach is known as the "pre-trained model starting point." TL refers to the information obtained by employing a model that has been trained in the past and which can be modified to examine different datasets. The primary purpose of the TL is to improve one's capability to grow in the target domain (Dt) by using prior knowledge of the source domain (Ds), the corresponding instructional assignment (Ts), and the source learning task within the same domain as the related learned task [33].

From a systems theoretical point of view, the current TL frameworks need to be improved in certain essential aspects. They are preoccupied with the domain and the work at hand, but they ignore the different points of view that might be gained by explicitly taking into account the conduct and framework of the system [34].

Making sequential decisions is a significant task in the field of artificial intelligence. This problem is sometimes formally called Markov decision process (MDP) optimization. Scheduling and reinforcement learning (RL) are two essential methods that may be used to solve this challenge. This book presents an overview of model-based RL, a well-recognized merger of the two domains.

Transferring the information gained from an image synthesis model that has been trained using a large dataset is necessary for effectively learning generative picture models from various domains. This chapter provides a formula for learning vision transformers using creative knowledge transfer. Our system is based on generative vision transformers, which depict a picture as a series of visual tokens and may be either self-regressive or non-autoregressive.

TL is a method that involves the information obtained by a mathematical model that has previously been trained and is used in the process of learning another data set. TL makes it possible to use a pre-trained CNN model that was created for another application that is closely linked to this one. Acquisition via transfer has demonstrated its usefulness in diagnosing and treating medical issues. Augmentation [30] is the most effective method for developing a classification model that can be used to learn from the data at hand and produce further data. A finite number of photos are available for training and testing the datasets. Creating duplicate data and its subsequent addition to the training set is one approach to resolving this problem.

3.8 CONCLUSION

Around the process of TL, domain revision is used to adapt to the comparable characteristics of the source and target domains and the DL method is applied to extract robust features to create an effective classifier. This study improved TL using a deep learning strategy, which optimally used a marginal probability-based domain adaption procedure. When both the source and destination domains display significant data dispersion, the novel TL framework can resolve the problem of comparable multi-domain problems. The suggested framework used the marginal probability distribution among the basis domain and the target domain to choose like characteristics time-efficiently to bridge the significant discrepancies between the source domain and the target domain. Domain-adapted TL with deep autoencoder is the name of the classification model. TL adaptive 1 and TL adaptive 2 utilizing SoftMax regression are the names given to the two different iterations of this feature representation approach that are recommended to be combined with deep autoencoder.

Additional recognized TL approaches were not as successful as Adaptive 2. In the future, researchers intend to implement the suggested method to large datasets such as the Galaxy Dataset and the Leaf Dataset, amongst others, to determine an analysis of the future system's accuracy compared to previous TL methodologies.

3.9 FUTURE WORK

In future work, a training set consisting of both pictures created by the system and photos acquired from the internet may be employed for training purposes. Adding noise to the training data might also assist in building a more varied dataset and bring the model closer to real-world applications. It's possible that the CNNs' training may benefit from a more in-depth hyperparameter adjustment, too. In addition, more approaches for extracting features may be employed, and additional kinds of charts can also be encompassed.

Researchers want to expand the use of the suggested TL approach to include extensive and varied datasets, such as the Galaxy Dataset and the Leaf Dataset, in their following study. The purpose of this extension is to comprehensively evaluate the performance and correctness of the framework for earlier TL approaches. The researchers want to thoroughly examine the complexities of data preparation, investigating the most effective strategies customized to the specific features of each dataset. In addition, they will take into account temporal characteristics, incremental learning, and ensemble techniques to adjust to changing data and improve the model's overall performance. The evaluation will include individual datasets and cross-domain tests, guaranteeing the model's resilience in managing a wide range of data domains. The focus will be on ensuring that the model can be easily understood, scaled up, and improved based on user input. The ultimate objective is to understand better how well the model can adapt, generalize, and be used in real-world situations. The primary aim of this comprehensive strategy is to enhance the comprehension of TL techniques on extensive datasets and make valuable contributions to the advancement of more efficient and adaptable models.

REFERENCES

1. Nareshkumar, R., Suseela, G., Nimala, K., & Niranjana, G. (2022). Feasibility and Necessity of Affective Computing in Emotion Sensing of Drivers for Improved Road Safety. Advances in Computational Intelligence and Robotics, 94–115. https://doi.org/10.4018/978-1-6684-3843-5.ch007.

2. Nareshkumar, R., & Nimala, K. (2022). An Exploration of Intelligent Deep Learning Models for Fine Grained Aspect-Based Opinion Mining. 2022 International Conference on Innovative Computing, Intelligent Communication and Smart Electrical Systems (ICSES). https://doi.org/10.1109/icses55317.2022.9914094.

3. Sirenjeevi, P., Karthick, J. M., Agalya, K., Srikanth, R., Elangovan, T., & Nareshkumar, R. (2023). Leaf Disease Identification Using ResNet. 2023 International Conference on Artificial Intelligence and Knowledge Discovery in Concurrent Engineering (ICECONF). https://doi.org/10.1109/iceconf57129.2023.10083963.

4. Nareshkumar, R., Agalya, K., Arunpandiyan, A., Vijayalakshmi, M., Ranjani, V., & Ramya, A. (2023). An Effective Deep Learning Based Recommender System with User and Item Embedding. 2023 International Conference on Artificial Intelligence and Knowledge Discovery in Concurrent Engineering (ICECONF). https://doi.org/10.1109/iceconf57129.2023.10083578.

5. Huang, J., Smola, A. J., Gretton, A., Borgwardt, K. M., & Schölkopf, B. (2007). Correcting Sample Selection Bias by Unlabeled Data. Advances in Neural Information Processing Systems, 19, 601–608. https://doi.org/10.7551/mitpress/7503.003.0080.

6. Pan, S. J., & Yang, Q. (2010). A Survey on Transfer Learning. IEEE Transactions on Knowledge and Data Engineering, 22(10), 1345–1359. https://doi.org/10.1109/tkde.2009.191.

7. Cao, X., Wipf, D., Wen, F., Duan, G., & Sun, J. (2013). A Practical Transfer Learning Algorithm for Face Verification. 2013 IEEE International Conference on Computer Vision. https://doi.org/10.1109/iccv.2013.398.

8. Wang, Z., Dai, Z., Poczos, B., & Carbonell, J. (2019). Characterizing and Avoiding Negative Transfer. 2019 IEEE/CVF Conference on Computer Vision and Pattern Recognition (CVPR). https://doi.org/10.1109/cvpr.2019.01155.

9. Redko, I., Habrard, A., Morvant, E., Sebban, M., & Bennani, Y. (2019). PAC-Bayesian Theory for Domain Adaptation. Advances in Domain Adaption Theory, 93–104. https://doi.org/10.1016/b978-1-78548-236-6.50006-4.

10. Sailesh, L. J., Kumar, V. K., Nimala, K., & Nareshkumar, R. (2023). Emotion Detection in Instagram Social Media Platform. 2023 International Conference on Artificial Intelligence and Knowledge Discovery in Concurrent Engineering (ICECONF). https://doi.org/10.1109/iceconf57129.2023.10083724.

11. Nareshkumar, R., & Nimala, K. (2023). Interactive Deep Neural Network for Aspect-Level Sentiment Analysis. 2023 International Conference on Artificial Intelligence and Knowledge Discovery in Concurrent Engineering (ICECONF). https://doi.org/10.1109/iceconf57129.2023.10083812.

12. Ling, X., Dai, W., Xue, G.-R., Yang, Q., & Yu, Y. (2008). Spectral Domain-Transfer Learning. Proceedings of the 14th ACM SIGKDD International Conference on Knowledge Discovery and Data Mining. https://doi.org/10.1145/1401890.1401951.

13. Arnold, A., Nallapati, R., & Cohen, W. W. (2007). A Comparative Study of Methods for Transductive Transfer Learning. Seventh IEEE International Conference on Data Mining Workshops (ICDMW 2007). https://doi.org/10.1109/icdmw.2007.109.

14. Chattopadhyay, R., Ye, J., Panchanathan, S., Fan, W., & Davidson, I. (2011). Multi-Source Domain Adaptation and Its Application to Early Detection of Fatigue. Proceedings of the 17th ACM SIGKDD International Conference on Knowledge Discovery and Data Mining. https://doi.org/10.1145/2020408.2020520.

15. El Zini, J., Rizk, Y., & Awad, M. (2020). A deep transfer learning framework for seismic data analysis: A case study on bright spot detection. IEEE Transactions on Geoscience and Remote Sensing, 58(5), 3202–3212. https://doi.org/10.1109/tgrs.2019.2950888.

16. Qiu, C., Zhang, S., Wang, C., Yu, Z., Zheng, H., & Zheng, B. (2018). Improving Transfer Learning and Squeeze- and-Excitation Networks for Small-Scale Fine-Grained Fish Image Classification. IEEE Access, 6, 78503–78512. https://doi.org/10.1109/access.2018.2885055.

17. Sohail, S. S., Himeur, Y., Amira, A., Fadli, F., Mansoor, W., Atalla, S., & Copiaco, A. (2023). Deep Transfer Learning for 3D Point Cloud Understanding: A Comprehensive Survey. https://doi.org/10.2139/ssrn.4348272.

18. Yu, Y., Lin, H., Meng, J., Wei, X., Guo, H., & Zhao, Z. (2017). Deep Transfer Learning for Modality Classification of Medical Images. Information, 8(3), 91. https://doi.org/10.3390/info8030091.

19. Lu, Z. (n.d.). Selective Transfer Learning for Cross Domain Recommendation (M.Phil. thesis), arXiv:1210.7056. https://doi.org/10.14711/thesis-b1240240.

20. He, M., Zhang, J., & Zhang, S. (2019). ACTL: Adaptive Codebook Transfer Learning for Cross-Domain Recommendation. IEEE Access, 7, 19539–19549. https://doi.org/10.1109/access.2019.2896881.

21. Pan, W. (2016). A Survey of Transfer Learning for Collaborative Recommendation with Auxiliary Data. Neurocomputing, 177, 447–453. https://doi.org/10.1016/j.neucom.2015.11.059.

22. Wang, Q., Oreilly-Morgan, D., Tragos, E. Z., Hurley, N., Smyth, B., Lawlor, A., & Dong, R. (2022). Learning Domain-Independent Representations via Shared Weight Auto-Encoder for Transfer Learning in Recommender Systems. IEEE Access, 10, 71961–71972. https://doi.org/10.1109/access.2022.3188709.

23. Alfa, A. A., Misra, S., Yusuf, A., & Agrawal, A. (2023). Comparative Analysis of Performances of Convolutional Neural Networks for Image Classification Tasks. Proceedings of International Conference on Recent Innovations in Computing, 179–190. https://doi.org/10.1007/978-981-19-9876-8_15.

24. Gaur, R., Prakash, S., Prasad, L. N., Kumar, S., Abhishek, K., & Guduri, M. (2023). A Secure and Efficient Scheme Based on Unlinkability and Anonymous Traceable Protocol for Cloud-Assisted IoT Environment. Journal of Circuits, Systems and Computers, 32(18), 2350316.

25. Raina, R., Ng, A. Y., & Koller, D. (2006). Constructing Informative Priors Using Transfer Learning. Proceedings of the 23rd International Conference on Machine Learning – ICML '06. https://doi.org/10.1145/1143844.1143934.

26. Dai, W., Xue, G.-R., Yang, Q., & Yu, Y. (2007). Co-Clustering Based Classification for Out-of-Domain Documents. Proceedings of the 13th ACM SIGKDD International Conference on Knowledge Discovery and Data Mining. https://doi.org/10.1145/1281192.1281218.

27. Blitzer, J., McDonald, R., & Pereira, F. (2006). Domain Adaptation with Structural Correspondence Learning. Proceedings of the 2006 Conference on Empirical Methods in Natural Language Processing – EMNLP '06. https://doi.org/10.3115/1610075.1610094.

28. Pradhan, J. D., Prasad, L. V. N., Dash, T. K., Guduri, M. & Panda, G. (2024) Cascaded PFLANN Model for Intelligent Health Informatics in Detection of Respiratory Diseases from Speech Using Bio-Inspired Computation. Journal of Artificial Intelligence and Technology. https://doi.org/10.37965/jait.2024.0435.

29. Hussain, M. M., Shanmugam, P., Moorthi, K., Sakthivelu, U., Rajasekar, A., & Kumar, R. N. (2023). "An Ensemble Deep Learning Model for Diabetic Retinopathy Identification," 2023 9th International Conference on Smart Structures and Systems (ICSSS), Chennai, India, pp. 1–7. https://doi.org/10.1109/ICSSS58085.2023.10407073.

30. Nareshkumar, R., & Nimala, K. (2024). An Enhanced BERT Model for Depression Detection on Social Media Posts. Lecture Notes in Networks and Systems, 53–64. https://doi.org/10.1007/978-981-99-8479-4_5.

31. Guduri, M., Chakraborty, C., Maheswari, U. and Margala, M., 2023. Blockchain-based federated learning technique for privacy preservation and security of smart electronic health records. *IEEE Transactions on Consumer Electronics*, 70(1), pp. 2608–2617.

32. Ganeshkumar, M., Ravi, V., Sowmya, V., Gopalakrishnan, E. A., Soman, K. P., & Chakraborty, C. (2022). Identification of Intracranial Haemorrhage (ICH) Using ResNet With Data Augmentation Using CycleGAN and ICH Segmentation Using SegAN. Multimedia Tools and Applications, 81(25), 36257–36273. https://doi.org/10.1007/s11042-021-11478-8

33. Awotunde, J. B., Chakraborty, C., & Folorunso, S. O. (2022). A Secured Smart Healthcare Monitoring Systems Using Blockchain Technology. Intelligent Internet of Things for Healthcare and Industry, 127–143. https://doi.org/10.1007/978-3-030-81473-1_6.

34. Jeberson, W., Kishor, A., & Chakraborty, C. (2021). Intelligent Healthcare Data Segregation Using Fog Computing With Internet of Things and Machine Learning. International Journal of Engineering Systems Modelling and Simulation, 1(1), 1. https://doi.org/10.1504/ijesms.2021.10036745.

4 Artificial Intelligence and Internet of Things Mechanism for Smart Healthcare 4.0

Ashima and Amit Kishor

4.1 INTRODUCTION

Society is progressing toward the fourth industrial revolution, characterized by integrating new technologies into healthcare to improve treatments and services. Medical technologies in the era of Healthcare 4.0 can provide timely and up-to-date information to healthcare professionals, enabling them to make informed decisions based on data analysis. Consequently, they are consistently associated with and kept up-to-date regarding the patients. Individuals with a sense of empowerment are equipped with the necessary resources and knowledge to carry out their most optimal tasks effectively. Although the prevalence of automation is anticipated to rise, it is imperative to acknowledge that human involvement will continue to be indispensable for its effective functioning. Information technology solutions further assist consumers by providing specific data or recommendations. Incorporating informed data, which encompasses the integration of automated and intelligent machinery inside intelligent manufacturing facilities, has demonstrated its ability to improve the effectiveness and output of goods across the complete value chain [1]. The enhancement of medical device manufacturers' adaptability is achieved through mass customization, which ultimately seeks to optimize efficiency by accommodating individual consumer demands, often resulting in a production size of one. The achievement of enhanced information transparency and more effective decision-making within a smart factory can be aided by gathering supplementary information and integrating it with other operational data within the company. The quality of decision-making is enhanced when individuals possess the requisite knowledge to base their conclusions on factual information. The manufacturing sector is experiencing an increased inclination toward innovation due to the ease of information sharing observed in the healthcare industry. Individuals' performance is generally expected to enhance when they can readily obtain comprehensive information without extensive search efforts. However, it is evident that many health sciences companies have yet to harness the capabilities of Industry 4.0 fully and are struggling to meet the specified standards. The implementation of Industry 4.0 is predictable to increase the effectiveness, and safety of production processes [2].

DOI: 10.1201/9781003603610-4

The increasing prevalence of digital touchpoints in patient interactions has enhanced the potential for predicting the likelihood of future illness severity. The massive quantity of data collected through medical devices aids in profiling patients and improves comprehension of their anatomical characteristics. The continuous endeavor to protect electronic health information has led to, and will further enable, the optimization of predictive health analysis. The utilization of real-time technology holds promise in assessing the demand for pharmaceuticals, devices, and other essential healthcare resources. Mobile technology will facilitate remote communication among physicians and specialists, enabling them to maintain contact irrespective of geographical constraints. Currently, a growing number of healthcare software solutions are being developed with primary objective of escalating health of patient and optimizing the communication medium between healthcare facilities and their patients [3].

Digital innovations aim to reduce time requirements, increase precision and efficacy, and incorporate technology in new ways within the healthcare industry. The potential exists for these breakthroughs to facilitate the integration of medical practices with other technologies, including the Internet of things (IoT), health, augmented reality, blockchain, medicine, and EMRs. The IoT application cases are diverse and extensive. Digital health tools provide the potential to enhance the ability to accurately identify and manage illnesses and strengthen the provision of personalized healthcare services. In addition, technological advancements such as cellular devices, online social platforms, and internet applications have introduced novel avenues for patients to effectively monitor their well-being and acquire relevant medical knowledge [4].

The concept of Industry 4.0 empowers consumers to produce intelligent products that are capable of monitoring and optimizing performance over time. These products are designed to satisfy the specific and individualized configurations of customers. Additionally, Industry 4.0 facilitates the development of intelligent factories that utilize data and intelligence to operate with a high degree of autonomy. Numerous organizations are compelled to swiftly transition to online platforms in order to sustain their momentum, primarily attributable to a need for more planning and foresight. Healthcare 4.0 represents the era characterized by intelligent, interconnected machinery and robotics, we must reassess our organizations, enhance our competencies, and reallocate our financial resources to adapt to and embrace emerging technologies [5] effectively. The objective of Medical 4.0 is to augment conventional manufacturing, industrial systems, and medical services and operations through the utilization of cutting-edge technology. The researchers have made a discovery that suggests an anticipated increase in expenditure on things falling under those specific categories in the upcoming years. However, investments in products that have a more extended income generation period can see a decrease or maintain a stable level. Efficient infection control and prevention can be facilitated by using telemedicine systems that leverage modern emerging technology. These technologies can identify and recognize any irregularities or abnormalities in patients during emergencies and initiate immediate communication with medical personnel [6].

Technicians can integrate preventive maintenance, management of assets, as well as supply chain data into their field of vision using an augmented reality headset or smartphone application. The collaboration between humans and machines offers a range of interconnected methods to enhance productivity and reduce expenses. VR headsets function as an interface that enables individuals to visit healthcare facilities from any location remotely. The implementation of a shared online platform for collaboration among individuals, organizations, and customers located in different geographical locations holds the promise of enhancing communication and customer service quality. Throughout history, manufacturing enterprises have demonstrated a need for comprehensive recognition regarding the importance of cyber attacks and cyber-physical systems. Nevertheless, incorporating factory and field operational equipment enables improved operational efficiency through adopting a digital transformation toward Industry 4.0. The development of a thorough cyber security strategy that contains both information technology (IT) and operational technology (OT) devices is crucial. The author achieved the accuracy of 96% [7].

In numerous modern organizations, there needs to be more certainty on the exact state of an health asset's, as data being collected and processed in separate systems. Consequently, many unnecessary periods of inactivity and inefficiency are observed. The synchronization between maintenance efforts and manufacturing processes often needs more efficiency, leading to the inefficient utilization of capacity and missed opportunities to fulfill high-priority orders. The transformation beyond reactive asset administration to proactively data-driven asset performance is achieved through the utilization of intelligent assets. The management and integration of intellectual assets are actively upheld and linked to all operational procedures [8]. The advent of Industry 4.0 has facilitated the electronic transformation of businesses, allowing them to create digital replicas, commonly referred to as digital twins, of their operational processes, manufacturing systems, physical infrastructure, and supply chains. Data derived from the IoT sensors, Programmable Logic Controllers, and other interconnected devices is employed to create a digital representation.

Within the realm of industry, the employment of sensors that are embedded and its associated gear results in significant quantities of data commonly referred to as big data. Manufacturers utilize data analytics as a vital instrument to analyze past trends, detect patterns, and augment their decision-making capabilities. To enhance their comprehension, intelligent factories have the potential to integrate data from various divisions within the firm and its wide range of vendors and distributors [9].

The major contribution of the chapter is to provide extensive review of the technologies such as IoT, CC and AI implementation in Healthcare 4.0. Also review the operational mechanism of their applications and find the feasible solution to current challenges in Healthcare 4.0 which have impact on healthcare sector in relation to industry 4.0.

4.2 HEALTHCARE 4.0

The objective of Medical 4.0 is to establish a strategic approach that facilitates the transformation of manufacturers into service providers. The advancement process is optimized to services for clients depending on their wants and preferences. Medical 4.0 leverage contemporary technology to facilitate communication and collaboration between healthcare and patients providers in terms of organizational aspects and therapeutic approaches. The technologies listed above are currently seeing a shift toward a patient-centric approach. This involves making the data accessible to industry stakeholders to improve innovation and healthcare service concepts [10].

The integration of virtual reality technology has substantially enhanced healthcare technology during the transition to the fourth industrial revolution in medicine. The virtual reality headset, wearable technology, enables patients to explore unexplored areas and virtually escape the monotonous hospital environment. This technology is utilized to simplify the patient's treatment experience. In addition to offering patients a means of psychological diversion, VR has also exhibited documented effectiveness in pain management. It has shown significant advancements in individuals suffering from chronic pain. In addition, individuals can acquire a headset for VR from commercial platforms. This allows them to engage in a pain-relief approach similar to a hospital setting while prioritizing self-care by home remedies and virtual remedy [11].

The breakthroughs in AI, machine learning (ML), robots, and BD substantially impact the field of digital healthcare. Major advancements have been achieved in the realm of digital healthcare, particularly pertaining to sensors, robotic caretakers, and remote monitoring devices for patients and applications. Furthermore, using sophisticated supply chain and manufacturing techniques would ensure the punctual provision of suitable medication and interventions to patients. Medical 4.0 technologies cover various gadgets, including smart watches, wearable devices, and mobile technologies, which enhance accessibility to healthcare assistance and monitoring. These technologies have garnered considerable attention, particularly in managing chronic and enduring medical diseases. The wearable device integrated various physiological monitoring capabilities, such as variability in heart rate evaluation, pulse oximetry, electro-cardiography (EC), and continuous glucose level monitoring. The utilization of comprehensive data analysis is of utmost importance in determining patient features and formulating preventive strategies to mitigate the probability of their readmission. Predictive analytics has promise in aiding hospitals and clinics in precisely estimating admission rates and enhancing the efficacy of scheduling employees [12].

The emergence of Medical 4.0 technology has brought about a substantial transformation in the healthcare sector. Technologies encompass a range of innovations, including mobile medical software and applications that leverage AI to aid clinical decision-making by physicians. In addition, hospitals have the potential to employ sensors to manage supply stocks effectively. This utilization can optimize resource utilization and expenditure on essential items such as gases, chemicals, masks, and gloves. Healthcare personnel are responsible for safeguarding patients' sensitive personal information. Furthermore, it is imperative for IoT devices to demonstrate reliability in various aspects, including connectivity, performance, and the transmission of real-time data. The utilization of electronic health record (EHR) technologies enables physicians to improve both the accuracy and effectiveness of patient diagnoses.

Additionally, these technologies facilitate integration with other physician networks, allowing for effective management of referrals and seamless communication of prescriptions to pharmacies. The application of patient interaction innovations has the potential to decrease unnecessary healthcare costs significantly. This data empowers individuals to cultivate a more robust connection with their well-being and evaluate the financial implications of pharmaceutical products or healthcare provisions that they can necessitate. The digital revolution has the potential to be advantageous for emerging pharmaceutical companies, as it allows the pharmaceutical sector to establish communication and interaction with prospective patients through online platforms while they are exploring the advantages of different products.

4.2.1 Need for Healthcare 4.0 for Medical

Streamlining specialists' methods for considering chronic patients should be enhanced by using the latest breakthroughs in biology and technology based on current research. The implementation of Medical 4.0 technologies enhances the provision of tailored treatment, expedites the management of symptoms, and enables real-time monitoring of patient health on a minute-by-minute basis. The focal point of this technological revolution revolves around the monitoring and analysis of technical advancements that have the potential to provide reliable and consistent patient data, a crucial element for the effective implementation of therapy. The concept of Medical 4.0 is gaining prominence within the healthcare industry as it explores the potential benefits of using CC and AI technologies. CC offers numerous benefits that contribute to improving personalized purchase experiences. The system can identify patterns in clients' browsing and purchasing behaviors. AI has the potential to deliver exact products to individual clientele. The process of automating customer interactions is achieved by employing AI techniques. AI-driven chat bots can communicate simultaneously with several clients, replying to and initiating discourse [13].

AI is another way to provide prompt and real-time help. Data mining is a crucial use of AI that efficiently identifies significant and pertinent insights while analyzing large datasets. This technology plays a vital role in operational automation and other corporate technologies for automation. The convergence of data from many different areas within the healthcare system is an opportunity to harness and utilize this information to develop innovative solutions that span multiple sectors. The exponential growth of medical research can be attributed to the availability and analysis of extensive data. Hence, the ability to collect and analyze vast quantities of data suggests that advancements in medical research will occur at a significantly accelerated pace compared to previous periods. Patients will have a more comprehensive understanding of their medical state as a result of engaging in ongoing communication with their healthcare provider, which facilitates personalized information delivery through real-time monitoring. Medical 4.0 enable for early patient detection and individualized treatment plans. Biometric devices have the potential to be developed to conduct scans on patients during intervals between sessions to identify and address diseases at the earliest possible stage. With the advancement of technology, an increasing number of individuals can avail of high-quality healthcare services at a reduced expense. The outcome is typically associated with improved population health, suggesting a subsequent expense reduction [14].

4.2.2 USING MEDICAL 4.0 TOOLS IN THE HEALTHCARE INDUSTRY

Incorporating Medical 4.0 technology in the healthcare sector facilitates numerous innovative methods for monitoring individuals' health and well-being, granting increased accessibility to their data. One of the primary benefits of telehealth, as opposed to conventional in-person alternatives, is its ability to minimize interactions among patients, healthcare professionals, as well as other patients, while simultaneously providing a substantial patient experience. The application of blockchain technology possesses the capacity to enhance the healthcare sector to a considerable extent. The healthcare sector greatly benefits from the interoperability feature offered by blockchain technology. The application of public-private strategies improves the reliability of healthcare data. Wearable gadgets provide healthcare practitioners with the capability to remotely access real-time patient data. Advancements in medical technologies have significantly facilitated communication between healthcare practitioners and patients [5].

Healthcare professionals can communicate using various electronic platforms such as email, telephones, text messaging, and other similar methods. Medical professionals can produce webinars and films and interact with other specialists through websites and social media. The introduction of teleconferencing has enabled the exchange of information and ideas despite geographical barriers. The deployment of electronic medical records enables the efficient management of patient data, encompassing health histories, outcomes of tests, diagnoses, and other relevant information. The incorporation of data enables the delivery of healthcare services that exhibit improved precision and reliability, as well as the capacity to identify patterns in individual well-being. The implementation of medical billing systems has been found to greatly improve the operational efficiency of various healthcare facilities such as clinics, hospitals, and medical offices. These healthcare professionals possess the ability to provide personalized treatment plans to prevent the need for hospitalization and unnecessary appointments. Medical technologies enable the acquisition of a substantial amount of data, enhance communication, and furnish crucial information for research purposes. Patients can utilize their mobile devices to submit inquiries from any location and at any given moment, while healthcare professionals may readily provide responses. It is argued that this practice enhances self-assurance, fosters reliance, and ensures prompt assistance for patients across various medical conditions [15].

4.2.3 TELEMEDICINE

Telemedicine, also called telemedicine or e-medicine, encompasses providing healthcare services, including diagnostic tests and consultations, by remote means. Telemedicine allows healthcare professionals to remotely assess, diagnose, and treat patients without needing in-person consultations. This technical development makes it easier for patients to obtain a number of health-related data, such as blood pressure, temperature, blood sugar, and other important markers. Utilizing telecommunication technology, telemedicine is a relatively new framework that offers therapeutic services like treatment, therapy, and medical diagnosis [16].

The word "Telehealth" is broad and covers both clinical and non-clinical services. For instance, individual medical training is provided, and patients can be observed from a distance. The utilization of telehealth services has experienced a surge in popularity over the past few years, driven mainly by global concerns about general health due to the COVID-19 pandemic [17]. Individuals have increasingly engaged in self-isolation and tried to mitigate the risk of infection, resulting in challenges when seeking medical attention. The utilization of telemedicine applications has become essential for a significant number of individuals globally to promote health and prevent illnesses. This technology has the capability to deliver healthcare services to persons who are unable to physically access a medical center. Telehealth applications are utilized by healthcare practitioners to enhance the process of diagnosing and treating patients [18].

4.3　HEALTHCARE 4.0 WITH AI

AI has made significant contributions to the healthcare sector. The consequences of the apps have had a considerable influence on the healthcare sector. The use of AI has been crucial in reducing the severity of the COVID-19 epidemic. In its early stages, AI has been utilized to automate routine and monotonous tasks, minimizing the need for manual paperwork. The prominence of the function of digitalization in health data and information requirements may be observed in its utilization by insurance companies, hospitals, and patients. AI applications are significantly transforming various aspects of the healthcare industry, including hospital care, clinical research, prescription development, and insurance. The objective of these improvements is to improve patient outcomes while concurrently lowering costs. The healthcare sector has observed the potential of ML in making significant contributions. The utilization of this technology spans across various domains, encompassing the detection of associations among genetic codes, the augmentation of robots for surgery, and the optimization of the effectiveness of hospitals [19]. AI exhibits the capacity to analyze huge volumes of data. One potential use involves the utilization of knowledge databases to facilitate the assessment and guidance provided to individual patients, enhancing the effectiveness of clinical decision support. Medical professionals have the potential to utilize this technology as a means of identifying potential risk factors within unstructured medical documentation. AI plays a crucial role in primary care automation, allowing doctors to allocate their time more effectively toward essential cases. Using AI-driven medical chat bot services can promptly address patients' inquiries regarding their health and offer guidance on potential issues, reducing unnecessary visits to healthcare facilities and medical practitioners. AI may help surgeons save time and reduce surgical errors by facilitating more precise incisions [20]. Figure 4.1 represents the flowchart of the chapter. The data of the patient is collected through IoMT devices such as smart lens, smart jacket, etc., and the data is sent to cloud using internet. Finally the data is analyzed by AI application and to find the possible feasible solutions.

AI systems can leverage data obtained from prior surgical procedures to develop novel surgical methodologies. The precision of this apparatus mitigates the potential for tremors or other unintended or inadvertent movements during surgical

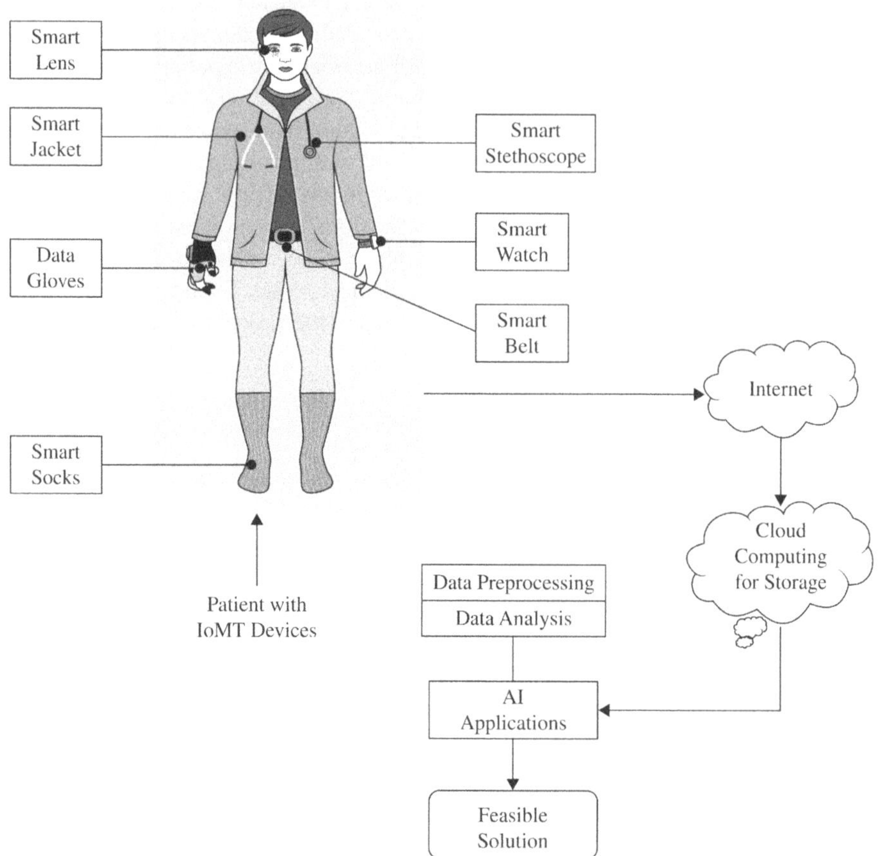

FIGURE 4.1   Flowchart of the work.

procedures. AI technologies facilitate the utilization of virtual nursing assistants for various tasks, including patient communication and directing them to the most suitable and efficient care facilities. The literature discusses the availability of virtual nurses at all times, as they are capable of responding to inquiries, assessing patients, and providing timely interventions. The utilization of AI has promise in augmenting the proficiency of medical practitioners by its ability to enable more precise and efficient identification, anticipation, and assessment of medical conditions. Similarly, AI algorithms demonstrate a notable level of accuracy and precision in the diagnosis of specific medical disorders, such as diabetic retinopathy.

Moreover, these algorithms offer a cost-effective approach to identifying and detecting this ailment. One of the primary benefits linked with the implementation of AI and healthcare technology lies in their ability to provide timely and accurate results. The active participation of humans is crucial in guaranteeing the suitability for treatment and its emotional consequences [21].Healthcare institutions that effectively analyze data have the capacity to draw insights that have a substantial impact on patient outcomes, ultimately leading to life-saving interventions. The integration of AI technologies within healthcare institutions involves the progression of

ML techniques, the implementation of techniques for processing natural language (NLP), and the cultivation of expertise in deep learning. These technologies are utilized to analyze and process vast amounts of data within the healthcare domain. Firms can enhance the quality of healthcare provision by utilizing medical history and test results analysis to identify prevailing health patterns. AI has the potential to serve as a valuable device in healthcare by facilitating medical diagnoses. In healthcare, using ML and AI has become increasingly prevalent. These technologies are employed to analyze vast quantities of data, enabling the delivery of precise medical diagnoses promptly, hence preventing the occurrence of delayed treatment. This facilitates physicians to initiate treatment before the event of any significant complications. AI technologies in cancer detection demonstrate their potential to save lives globally. These interventions are progressively expanding in efforts to mitigate diseases and enhance the preservation of human life [22].

Medical professionals and researchers commonly conduct tests and investigations with the aim of identifying pharmaceutical interventions that can enhance the speed and efficacy of patient healing. It comprises determining the appropriate chemicals for a drug's composition and impact. ML and AI can be employed by healthcare researchers to generate diverse designs and evaluate their feasibility, while ensuring the safety of human participants [23]. AI software has the capability to collect health data and continuously update it through the utilization of smart gadgets and wearable's. This enables healthcare professionals to access the data and make well-informed assessments and decisions. AI systems have the capability to analyze a patient's previous medical records, merge them with medical imaging and scans, and generate a precise assessment of the individual's health status. It has the capability to provide information regarding potential future diseases that may afflict the patient [24].

Advancements in AI have facilitated the utilization of virtual assistants by healthcare practitioners to provide assistance during surgical and nursing procedures. Using AI to analyze data before surgery and make suggestions for the best way to proceed shows promise for improving medical procedures. The utilization of AI in the healthcare industry is increasingly observed as a novel approach. In present-day healthcare environments, human personnel remain integral to the functioning of hospitals. Nevertheless, there has been a significant increase in the incorporation of artificially intelligent programs, which are gradually taking on diverse roles and helping to the improvement of healthcare delivery. AI possesses the capacity to become a revolutionary technology that presents substantial advantages to individuals. Numerous firms actively engage in diverse committees as well as groups that have been established to facilitate the advancement of standard and regulatory frameworks. Furthermore, it is crucial to emphasize that during the development and implementation of AI-based solutions, numerous enterprises establish strong collaborations with local governmental entities [25].

4.3.1 Applications of Artificial Intelligence in Healthcare 4.0

The author research [4] examined the implementation of Industry 4.0 applications for healthcare as a strategy to tackle the issues caused by the COVID-19. The main aim of this study was to investigate the incorporation of suitable technology, including intelligent machines, as a strategy for resolving the aforementioned challenge.

Discussions on the identification and evaluation of COVID-19 were additionally noted. The aim of this study was to examine the integration of Industry 4.0, also known as Healthcare 4.0, and its many technical breakthroughs in the context of the COVID-19. The implementation of virtual reality technology holds promise in enhancing the administration of robotically assisted therapy to patients, while mitigating the hazards encountered by medical practitioners [26].Healthcare 4.0 technologies, including AI, can promptly detect any medical concerns experienced by patients by utilizing sensors in emergencies. Now, China is implementing AI-based video monitoring, utilizing Healthcare 4.0 technology, to observe the actions of individuals infected with COVID-19 and mitigate the transmission of the virus. The work has achieved the accuracy of 99.31% [27]. The utilization of AI-based technology can potentially enhance the efficacy of clinical studies on antiviral drugs and vaccines [4]. AI has been utilized in managing supply chains within the medical industry throughout the outbreak [28]. CT scans (computed tomography) and AI has been shown to be useful in identifying cases of viral pneumonia. In the circumstances surrounding the COVID-19 pandemic, a robot powered by AI might be used to perform the tasks of a law enforcement officer throughout a lockdown in order to ensure that the approved protocols are followed. For example, in the context of a pandemic, AI may be used to monitor and manage big gatherings, making it easier to exert authority over people's relationships with one another.AI has enabled the distant accomplishment of tasks. Figure 4.2 shows several AI applications in the ongoing battle against the COVID-19 pandemic.

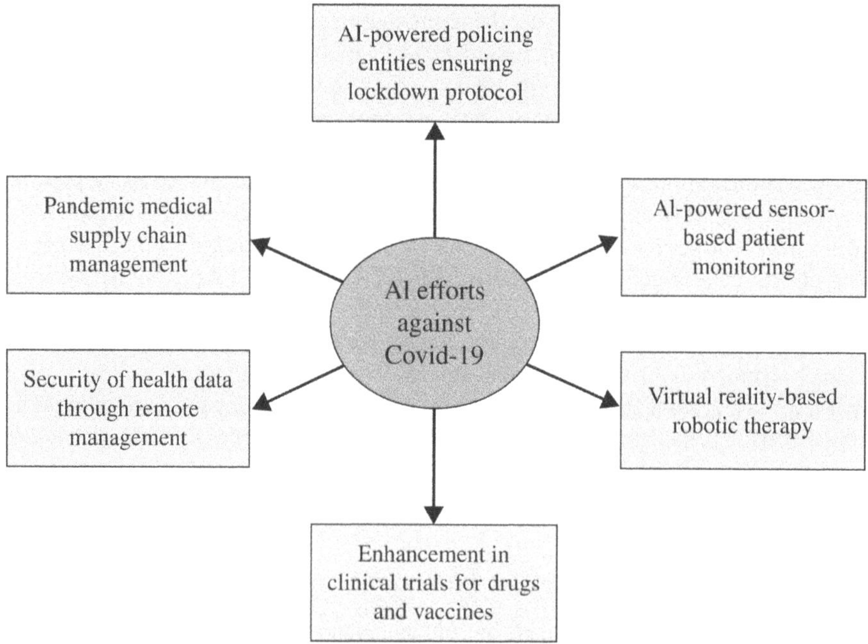

FIGURE 4.2 AI efforts against COVID-19.

Health information of individuals is well managed and shared among multiple authorities in different countries. Privacy serves as a safeguard against the unauthorized access to an individual's personal information. The use of IT structures played a key part in the establishment of Healthcare 1.0. The later 2.0 iteration, Healthcare 2.0, placed an emphasis on easy accessibility and storage. EHR data was retrieved with the use of WDs. From here, the idea of Healthcare 3.0 developed. Significant changes have occurred in the healthcare sector as a result of the fourth industrial revolution, sometimes known as "Healthcare 4.0." The IoT, computing via the cloud, and blockchain are just a few of the technologies that come together to form "Healthcare 4.0." The shown work achieved an accuracy of 96.62% [29]. By combining these many forms of technology, breakthroughs in healthcare are made possible. Utilizing WDs and IDs in the telehealthcare network to promote traffic between patient associations and doctor groups could lead to the creation of a new trademark [30]. Data security is of the utmost importance because of the massive amount of information at risk. The maintenance of an individual's record permissions is accomplished through the implementation of security protocols, which serve the primary purpose of protecting it from unauthorized access. Security can be attained by utilizing operational controls.

4.3.2 Cutting-Edge Artificial Intelligence in the Healthcare 4.0

AI has significantly impacted Healthcare 4.0 as AI-based technology has improved over time. The biomedical business has witnessed the introduction of contemporary advancements. In alternative terms, AI is commonly employed in the analysis of biomedical data types. After assembly, these are examined. The interconnected biological processes can be characterized using several omics data resources [31]. Model-based integration is the subsequent strategy. Various data views are employed to generate distinct models, and the resulting model output is consolidated as outlined in reference. Construction and development of neural networks and models are largely dependent on each omic data type throughout the integration phase. The edges of several conventional weighted network types are augmented in situations involving multi-omic data. The utilization of AI techniques has shown significant promise in examining multi-omics networks [32].

AI technology has been used to analyze clinical data, EHRs, medical pictures, and physiological signals. Feature engineering is a method that is frequently used to classify descriptors that are derived from pictures into several segments or classes. This approach is often utilized for doing such analyses. EHR are used to keep track of patients' medical histories. Structured health data includes dictionaries with information on patients, medical professionals, procedures, tests, and diagnoses. In contrast, medical records written by doctors and nurses are examples of unstructured health data. The advancements in AI techniques for the analysis of EHRs have demonstrated notable progress. To assess structured data, vector-based ML techniques are employed to transform patient records into vector representations [33]. This technology facilitates the assessment of several elements of a patient's features and provides comprehensive summaries. EHR data format has been determined using recurrent neural networks. ECGs are simply one type of invariant data set that can be categorized under the general phrase "physiological data." Modern deep learning techniques were applied in a recent study by the author [34] to detect and classify heart arrhythmias. In this investigation, a growing number of state-of-the-art methods are employed. To convert electrocardiogram (EKG) information into distinct rhythm classes, they used a network of convolutional neural networks (CNN) model with 34 layers.

An interactive chatbot was created by Tang et al. [35] using transcript from Tencent's clinical trials. Unlike supervised models, the aforementioned agent was capable of to optimize the precision of MCI detection with a limited amount of conversational events.

4.3.3 CHALLENGES IN IMPLEMENTATION OF AI

Once the medical records have been converted into digital format, they can be accessed and stored in a cloud server. Cybercriminals or malicious actors have the capability to infiltrate the cloud server, gain illegal entry, and readily compromise an individual's personal and medical information. Hence, persistent obstacles and struggles continue to exist. The prioritization of ethical concerns is of utmost importance. Many of the issues that surface in this specific paradigm concern privacy, access control, ownership, and governance, among other things. Ethical quandaries are a subset of the difficulties and complications listed above. The principal challenge in this particular situation is guaranteeing the timely retrieval or complete preservation of the patient's data. Individuals with the appropriate authorization are granted access to patient records stored in the EHR system. The issue at hand pertains to the vulnerability of a user's identity being compromised by an attacker or hacker, resulting in unauthorized access to their personal information. This poses a significant danger and may lead to the mishandling or misuse of this information. However, the identification of unauthorized access is a relatively challenging task. Confidentiality serves to conceal vital information in the case of an illegal intrusion. Hence, the maintenance of confidentiality is a crucial undertaking. The fidelity of data ensures its accuracy. The potential for data inaccuracy arises when an attacker is able to manipulate information. The task of safeguarding against unauthorized access or theft of data presents significant difficulties [30]. It is conceivable that hackers may possess the requisite level of access to get ownership details and subsequently manipulate them to assert ownership. They may make the authorized entry unavailable. Maintaining policy at a high standard of care is essential. To guarantee the protection of health diagnosis data, it is essential to put strong security measures in place and follow strict administrative procedures. In order to mitigate the risk of theft, it is advisable to design an EHR system using a layered approach, incorporating many indemnity patterns. Certain websites offer online EHR systems that provide users with a certain amount of complimentary storage capacity, a practice that has inherent risks. There exists a potentiality for the sale of said information, which could result in significant ramifications for both the patient and the employees involved. Ensuring that information is appropriately disseminated poses a considerable challenge [36]. AI has great potential for usage in the healthcare industry, particularly in the fight against viruses. Nevertheless, it is crucial to remember that AI systems are still in their infancy, therefore more time will pass before the results of these AI interventions are apparent [27]. The deployment of Healthcare 4.0 technologies will aid in the future battle against pandemics similar to COVID-19. AI is one cutting-edge technology in which the medical industry can leverage to help create a more intelligent healthcare system.

4.4 CLOUD COMPUTING IN HEALTHCARE 4.0

Cloud computing is an important part of the current industrial revolution, which is sometimes called "Industry 4.0." It has the ability to make huge changes in the healthcare field. Cloud computing saves healthcare companies a lot of money because they don't have to pay for and manage expensive and time-consuming servers on-site.

There are three main service models that define cloud computing. Among the three primary service models, Software as a Service (SaaS) has emerged as the clear frontrunner. Customers use it in a wide variety of contexts, including but not limited to e-mail, social networking apps, literary content, and data storage. Using the Platform as a Service (PaaS) model, clients can take advantage of the provider's infrastructure, programming tools, and language support to create and manage their own applications. The PaaS model restricts user agency by preventing them from directly controlling the underlying cloud architecture. Whereas the Infrastructure as a Service (IaaS) model offers users with the capacity to manage storage, distributed apps, operating systems, and specialized networking components. The four deployment models used in cloud computing include:

Private cloud – A cloud infrastructure is utilized by a collective group of clients who share exclusive access to a single entity.

Public cloud – The term "public cloud" is used to describe a platform that is freely accessible by everyone.

Community cloud – Community clouds are hybrid environments that combine elements of both private and public clouds. On a shared infrastructure, multi-tenant platforms enable collaboration among multiple organizations.

Hybrid cloud – The cloud architecture comprises many autonomous infrastructures, such as private, communal, or public, maintained as distinct entities but interconnected utilizing standardized techniques to enable seamless data and device mobility. The cloud contains distinct characteristics and frameworks [37].

Demand-based self-service clients have the ability to autonomously distribute computational resources, including network storage and server time, without necessitating direct engagement with individual service providers. Wide-ranging network standard frameworks facilitate the effective use of network capabilities, thereby encouraging the connection of diverse consumer channels, including thin or thick laptops, tablets, workstations, and mobile phones.

4.4.1 Resource Pooling

The provider employs a multi-tenant architecture to efficiently manage its computer resources, allowing for the simultaneous utilization of these resources by numerous clients. This architecture involves the pooling of both physical and virtual resources, which are dynamically distributed and reallocated as per the specific requirements of each user. Typically, customers possess limited control and information regarding the precise location of the services provided. However, they may designate a broader degree of abstraction when defining the place, imbuing the location with a perception of autonomy, such as identifying it by nation, or data center. Bandwidth, memory, and network storage are illustrative examples of technological resources.

4.4.2 Rapid Elasticity

Flexibility in providing and withdrawing capabilities allows for their dynamic expansion and contraction, responding promptly to external and internal demands. The user believes that the abilities required for provisioning are boundless and may be accessible without limitations in terms of time or quantity. Measured service Cloud systems employ metering capabilities at various levels of abstraction to effectively monitor and optimize resource utilization in an automated manner. Tracking, managing, and recording service consumption is essential to establish accountability for both the service provider and the service recipient.

4.4.3 Cloud Computing Applications in Healthcare 4.0

Industry 4.0 has led to significant technological improvements in the healthcare sector, particularly in cloud computing. As a result, cutting-edge medical innovations have been created. The concept of "cloud computing" pertains to providing computer services on demand, encompassing a wide range of offerings such as applications, storage, and processing power. The Pay-As-You-Go (PAYG) operating system is an additional system that is employed. The operational mechanism of this system can be likened to a usage-based payment model for cloud computing. The PAYG technique ensures that users are only charged for services that have been requested and are prepared, hence preventing any loss of data. Three different types of cloud computing services fall under different PAYG model subcategories. The three main categories in cloud computing, namely Infrastructures as a Service, or IaaS, PaaS, and SaaS, are each separated into three subcategories. Users or consumers in the IaaS do not have a specific time limit or restriction. They can choose to pay per-use, monthly, weekly, or hourly. Cloud companies have been observed to levy charges for the utilization of Virtual Machines (VMs). In the context of this specific category, there exist no explicit prerequisites or criteria pertaining to hardware or software. Prominent providers of IaaS include IBM, Microsoft, Hewlett-Packard and Amazon Web Services.

The PaaS is delivered through a pricing model that is determined by an allocation of bandwidth or application usage on an hourly basis. PaaS refers to a cloud computing service offered by Google. The pricing and usage of SaaS are influenced by several aspects,

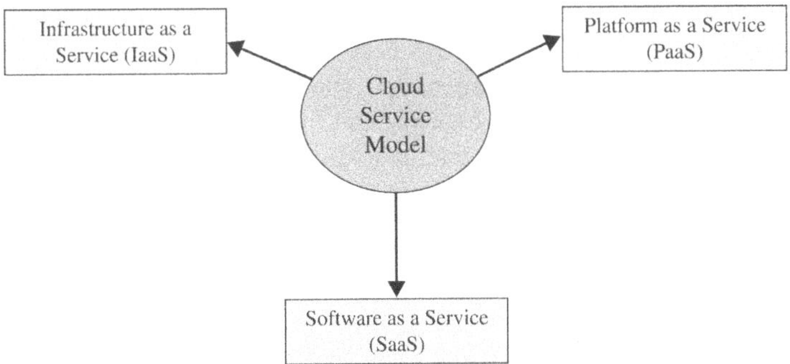

FIGURE 4.3 Versions of cloud services.

such as the quality of the service, the inclusion of the latest features, and the available storage capacity. SaaS solutions comprise a diverse array of apps, including but not limited to Office 365, Gmail, Trello, and Slack. The cloud Foundry, Heroku, which operates and OpenShift represent instances of PaaS components. IaaS encompasses a range of services, such as Azure, Amazon Web Services (AWS), the VMware (which offers dual operating system compatibility), and Stack scale. Figure 4.3 illustrates the aforementioned services within the context of the cloud-based service paradigm.

The most important achievements in cloud computing are rare and tend to center on cutting-edge technologies. A new age of innovation is being proposed by the extraordinary contribution of cloud computing to preserving healthcare integration. Before switching to cloud computing, firms with insufficient resources were experiencing a variety of issues. At the moment, cloud computing makes it simple to access anywhere. The utilization of cloud technology enables the availability of diverse information, encompassing data about patients, physicians, several healthcare facilities, and health institutions, with the convenience of accessibility from any location and at any given moment. The most recent approach, a delivery model, has improved the healthcare industry and reduced expenses. The primary concept of computing in the cloud is to ensure the secure and efficient storage of vast quantities of data and computational resources. Medical organizations and healthcare professionals are not required to get the essential servers and hardware. Data storage in the cloud is free of charge upfront. Hospitals and healthcare institutions only have to pay for resources that are really used, which results in significant cost savings. The ecosystem of healthcare is extremely complicated. The primary concerns revolve around health insurance and the networks of hospitals and physicians. All healthcare-related activities must conform to a multitude of laws and regulations.

Regarding the cloud's assistance, information must be provided as quickly as feasible and be secured. The key point in this situation is protecting a patient's data. Due to security concerns, the private cloud is used initially, and then public infrastructure as a service is introduced. The software has features like scalable architecture, suitable data centers, top-notch security models, and quick data retrieval. Maintaining stability in the face of change is the goal of both infrastructure and dynamic scalability. Corporations reinvest in a growing business as a means to maintain its viability. Because of this, there is a scarcity of storage space, necessitating an increase in both processing power and information technology. Organizations can also have a substitute with the help of the cloud, allowing them to discover the capacity problem. The cloud hosts the platform as a service model. Alternatively, it can offer infrastructure as a service [38], letting businesses make use of the existing infrastructure while tailoring it to their specific operational and functional requirements. When you put your data on the cloud, you can access it from anywhere with an internet connection. Setting up servers may be done more quickly to reduce downtime. Healthcare services include the interchange of a considerable amount of information.

4.4.4 Cutting-Edge Cloud Computing in the Healthcare 4.0

A hospital's paper-based information is represented numerically in electronic medical records (EMRs). Patients' personal information, medical conditions, and other data are provided through and stored in EMRs. Patients can be readily recognized and carefully tracked because of the EMRs' ability to track data over time. A physician or other healthcare professional inside a single healthcare institution can construct, collect, manage, and evaluate a person or individual in an EMR, which is, in a nutshell, an electronic record of health-related information. An EMR comprises five stages, according to the Health Institute: a provider-based computerized medical record, an Electron A hospital's paper-based information is represented numerically in EMRs, Basic Electronic Medical Record, Advanced Electronic Medical Record, and Integrated Electronic Health Record (EHR). Patients' personal information, medical conditions, and other data are provided through and stored in EMRs. Patients can be readily recognized and carefully tracked because to the EMRs' ability to track data over time. A physician or other healthcare professional inside a single healthcare institution can construct, collect, manage, and evaluate a person or individual in an EMR, which is, in a nutshell, an electronic record of health-relic Patient Record (EPR), an EMR, an automated medical record, and eventually an EHR. Many regiments and medical professionals in the healthcare industry have started using the terms EHR and EMR interchangeably. Both EMR and EHR present significant challenges in the broader context of healthcare digitalization, aiming to enhance the security and efficiency of patient care. However, they have the potential to reduce healthcare delivery operating expense. EMRs are the property of specific healthcare professionals. However, some subsets of EMRs are generally included in EHRs. There are no alternatives to EHRs that can offer high-quality items at a reasonable price. A personal health record (PHR) refers to an individual's health record that is maintained or utilized by the person themselves. The patient's or an individual's medical history and health summary can be found in the PHR. A patient's or a staff member's treatment of others is documented in an EMR. For the purpose of looking up health information and providing counseling, healthcare providers create, use, and maintain an electronic medical record, or EMR [39].

4.4.5 Challenges in Implementation of Cloud Computing

Within the last few years, cloud-based computing has become a lot more common. The healthcare sector has been significantly impacted by the fourth industrial revolution. Cloud computing has made a substantial contribution to this situation to ensure the optimal performance of cloud services.

Numerous obstacles exist, despite the relatively low acceptance rate of cloud computing in the medical and healthcare industries, the primary obstacles that hinder its implementation are privacy and interoperability [38]. The protection of healthcare data should adhere to stringent protocols to ensure its confidentiality and privacy. Failure to do so increases the likelihood of data breaches or the potential for unethical utilization of the data. The advent of cloud computing has simplified the process of data storage, hence necessitating enhanced security measures [40]. The act of moving a significant amount of data to a third-party company poses a challenging endeavor. Ensuring the safeguarding of healthcare data is of utmost importance owing to its criticality and the high level of sensitivity associated with it. The establishment of mechanisms ensuring the prevention of illegal access, authentication, transmission security, and authorization is of paramount importance. The second concern revolves around interoperability, a concept that pertains to the ability of software or hardware to permit the seamless transfer and utilization of information. Cloud storage in the healthcare industry has been a prominent feature throughout the fourth industrial revolution. Interoperability across healthcare systems can be achieved through several means, including provider-level, software-level, computer-level, data-level, and transfer-level approaches [41]. Cloud providers typically store their separate datasets. In order to safeguard or optimize the cloud infrastructure, healthcare organizations should execute their remaining protocols utilizing cloud-based solutions.

4.5 IoT IN HEALTHCARE 4.0

The incorporation of IoT technology within the healthcare industry offers numerous advantages, including enhanced interoperability, machine-to-machine connectivity, efficient information interchange, and seamless data migration. These aspects greatly improve the effectiveness and efficiency of healthcare service provision. IoT devices have the capability to gather, transmit, and evaluate data in real-time, hence obviating the need to retain raw, unprocessed data. Health IoT devices have the capability to collect essential health indicators associated with diverse medical conditions. The aforementioned data is thereafter supplied to healthcare specialists for the purpose of continuous real-time monitoring. Additionally, mobile applications and intelligent sensors are utilized to inform individuals about essential aspects of their health. The cost of healthcare services has reached unprecedented levels, coinciding with a global population that is experiencing an aging trend. Moreover, the prevalence of chronic diseases is on the rise, partly due to technological advancements. The utilization of technology-based healthcare strategies offers unparalleled advantages that have the potential to enhance the quality and efficiency of treatments, hence improving the health outcomes of elderly individuals. The utilization of interconnected devices for remote health monitoring has the potential to be life-saving during medical emergencies, including instances of heart failure, diabetes, asthma attacks, and other related conditions [6].

An advanced medical device connected to a smartphone app can be used to track a person's health in real time. Medical devices can collect important medical and health data in this way. The data connection on the smartphone could then be used by these gadgets to send the data to a doctor or a cloud platform. As healthcare gets better in the future, it will use healthcare mobility options and other cutting-edge IoT technology.

Integrating IoT technology can automate various aspects of patient care workflow within healthcare facilities. Furthermore, it aids healthcare professionals in making well-informed assessments and delivering prompt medical interventions. Consequently, the IoT provides the capability of delivering real-time alerts, tracking, and monitoring, enabling interactive interventions, enhanced precision, prompt medical interventions, and improved outcomes in the provision of patient care. Healthcare IoT applications can also be employed for research purposes. IoT enables the collection of extensive data about a patient's illness. This process would have required significant time if done manually [4].

The IoT is employed in a diverse range of devices to enhance the healthcare services rendered to patients. The IoT is improving existing equipment by install smart healthcare device chips. This microelectronic device amplifies the patient's requirement for assistance and attention. Data security and privacy pose significant challenges for the healthcare sector's IoT. The security equipment utilized in the IoT can capture and transmit data in real time, as evidenced by scholarly sources [39]. There exist several rationales for the utilization of linked devices in the monitoring of health vitals, data routing, alert provision, medication dispensation, and automation of crucial procedures. The healthcare sector effectively integrates IoT technology in various domains, encompassing medical wearable's, patient monitoring systems, and pharmaceutical temperature monitoring mechanisms. The primary objective of this integration is to augment accuracy, streamline operational effectiveness, minimize costs, adhere to regulatory obligations, and boost health and safety protocols [42].

The current uses of the IoT in the healthcare sector cater to a diverse range of significant requirements. The monitoring and regulation of pharmaceutical substances and the enforcement of proper adherence to prescribed medications present persistent challenges within clinical, hospital, and care facility settings. The integration of IoT technology in the healthcare sector has enhanced application processor performance, leading to improved capabilities in rendering and providing medical images at higher resolutions [43]. IoT devices have the capability of tracking patients and wearable IoT gadgets are increasingly being utilized in the healthcare industry. Remote patient monitoring is a promising field for the utilization of IoT devices. These devices are capable of gathering crucial health information from persons who are not present in a healthcare setting [44].

4.6 BIG DATA ANALYTICS IN HEALTHCARE 4.0

BD is widely employed across various industries, with healthcare being particularly advantageous. The advent of the big data revolution has significantly transformed various aspects of our daily lives. In recent years, there has been a notable proliferation of data that has profoundly impacted several aspects of our everyday existence. Nevertheless, it is imperative for the healthcare industry to effectively utilize the vast potential of this data. The field of big data endeavors to collect data along the entire continuum of healthcare, spanning from the early stages of therapy and diagnosis to the culmination of the process. The feasibility of forecasting cancer care can be enhanced by integrating clinical and diagnostic information with the available data [45]. The application of big data enables the prediction of disease transmission. The utilization of GPS trackers can enhance the ability to forecast population movements, thereby contributing to the effective management of disease transmission. This report presents data regarding the places that have been most significantly affected, facilitating the optimization of treatment center design and the implementation of mobility constraints in these regions. Using trends and forecasting technology has resulted in a tenfold increase in growth. Given the text, the user intends to have it rewritten academically.

The utilization of big data plays a crucial role in assessing the effectiveness of medical treatments. The recommendation of a suitable action plan is facilitated through the analysis and comparison of causes, symptoms, and treatment modalities. The utilization of big data also facilitates the identification of effective and standardized treatments for specific medical conditions. Additional applications associated with the facilitation of effective therapy encompass the examination of various drug side effects in relation to one another, the categorization of shared symptoms to assist in the diagnosis process, and the identification of efficacious medicinal products and combinations tailored to distinct demographic groups. The utilization of big data plays a significant role in the governance of the healthcare system, contributing to cost reduction. It enhances outcomes and reduces expenses by implementing enhanced strategies for disease management.

Moreover, it plays a pivotal role in facilitating the management of healthcare by enabling the development of improved diagnostic and treatment processes. At a higher level, the utilization of big data enables the analysis of practice patterns, allocation of resources, and expenditures in hospitals across various healthcare cohorts, among other features. The utilization of big data facilitates the methodical retention of a significant volume of data [46]. Healthcare professionals, such as physicians, now possess a considerable volume of data, which empowers them to make decisions that are well-informed.

The utilization of big data significantly enhances the efficiency of healthcare management. It facilitates the reduction of expenses associated with measuring care while offering optimal clinical support and guidance for the group of at-risk patients. This technology aids healthcare professionals in examining and interpreting data derived from diverse sources. The utilization of big data plays a crucial role in mitigating various faults among health managers, encompassing inaccuracies in dosage administration, prescription blunders, and other human-related mistakes.

Furthermore, insurance companies will derive significant benefits from this as well. The implementation of these measures has the potential to mitigate a wide range of fraudulent insurance claims effectively. Clinical data encompasses the large volume of data generated by healthcare institutions, including but not limited to medical imaging and clinical records. Incorporating big data in the field of medicine derived from primary clinical operations significantly influences the medical industry.

4.7 STATE-OF-THE-ART OF IoT AND BD IN HEALTHCARE 4.0

Remote monitoring systems are made possible by IoT, which has a significant positive impact on healthcare. New advancements in health sensing technology have been made to, among other things, measure patients' heart rates and blood pressure. There are many cutting-edge IoT technologies. The utilization of technological advancements in the healthcare sector, stemming from the fourth industrial revolution, is incredible. Technologies already in existence are used quickly in healthcare. The procedure can be seen on the IoT healthcare network. The IoT network is used for both data transmission and reception. The topology, architecture, and platform comprise IoT healthcare. The topology supports numerous use cases, application situations, and activities. The healthcare architecture reflects the hierarchical concept, which displays how the system's software is organized overall [47]. The platform is made up of environment, framework, and libraries. Systems for wearable remote health monitoring are already in use in the healthcare industry. IoT devices have sensors built in that can deliver precise data. These wearable gadgets, such as smart watches and smart bands, can monitor chronic illnesses. Data from ECG sensors can be detected using AI-based data processing methods. Steps, heart rate, blood pressure, calories, and a number of other metrics can be tracked using smart bands, such as wristbands. As a result, IoT devices can be used to detect health issues.

The Apple and Google Play app stores offer mobile smartphone applications, such as mHealth apps that provide user health details. The sensors built inside the phone are used by these applications to function. Medication adherence is another application area, but it is expensive and sometimes out of reach for consumers, medical professionals, and healthcare service providers. IoT healthcare systems have been proposed in some instances. One is a smart hospital system (SHS) architecture built on a 6LoW- PAN design. IPv6 internet protocol over wireless personal networks is referred to as 6LoWPAN. A SHS can gather information in real-time about environmental circumstances, including patient physiological indicators. The entire system suggests a new functional architecture. This system collects data and sends it to the main control center. The monitoring program then examines the data it has received and, in the event of an emergency, sends alert messages [48]. A 6LoWPAN Border Router can be used with an RFID-enhanced door. A 6LBR can provide a link between remote users and wireless sensor network (WSN) nodes. The monitoring application acquires the data, which then stores it in a database. Access to local and distant control is made simple by the REST web-based paradigm. Network and communication operators can manage the ambient characteristics of sensors using a website-based graphical user interface (GUI).

The authors represent a cloud-based architecture for the IoT as the dominant paradigm for neuroscience technology. The architecture in question is commonly known as the "secure cloud-based IoT framework designed for neuroscience applications." The main approaches utilized in the development of collaborative frameworks for the integration of brain signals, including the electroencephalogram (EEGs), electrocochleography (ECoG), anterior-posterior (AP), local field potential (LFP), and similar methods, involve the application of big data and cloud computing technologies. Various techniques can be employed to get brain imaging, including magnetic resonance imaging (MRI), functional magnetic resonance imagery (fMRI), and positron emission tomography (PET). Various technological advancements, such as cloud computing, edge computing, and fog computing, can potentially facilitate the remote provision of essential medical treatments to patients [49]. A safe cloud-based framework for neuroscience in the context of IoT consists of three main components: the IoT end, the cloud component, and processing and analysis. The framework illustrates the integration of several neuro technologies to facilitate the collaboration of devices, hence enabling the implementation of advanced methodologies that are highly effective in neuroscience and medical studies.

Cyber-physical systems (CPS) encompass the integration of physical and computer elements. As exemplified by scholarly research, cyber-physical systems contain robots and sensors [50]. The convergence of fiction and reality has been made possible by the emergence and advancement on the IoT.

Projections made with electronics have been a subject of several agendas. The idea of smart manufacturing management is the next one. The nucleus of Industry 4.0 might be referred to as smart factories. Industry 4.0 guarantees the capability to automate tasks and assist individuals in achieving their engaged task objectives. Context awareness has also been introduced by Industry 4.0 [51]. Data for patients have been amassing quickly due to the rapid development of the IoT rapid development. The predictive potential of cognitive systems aids in improvements to secure databases. Deep learning can assist cognitive system algorithms in employing self-learned data. Cognitive system methods are used in ML and pattern recognition. The algorithm is often content-based, but occasionally it takes the form of collaborative filtering. These algorithms may use memory or be model-based. Two fundamental principles of the field of CPS are e-Health and M-Health. E-Health encompasses the integration of technology into healthcare, encompassing many activities such as the collection of insurance coverage data. However, M-Health can be utilized as an illustration of Industry 4.0. Any sophisticated or intelligent environment can use ML concepts. Currently, automation is prioritized in the "smart factory" concept that most sectors are pursuing. Industry 4.0 has a significant impact and is now widely used in engineering to create smarter, more intelligent robots that can perform tasks more quickly and effectively, among other things.

Big data is a broad term for a lot of structured and unstructured data. Five characteristics are used to describe big data: volume, velocity, diversity, truth, and value [52]. Enterprise data is currently a source of big data. Businesses generate and handle large amounts of data since they are in charge of keeping track of employee information, internal communications, and accounting. Information on scheduling, administration, and billing for healthcare is also applicable. The existing research classifies several use cases of big data in the healthcare industry, including clinical decision assistance, consumer behavior, support services, and administration [50].

4.7.1 Challenges IoT and BD in HealthCare 4.0

The IoT has instigated a substantial transformation within the medical sector, resulting in notable benefits for the healthcare business. The advent of the fourth industrial era has underscored the astonishing capabilities of technology employed across various sectors, including healthcare, particularly in data storage and analysis. The healthcare sector has witnessed notable advancements facilitated by the IoT. However, despite these good developments, certain difficulties persist that, if effectively addressed, can bring about substantial improvements. The ability to adapt to varying performance requirements and effectively handle large amounts of data is a significant obstacle in the IoT field. Managing the variability in scale poses a significant problem. If a hospital offers IoT services through sensor-equipped equipment, it is imperative to ensure appropriate diversity in the data collected. The data obtained from the sensors should consist of accurate and relevant information. The presence of device damage or inaccurate data may be observed.

The hospital or healthcare institution runs the risk of experiencing a decrease in patient and employee retention. Data transfer serves several objectives, and it is imperative to prioritize privacy as a primary ethical consideration. The presence of inaccurate information can potentially result in significant negative consequences. The successful handling of large-scale data necessitates the presence of appropriate infrastructure. Substantial network bandwidth is required to effectively process the vast volume of data generated by multiple devices. It is widely recognized that IoT devices are commonly linked to sensors. When the size of the server is enormous, it poses challenges in retrieving all the data, particularly when utilizing a network with limited bandwidth. Hence, there exists a requirement for a substantial amount of network capacity. Acknowledging the potential vulnerability of interconnected IoT devices to hacking and unauthorized information disclosure is imperative.

Therefore, it is imperative to give priority to the implementation of rigorous mechanisms for ensuring the security of data transit. Implementing a secondary network, employing unique passwords resistant to guessing, regularly updating all devices, and minimizing reliance on cloud technologies can effectively mitigate the risk of unauthorized access. Maintaining the foundation of IoT can provide challenges due to the substantial volume of data it saves and transfers. Certain technical issues can be encountered in healthcare institutions and hospitals, including signal strength and electromagnetic effects' impact [53]. Hospitals' fundamental goal is to ensure health and safety maintenance.

The primary issues can be succinctly categorized as security, trust, and privacy concerns. The topic of security was initially addressed, and numerous researchers have dedicated their efforts to enhancing the security of IoT gadgets and systems. Given the inherent limitations of every system, it is imperative for specialists to undertake the task of identifying and quantifying potential security risks. The primary focus in this context is on privacy, as patients have an expectation of maintaining the confidentiality and privacy of their information. It is the duty of an institution of healthcare or medical institution to uphold and guarantee the maintenance of confidentiality. Managing and overseeing a huge volume of data can provide challenges and complexities. Consequently, it can be arduous at times. Legislation pertaining to the safeguarding of healthcare data in the context of IoT implementation is in place. The issue of trust is a substantial challenge for the IoT as well. The capability for data transfer is facilitated within IoT gadgets. During the process of data transmission, there is a possibility of data corruption or the introduction of malicious software. Unauthorized access may potentially occur. Given that the transmitted data is utilized to influence critical decisions with potential life-or-death implications, any type of corruption within the data has the potential to provide unfavorable consequences for patients. This particular issue remains unresolved. It is well understood that the concept of caring pertains to the act of bringing about happiness in an individual. Patients and individuals experiencing illness consistently anticipate receiving appropriate medical attention and being treated with a sense of trust. In the context of the 4th industrial revolution, technological advancements have extended to the immediate vicinity of a patient's bedside.

4.8 SENSORS AND WEARABLE TECHNOLOGY

Care for patients can be improved outside of traditional healthcare facilities, including at home or in the community, by implementing cutting-edge technological solutions. Wearable devices are employed for monitoring diverse aspects of health, including weight, sleep patterns, exercise, and dietary habits. By providing users with factual data, these devices enable them to make informed health decisions, surpassing the reliance on simply calorie counting and step tracking. Specific patient advocacy organizations are employing this technology to assist individuals residing in remote areas or outside of healthcare facilities facing weight and health challenges. The use of wireless sensors manufactured by Sensor MetriX is prevalent in hospital settings, specifically refrigerators, freezers, and laboratories. These sensors are crucial in maintaining optimal temperature conditions for various goods such as blood samples, medications, and other relevant substances [54]. Integrating wearable monitors with additional data sensor sources enables cost and time savings, facilitating effective monitoring of progress and challenges for older patients and individuals with chronic health conditions. This sensor can detect irregularities related to bowel dysfunction and colon cancer as an alternative to more invasive procedures. Wireless medical equipment has existed for a considerable period, mostly serving as aids to clinicians in conducting evaluations and monitoring essential patient information. There is a growing trend toward integrating facilities and organizations, which facilitates enhanced accessibility and streamlined administration. The effective processing and exchange of data with service providers is made possible by a cross-device connection.

Implementing intelligent monitoring systems can contribute to the early identification of sickness signs, leading to improved treatment strategies and preventive measures. Additionally, the device provides updates on medical illnesses such as diabetes and prostate cancer, as well as transmitting this data to healthcare professionals, thereby aiding in managing these ailments. The aforementioned service offers location-as-a-service capabilities for the purpose of tracking patients and medical devices. The proposed system aims to enhance both staff and patient happiness while also optimizing handling assets and patient flow [55]. These devices collectively assist in creating an environment that enables more efficient monitoring and management of health conditions, whether in clinical settings, at home or for general health tracking purposes. Currently, a significant proportion of patient interactions with the healthcare system involve using medical technology and devices.

Each user's health is closely intertwined with the reliability and quality of these medicinal devices. The maintenance of vaccine safety is crucial during all stages of the vaccine's lifecycle, encompassing research, development, manufacture, transportation, and usage. The monitoring system serves an essential role in the surveillance of temperature and humidity conditions about vaccines, as well as in the provision of timely alerts in the event that these conditions go beyond the permissible thresholds. Similar to other vaccines, the efficacy of a COVID-19 vaccine necessitates the establishment of optimal conditions at low temperatures. A data recorder, integrated with sensors, possesses the capability to detect instances of cold chain disruptions subsequent to the vaccine's departure from the manufacturing facility and prior to its arrival at the end user. This enables timely notification to the user, thus mitigating the occurrence of irreversible damage. Patients exhibit diverse needs and require a range of care interventions. This principle is equally applicable to the monitoring of patients. It may be necessary for individuals with heart conditions to have regular blood pressure assessments. Therefore, a handheld stethoscope can be employed for the purpose of monitoring the heart rate. The effective management of a rare ailment necessitates regular consultations with several healthcare professionals and meticulous strategic planning. Remote patient monitoring (RPM) has been shown to have significant potential in improving patient outcomes and potentially saving lives [56]. By utilizing RPM, healthcare providers are able to monitor patients and stay ahead of potential treatment choices proactively. Implementing this proactive approach can facilitate the early identification of health concerns, prompt intervention, and ultimately enhance patient outcomes. Continuous glucose monitoring (CGM) is an innovative approach utilized by individuals with diabetes to check their glucose levels in real-time. These gadgets can track a person's blood sugar and relay that information to a pump that can pause insulin delivery on its own. Glucose data might be collected and stored in an information system for healthcare using the proposed system design. This technology facilitates the ability of healthcare professionals to retrieve and examine real-time data that has been gathered from their patients. Patients have the ability to consume devices that contain sensors in the style of pills. After the ingestion of the sensors, they transmit data to a mobile application utilized by the patient, facilitating adherence to the appropriate medication dosages. Most medications are not used according to prescribed instructions due to factors such as forgetfulness or human error. Using an ingestible sensor guarantees that patients adhere to the accurate medication regimen by consuming the appropriate medications at the designated time and in the prescribed dosages. In addition, there is a current utilization of ingestible sensors in the medical field to enhance the accuracy of identifying patients with illnesses like irritable bowel disorder and colon cancer [57]. The researchers' proposed for advancing healthcare via wearable devices and AI is exhaustively covered in this article. Detailed discussion follows of the methods utilized by the researchers to enhance the healthcare system's overall precision, efficacy, and security. Furthermore, the limitations and prospects associated with the advancement of IoT-based healthcare systems powered by AI are elucidated in this article [58].

TABLE 4.1
Summary of Wearable Devices Implanted with AI and IoT

Wearable Device	Application Position	Monitoring Parameters
Smart thermometer (Monitoring)	Armpit, chest, ear	Fever monitoring, COVID-19
Smart watch	Wrist	Body temperature, chronic disease, viral diseases fitness, fall detection, pulse rate.
Smart jacket	Chest, arm	Pneumonia, lungs sounds, safety of workers, body temperature, oxygen saturation
Data gloves	Fingers, hands	Rheumatoid arthritis, COVID-19, Parkinson's
Smart stethoscope	Chest, ears, neck	Sound of heart beat, breathing, flu, stomach sound, pneumonia, influenza.
Smart belt	Waist, chest	Monitor movements, body temperature, heartbeat, breathing rate, ECG, respiratory rate
Smart lens	Eyes	Allergies, glaucoma, vision enhancement.
Smart mood monitoring system	Wrist	Pulse rate, monitor mood
Smart helmet	Head	Location monitoring, head safety, imaging, crowds monitoring
Smart glasses	Eyes, head	Crowd monitoring, body temperature, ebola
Smart socks	Feet	Pulse rate, oxygen saturation, injury, Parkinson's, diabetic infection

The Table 4.1 presents the summary of some of the most important wearable devices that are placed on the human body to monitor health and provide the health data for further processing which are implemented using AI and IoT.

4.8.1 Internet of Medical Things (IoMT)

The process of gathering and examining data for medical research and monitoring crucial elements of the IoMT involves the application of the IoT in the context of medical and healthcare objectives. The term "Smart Healthcare" has become a popular way to describe the IoMT, which enables the establishment of a digitalized healthcare system and the incorporation of diverse healthcare resources and services. IoMT is a nascent concept that aims to tackle diverse healthcare concerns [56]. The medical industry still faces challenges in effectively using the information created by the IoMT, despite its significant impact on the dynamic nature of contemporary global society [59]. The objective is to oversee an individual's physical condition and welfare by introducing a substantial assortment of groundbreaking wearable or interconnected medical equipment into the consumer market. The use of AI in the field of the IoMT industry has presented a multitude of opportunities for the instantaneous, remote assessment and examination of patient information. This development has paved the way for the emergence of other technologies and enhanced accessibility to healthcare through improved connectivity. The IoMT leverages AI, ML, and data mining techniques to categorize health data and uncover latent trends effectively.

The IoMT enables healthcare professionals to systematically manage patients by supplying them with real-time patient data. IoT technologies facilitate the interconnection of numerous devices with one another. These interconnected gadgets generate a substantial volume of data. Medical professionals typically ascertain health threat trends through the analysis of relevant information. Furthermore, it aids in determining the impact of various medications on individuals.

The IoMT is an interconnected system comprising various medical devices and software applications. The IoMT offers a data gathering service. The data obtained from patients is subsequently transmitted to healthcare practitioners. The use of IoMT has significantly revolutionized the communication between patients and healthcare professionals, facilitating enhanced provision of personalized care to patients and concurrently fostering the promotion of preventive healthcare measures. IoMT is gaining popularity in the healthcare sector as a means to increase productivity. To this end, we employ apparatus and tools that can link to the IoT. Healthcare providers and other organizations are increasingly relying on technological solutions for efficient patient data management and remote monitoring of patients' health. Data from IoMT medical devices is invaluable to the healthcare industry. The use of conventional approaches for analyzing, storing, and managing vast volumes of data presents significant difficulties. In the healthcare IoT space, the combination of computing via the cloud, ML, and analytics for big data is becoming more and more important as a means of addressing the aforementioned issues. In the healthcare industry, cloud-based computing technologies and ML techniques are used to predict epidemics, avert preventable deaths, and maximize the delivery of high-quality patient care. The healthcare IoT framework will encompass any device that can create health data and upload that data to the cloud. It's generally agreed that wearable devices are the most noticeable IoMT-related medical hardware. Establishing a platform that effectively supports the integration of the digital health ecosystem is of utmost importance. This platform should enable the creation, management, and assessment of diverse applications. The term "connected health" is employed within digital health to delineate the increasing interconnectivity observed in the healthcare domain. In the realm of digital healthcare, the implementation of a connected health system holds the potential to optimize healthcare resource utilization. This is achieved by the provision of enhanced communication channels between patients and healthcare professionals, granting customers greater flexibility in their interactions. Consequently, individuals are empowered to exert more control over their own healthcare management. The establishment of a linked healthcare system serves a pivotal role in facilitating the advancement of the digital health industry. This study examines the necessity of introducing recent developments, trends, and trends in Healthcare 4.0 and IoMT. This chapter examines the ultimate demands that these networks will face in the era of 5G and subsequent generations of networks. Furthermore, the design complexities and ongoing areas of research pertaining to these networks. The author examines the fundamental enabling technologies of distributed edge computing and AI [60].

Cloud technologies are utilized to store and handle a huge quantity of health-related information generated by IoMT medical equipment. Cloud computing presents challenges such as response time, which can have severe consequences in the healthcare sector because even little delays might potentially result in the loss of life for critically ill patients. The author achieved an accuracy of 92% [61]. Fog computing is used to process the data via the IoMT healthcare sensors in order to allay this worry. To accelerate cloud computing adoption, fog computing is used. Fog computing offers a superior response rate in comparison to cloud computing due to its proximity to the patient. The computed results are transmitted to the cloud server, facilitating their retrieval at a subsequent stage. Fog computing employs ML methods for the purpose of analyzing healthcare data [62]. ML techniques are used to analyze data, identify patterns, extract insights, and make informed decisions based on the acquired knowledge. ML algorithms autonomously analyze the data and make informed decisions regarding the patient's progression, distinguishing between deterioration and improvement. They achieved an accuracy of 92.3% [63–65]. The goal of this change is to deliver healthcare services that are more effective, convenient, and individualized. The idea of intelligent healthcare was covered by the author in this chapter. Scholars enumerate the primary technologies that facilitate smart healthcare and deliberate on the present state of smart healthcare in many domains. In addition, he discusses possible answers and addresses the difficulties smart healthcare faces. Finally, researchers assess the potential implications of smart healthcare and look forward to its future [66]. These strategies have the potential to mitigate the likelihood of severe issues and ensure the preservation of human life when implemented promptly.

4.9 RESEARCH GAP TO EXISTING WORK

The use of technology has grown dramatically in the last few years. The healthcare industry has been greatly impacted by the fourth industrial revolution. Interoperability and security present the biggest obstacles. Medical records ought to be rigorous, private, and confidential. If not, there's a good chance the information could be misused or compromised for nefarious purposes. Managing data volume and performance flexibility is a major challenge. The sensors need to be receiving genuine, meaningful truths as data. The hospital or healthcare provider may lose staff members or patients if the gadget is damaged or the information it holds is inaccurate. The sensors must be receiving genuine, meaningful truths as data. The hospital or healthcare provider may lose staff members or patients if the gadget is damaged or its data is inaccurate. Another issue is that a large server can make it challenging to access all of its data over a slow network. High network bandwidth is therefore required. In hospitals and other healthcare facilities, there are a few technological issues, such as electromagnetic impacts and issues with signal strength.

4.10 CONCLUSION

This chapter highlighted the sophisticated approaches for analytics of healthcare data. AI opens the gate of approaches and put forward the attention of researchers. Initially the chapter introduces about the various latest technology used to upgrade the healthcare system. The extensive overview of the AI, IoT, big data, and wearable devices challenges are presented in this chapter. Wearable devices are used to connect the health data of the patients. The data is processed by emerging technologies such as AI, cloud computing, and big data. The IoT is used to establish the interconnection among the wearable devices. IoMT technology supports the Healthcare 4.0 system to provide the better results. AI support mechanism empowered the Healthcare 4.0 and collects the data from various sources. Healthcare 4.0 is a revolution in healthcare industry. It makes the system smooth, faster, and effective. These technologies are more effective to keep the track health on real-time. In future we can enhance the quality and durability of wearable devices that increase the efficiency with low power consumption of the smart healthcare.

REFERENCES

1. Qiu, H., Qiu, M., Liu, M., & Memmi, G. (2020). Secure health data sharing for medical cyber-physical systems for the Healthcare 4.0. IEEE Journal of Biomedical and Health Informatics, 24(9), 2499–2505.
2. Au-Yong-Oliveira, M., Pesqueira, A., Sousa, M. J., Dal Mas, F., & Soliman, M. (2021). The potential of big data research in healthcare for medical doctors' learning. Journal of Medical Systems, 45, 1–14.
3. Pang, Z., Yang, G., Khedri, R., & Zhang, Y. T. (2018). Introduction to the special section: Convergence of automation technology, biomedical engineering, and health informatics toward the healthcare 4.0. IEEE Reviews in Biomedical Engineering, 11, 249–259.
4. Javaid, M., Haleem, A., Vaishya, R., Bahl, S., Suman, R., & Vaish, A. (2020). Industry 4.0 technologies and their applications in fighting COVID-19 pandemic. Diabetes & Metabolic Syndrome: Clinical Research & Reviews, 14(4), 419–422.
5. Chakraborty, C., & Kishor, A. (2022). Real-time cloud-based patient-centric monitoring using computational health systems. IEEE Transactions on Computational Social Systems, 9(6), 1613–1623.
6. Kumari, A., Tanwar, S., Tyagi, S., & Kumar, N. (2018). Fog computing for healthcare 4.0 environment: Opportunities and challenges. Computers & Electrical Engineering, 72, 1–13.
7. Teng, F., Ma, Z., Chen, J., Xiao, M., & Huang, L. (2020). Automatic medical code assignment via deep learning approach for intelligent healthcare. IEEE Journal of Biomedical and Health Informatics, 24(9), 2506–2515.
8. Winter, A., Stäubert, S., Ammon, D., Aiche, S., Beyan, O., Bischoff, V., & Löffler, M. (2018). Smart medical information technology for healthcare (SMITH). Methods of Information in Medicine, 57(S 01), e92–e105.
9. Misztal-Okońska, P., Goniewicz, K., Hertelendy, A. J., Khorram-Manesh, A., Al-Wathinani, A., Alhazmi, R. A., & Goniewicz, M. (2020). How medical studies in Poland prepare future healthcare managers for crises and disasters: Results of a pilot study. Healthcare, 8(3), 202.
10. Yang, G., Pang, Z., Deen, M. J., Dong, M., Zhang, Y. T., Lovell, N., & Rahmani, A. M. (2020). Homecare robotic systems for healthcare 4.0: Visions and enabling technologies. IEEE Journal of Biomedical and Health Informatics, 24(9), 2535–2549.
11. Quintero, G. A. (2014). Medical education and the healthcare system – Why does the curriculum need to be reformed? BMC Medicine, 12(1), 1–4.
12. Chanchaichujit, J., Tan, A., Meng, F., Eaimkhong, S., Chanchaichujit, J., Tan, A., & Eaimkhong, S. (2019). An introduction to Healthcare 4.0. Healthcare 4.0: Next Generation Processes with the Latest Technologies (1–15).

13. Awan, K. M., Ashraf, N., Saleem, M. Q., Sheta, O. E., Qureshi, K. N., Zeb, A., & Sadiq, A. S. (2019). A priority-based congestion-avoidance routing protocol using IoT-based heterogeneous medical sensors for energy efficiency in healthcare wireless body area networks. International Journal of Distributed Sensor Networks, 15(6), 1550147719853980.

14. Tortorella, G. L., Saurin, T. A., Fogliatto, F. S., Rosa, V. M., Tonetto, L. M., & Magrabi, F. (2021). Impacts of Healthcare 4.0 digital technologies on the resilience of hospitals. Technological Forecasting and Social Change, 166, 120666.

15. Allen, M. (2020). Big healthcare data analytics in internet of medical things. American Journal of Medical Research, 7(1), 48–54.

16. Martínez, A., Villarroel, V., Seoane, J., & Pozo, F. D. (2004). Rural telemedicine for primary healthcare in developing countries. IEEE Technology and Society Magazine, 23(2), 13–22.

17. Leite, H., Hodgkinson, I. R., & Gruber, T. (2020). New development: 'Healing at a distance'—Telemedicine and COVID-19. Public Money & Management, 40(6), 483–485.

18. Guduri, M., Chakraborty, C., & Margala, M. (2023). Blockchain-based federated learning technique for privacy preservation and security of smart electronic health records. IEEE Transactions on Consumer Electronics. 70(1), 2608–2617.

19. Yu, K. H., Beam, A. L., & Kohane, I. S. (2018). Artificial intelligence in healthcare. Nature Biomedical Engineering, 2(10), 719–731.

20. Rong, G., Mendez, A., Assi, E. B., Zhao, B., & Sawan, M. (2020). Artificial intelligence in healthcare: Review and prediction case studies. Engineering, 6(3), 291–301.

21. Asha, P., Srivani, P., Ahmed, A. A. A., Kolhe, A., & Nomani, M. Z. M. (2022). Artificial intelligence in medical imaging: An analysis of innovative technique and its future promise. Materials Today: Proceedings, 56, 2236–2239.

22. Laï, M. C., Brian, M., & Mamzer, M. F. (2020). Perceptions of artificial intelligence in healthcare: Findings from a qualitative survey study among actors in France. Journal of Translational Medicine, 18(1), 1–13.

23. He, J., Baxter, S. L., Xu, J., Xu, J., Zhou, X., & Zhang, K. (2019). The practical implementation of artificial intelligence technologies in medicine. Nature Medicine, 25(1), 30–36.

24. Asan, O., Bayrak, A. E., & Choudhury, A. (2020). Artificial intelligence and human trust in healthcare: Focus on clinicians. Journal of Medical Internet Research, 22(6), e15154.

25. Lee, D., & Yoon, S. N. (2021). Application of artificial intelligence-based technologies in the healthcare industry: Opportunities and challenges. International Journal of Environmental Research and Public Health, 18(1), 271.

26. Riffat, M., Yasir, A., Naheen, I. T., Paul, S., & Ahad, M. T. (2020, April). Augmented Reality for Smarter Bangladesh. In 2020 IEEE Green Technologies Conference (GreenTech) (pp. 217–222). IEEE.

27. Poongodi, M., Hamdi, M., Malviya, M., Sharma, A., Dhiman, G., & Vimal, S. (2022). Diagnosis and combating COVID-19 using wearable Oura smart ring with deep learning methods. Personal and Ubiquitous Computing, 1–11.

28. Ruan, Q., Yang, K., Wang, W., Jiang, L., & Song, J. (2020). Correction to: Clinical predictors of mortality due to COVID-19 based on an analysis of data of 150 patients from Wuhan, China. Intensive Care Medicine, 46(6), 1294.

29. Kishor, A., & Chakraborty, C. (2022). Artificial intelligence and internet of things based Healthcare 4.0 monitoring system. Wireless Personal Communications, 127(2), 1615–1631.

30. Hathaliya, J. J., & Tanwar, S. (2020). An exhaustive survey on security and privacy issues in Healthcare 4.0. Computer Communications, 153, 311–335.

31. Wang, F., & Preininger, A. (2019). AI in health: State of the art, challenges, and future directions. Yearbook of Medical Informatics, 28(01), 016–026.
32. Baytas, I. M., Xiao, C., Wang, F., Jain, A. K., & Zhou, J. (2018, November). Heterogeneous hyper-network embedding. In 2018 IEEE International Conference on Data Mining (ICDM) (pp. 875–880). IEEE.
33. Chakraborty, C., Kishor, A., & Rodrigues, J. J. (2022). Novel enhanced-grey wolf optimization hybrid machine learning technique for biomedical data computation. Computers and Electrical Engineering, 99, 107778.
34. Hannun, A. Y., Rajpurkar, P., Haghpanahi, M., Tison, G. H., Bourn, C., Turakhia, M. P., & Ng, A. Y. (2019). Cardiologist-level arrhythmia detection and classification in ambulatory electrocardiograms using a deep neural network. Nature Medicine, 25(1), 65–69.
35. Tang, F., Lin, K., Uchendu, I., Dodge, H. H., & Zhou, J. (2018). Improving mild cognitive impairment prediction via reinforcement learning and dialogue simulation. arXiv preprint arXiv:1802.06428.
36. Strielkina, A., Kharchenko, V., & Uzun, D. (2018, May). Availability models for healthcare IoT systems: Classification and research considering attacks on vulnerabilities. In 2018 IEEE 9th international conference on dependable systems, services and technologies (DESSERT) (pp. 58–62). IEEE.
37. Nazneen, F. (2021). Cloud computing and the legal arena: digitization of courts during Covid-19. *International Journal of Legal Science and Innovation*, 3(3), 412–429.
38. Zhang, R., & Liu, L. (2010, July). Security models and requirements for healthcare application clouds. In 2010 IEEE 3rd International Conference on cloud Computing (pp. 268–275). IEEE.
39. Garets, D., & Davis, M. (2006). Electronic medical records vs. electronic health records: yes, there is a difference. Policy white paper. Chicago, HIMSS Analytics, 1.
40. Paul, S., Riffat, M., Yasir, A., Mahim, M. N., Sharnali, B. Y., Naheen, I. T., & Kulkarni, A. (2021). Industry 4.0 applications for medical/healthcare services. Journal of Sensor and Actuator Networks, 10(3), 43.
41. Tarouco, L. M. R., Bertholdo, L. M., Granville, L. Z., Arbiza, L. M. R., Carbone, F., Marotta, M., & De Santanna, J. J. C. (2012, June). Internet of Things in healthcare: Interoperatibility and security issues. In 2012 IEEE international conference on communications (ICC) (pp. 6121–6125). IEEE.
42. Rghioui, A., & Oumnad, A. (2018). Challenges and opportunities of internet of things in healthcare. International Journal of Electrical & Computer Engineering, 8(5), 2088–8708.
43. Adhikary, T., Jana, A. D., Chakrabarty, A., & Jana, S. K. (2020). The IoT augmentation in healthcare: An application analytics. ICICCT 2019–System Reliability, Quality Control, Safety, Maintenance and Management: Applications to Electrical, Electronics and Computer Science and Engineering, 576–583.
44. Shah, S. A., Ren, A., Fan, D., Zhang, Z., Zhao, N., Yang, X., & Abbasi, Q. H. (2018). Internet of things for sensing: A case study in the healthcare system. Applied Sciences, 8(4), 508.
45. Viceconti, M., Hunter, P., & Hose, R. (2015). Big data, big knowledge: Big data for personalized healthcare. IEEE Journal of Biomedical and Health Informatics, 19(4), 1209–1215.
46. Mathew, P. S., & Pillai, A. S. (2015, March). Big data solutions in healthcare: problems and perspectives. In 2015 International conference on innovations in information, embedded and communication systems (ICIIECS) (pp. 1–6). IEEE.
47. Jayaraman, P. P., Forkan, A. R. M., Morshed, A., Haghighi, P. D., & Kang, Y. B. (2020). Healthcare 4.0: A review of frontiers in digital health. Wiley Interdisciplinary Reviews: Data Mining and Knowledge Discovery, 10(2), e1350.

48. Durga, S., Nag, R., & Daniel, E. (2019, March). Survey on machine learning and deep learning algorithms used in IoT healthcare. In 2019 3rd international conference on computing methodologies and communication (ICCMC) (pp. 1018–1022). IEEE.

49. Kishor, A., & Chakraborty, C. (2023, June). Role of feature selection in Healthcare 4.0. In 2023 International Conference on IoT, Communication and Automation Technology (ICICAT) (pp. 1–4). IEEE.

50. Mishra, S., & Kishor, A. (2023). Convergence of artificial intelligence in sustainable human resource management for modern organizational growth. In *Disruptive Artificial Intelligence and Sustainable Human Resource Management* (pp. 247–269). River Publishers, Denmark.

51. Zawadzki, P., & Żywicki, K. (2016). Smart product design and production control for effective mass customization in the industry 4.0 concept. Management and Production Engineering Review, 7(3). 10.1515/mper-2016-0030

52. Aceto, G., Persico, V., & Pescapé, A. (2020). Industry 4.0 and health: Internet of things, big data, and cloud computing for healthcare 4.0. Journal of Industrial Information Integration, 18, 100129.

53. Laplante, P. A., & Laplante, N. (2016). The internet of things in healthcare: Potential applications and challenges. IT Professional, 18(3), 2–4.

54. Clauson, K. A., Breeden, E. A., Davidson, C., & Mackey, T. K. (2018). Leveraging blockchain technology to enhance supply chain management in healthcare: An exploration of challenges and opportunities in the health supply chain. Blockchain in Healthcare Today.

55. Luan, H., & Tsai, C. C. (2021). A review of using machine learning approaches for precision education. Educational Technology & Society, 24(1), 250–266.

56. Rodrigues, J. J., Segundo, D. B. D. R., Junqueira, H. A., Sabino, M. H., Prince, R. M., Al-Muhtadi, J., & De Albuquerque, V. H. C. (2018). Enabling technologies for the internet of health things. IEEE Access, 6, 13129–13141.

57. Gaur, R., Prakash, S., Prasad, L. N., Kumar, S., Abhishek, K., & Guduri, M. (2023). A secure and efficient scheme based on unlinkability and anonymous traceable protocol for cloud-assisted IoT environment. Journal of Circuits, Systems and Computers, 32(18), 2350316.

58. Subhan, F., Mirza, A., Su'ud, M. B. M., Alam, M. M., Nisar, S., Habib, U., & Iqbal, M. Z. (2023). AI-enabled wearable medical internet of things in healthcare system: A survey. Applied Sciences, 13(3), 1394.

59. Alamri, A. (2019, January). Big data with integrated cloud computing for prediction of health conditions. In 2019 International conference on platform technology and service (PlatCon) (pp. 1–6). IEEE.

60. Osama, M., Ateya, A. A., Sayed, M. S., Hammad, M., Pławiak, P., Abd El-Latif, A. A., & Elsayed, R. A. (2023). Internet of medical things and healthcare 4.0: Trends, requirements, challenges, and research directions. Sensors, 23(17), 7435.

61. Kishor, A., Chakraborty, C., & Jeberson, W. (2020). A novel fog computing approach for minimization of latency in healthcare using machine learning. International Journal of Interactive Multimedia and Artificial Intelligence, 1(1), 7–17.

62. Kishor, A., Chakraborty, C., & Jeberson, W. (2021). Intelligent healthcare data segregation using fog computing with internet of things and machine learning. International Journal of Engineering Systems Modelling and Simulation, 12(2–3), 188–194.

63. Kishor, A., & Jeberson, W. (2021). Diagnosis of heart disease using internet of things and machine learning algorithms. In Proceedings of Second International Conference on Computing, Communications, and Cyber-Security (pp. 691–702). Springer, Singapore.

64. Kishor, A., & Chakraborty, C. (2021). Early and accurate prediction of diabetics based on FCBF feature selection and SMOTE. International Journal of System Assurance Engineering and Management, 15, 1–9.

65. Ashima and M. Kapil. (2023). Hybrid Machine Learning Approaches for Multi Disease Prediction Utilizing Relief Feature Selection. 2023 International Conference on IoT, Communication and Automation Technology (ICICAT), Gorakhpur, India, 2023, (pp. 1–6), doi: 10.1109/ICICAT57735.2023.10263604.
66. Mishra, P., & Singh, G. (2023). Smart healthcare in sustainable smart cities. In Sustainable smart cities: Enabling technologies, energy trends and potential applications (pp. 195–219). Springer International Publishing, Cham.

5 Significance of Quality Attributes of IoT-Based Smart Devices in Healthcare Monitoring Systems

Leading Towards Success or Failure

Aleena Nadeem, Mahnoor Khan, Fahim Arif, Saddaf Rubab, and Ali El-Moursy

5.1 INTRODUCTION

The Internet of Things (IoT) is popularly known as a system of systems. It is a novel technology with a lot of social and technical impact. In IoT, hardware, information processing devices, and software are integrated over a network, which facilitates their communication, interaction, collection, and exchange of data.

IoT is an interconnection of billions of devices that are deployed just about everywhere; from our homes to cars to traffic signals to our alarm clocks to coffee makers and refrigerators, IoT aims to connect everything into one big complex network. Even our bodies are host to IoT devices in the form of wearable and ingestible sensors (Burkhalter, 2022). It is safe to say that very soon, we will have to entrust our lives to IoT.

While IoT intends to affect almost every area of human life, the health sector is among the most prominent of its applications. IoT has given way to endless possibilities in the world of medicine (Lu et al., 2023). Remote diagnosis and treatment with the help of IoT devices is already being experimented upon. IoT implants have the ability to diagnose diseases, detect fluctuations in blood pressure levels, measure pH and temperature, and manage pain (Burkhalter, 2022). Devices to monitor physiological and pathological markers help with the diagnosis of diseases at onset and monitor the patient's health according to the clinical needs (Lu et al., 2023), these and many others are underway in the field of medical IoT. These devices monitor your body consistently and communicate any abnormalities to your doctor without

DOI: 10.1201/9781003603610-5

you having to visit the doctor physically. The devices might even take appropriate action on their own without having to consult the doctor.

IoT in medicine aims to provide better accessibility to health services while keeping the costs and efforts minimal. But with all its perks, it has also raised a lot of concerns among the community. The arena of medicine IoT requires that we entrust the devices with our lives. Hence, the quality of the IoT devices becomes a major concern.

There exists a trust deficit among the medical community regarding IoT-based health care monitoring particularly when it comes to diagnosis through such systems; The main reasons for this unwillingness is limited accuracy, privacy, and interoperability (DeFranco et al., 2017) of sensory devices as well as related IoT systems. When there is ample availability of sensors, ambient assisted living (AAL) (Florea et al., 2022) is a reality of today's world. Adoption and usage of AAL technology accelerated during the COVID-19 pandemic. However, a gap needs to be bridged to cater for the existing trust deficit, the core reason for which is that in most of the cases, NFRs are not catered for. When designing a system of medical grade, quality requirements are to be achieved without any tolerance of failure. This research aims at achieving the above-mentioned requirements through improvement in accuracy, privacy, and interoperability while decreasing the trust deficit of the medical community regarding smart gadgetry.

5.2 BACKGROUND

There are hundreds of applications associated with IoT across different disciplines. One of the major application domains of IoT is the healthcare system, which works with the help of hardware, software, and physical devices like sensors to record important data related to the human body like body temperature, heartbeat, sugar, etc., and actuators.

IoT in healthcare provides virtual and distant interaction to doctors and caretakers, so that a patient can avoid the hitch of always visiting a doctor. In IoT healthcare systems multi-layer architecture is needed: integrated computing devices producing a variety of data, cloud to handle that data, speed, and latency, interactive and user-friendly mobile application (Domínguez-Bolaño et al., 2022). Application of IoT in healthcare systems ranges from assisted living, e-medicine, and warning generation systems, to disease monitoring systems.

Existing IoT-based healthcare system somehow lacks the critical or relevant quality attributes or non-functional requirements (NFRs) (DeFranco et al., 2017). This is the main reason behind the failure or crisis of many systems that they do not get accepted by aged people. There is an absence of quality attributes like interoperability, security, safety, and accuracy in existing systems which affects the acceptability adversely; since these attributes are critical to health systems (Karunarathne et al., 2021). Moreover, problem of management and storage of data e.g. issues of physical storage, availability and maintenance, privacy, permission control, data anonymity, etc. was also observed.

This chapter presents a model in which unfulfilled quality attributes/NFRs which are critical to the system, can be adhered to the functional requirements in order to make the IoT-based healthcare monitoring system acceptable to the users, hence making it a success. Furthermore, this chapter addresses the role of NFRs and map the NFRs to the success criteria or acceptance criteria of IoT-based healthcare monitoring system.

This chapter addresses the following three questions.

1. What is the significance of NFRs in success or failure of IoT-based healthcare systems?
2. How the acceptability of IoT-based healthcare monitoring system can be ensured/improved by enhancing other NFRs like interoperability, connectivity, and usability of the system?
3. How the gap between functional and NFRs can be reduced in design to ensure the adaptability of the system.

5.3 RELATED WORK

DeFranco et al. (2017) suggested that there are several research challenges for IoT healthcare systems. Most system failures are due to ineffective system design to satisfy NFRs. In accordance with the fact that functional requirements (FRs) get more attention as compared to NFRs during software development (DeFranco et al., 2017). This observable gap between FRs and NFRs is due to the fact that, NFs cannot be directly and explicitly implemented in software from beginning to end.

Paiva et al. (2022) conducted a thorough literature review on IoT with the aim of identifying the NFRs that have been considered for the evaluation of IoT systems. They also provided an overview of tools, methods, and processes that have been used for evaluating the NFRs of IoT systems. They identified a set 48 NFRs including acceptability, adaptation, availability, context awareness, ease of use, efficiency, interoperability, performance, reliability, security, etc.

In 2022, Florea et al. (2022) conducted research on IoT-based AAL and assisted care for patients and elderly. The chapter focused on the security challenges faced by AAL applications and reviewed blockchain solutions to tackle those challenges. Assisted care applications had widespread usage during the COVID-19 pandemic. This application uses sensors to monitor and record patient data, learns specific behaviors from this data, and disseminates patient information to relevant devices in the IoT network, hence making security and privacy a major concern. Blockchain technology helps in making IoT communication more secure but more research needs to be done in this area.

AAL is an application of IoT with significant usage in healthcare (Gimenez Manuel et al., 2022). It builds a safe environment around people with special needs like those suffering from dementia, by communicating with them. It tackles their healthcare needs and assists them in their everyday activities. This chapter analyzed the existing AAL systems and found that most of the focus of previous research is on secondary persons, i.e. caregivers, rather than the person who is suffering. (Gimenez Manuel et al., 2022) focused their solution on this limitation and designed a system that monitors real-time user activity continuously, and generates reminders and alerts to dementia patients when necessary. Their indoor localization system is context-aware and is able to distinguish users and generate user-specific alerts.

Karunarathne et al. (2021) studied the privacy and security challenges in smart healthcare. In IoT healthcare, static as well as dynamic patient information is at risk due to the use of sensors and the transmission of real-time data across the IoT network. Vulnerability of any of the IoT devices in the network can put the entire network at security and privacy risk. The heterogeneity of devices along with differences in implementation of security protocols poses a serious threat. To tackle these challenges, they have presented solutions using zone-based architecture, machine learning, deep learning, blockchain, biometric cryptography, nanotechnology, and fog or edge computing.

In 2021 Aghdam et al. (2021) conducted a survey on IoT healthcare research articles and investigated issues and challenges. They identified that parts of IoT healthcare technology is still in primary stages and need improvement. Interoperability, availability, privacy, security and effective data validation, data storage, costs, and quality of services have been identified as critical challenges that need to be addressed.

Finding the right balance between security and efficiency in IoT systems is crucial. In Das and Namasudra (2022), authors proposed an architecture to enhance the security of IoT healthcare, keeping in view resource constraints and special data security requirements. They proposed a hybrid encryption methodology that combines both symmetric and asymmetric encryption techniques, like elliptic curve cryptology, Advanced Encryption Standard, and Serpent.

Alshammari (2023) suggested that Message Queuing Telemetry Transport (MQTT) is the most critical protocol for communication in healthcare systems to ensure accuracy and reduce latency in data transmissions, hence fulfilling the performance requirements. It covers access control and authentication aspects in a modern healthcare system to ensure no data package loss. The proposed system provides healthcare providers with access to patient data anytime anywhere reducing time and costs.

In Khan (2021), the author highlighted the key challenges faced by IoT healthcare systems. Accuracy and information security are the most critical challenges faced by these systems. Al-Kahtani et al. (2022) mentions QoS, i.e. reliability and efficiency as major challenges. Patient mobility, heterogeneity of devices, performance, interoperability, cost of implementation and devices, and privacy and security have also been identified as challenges faced by IoT in the medical sector.

Azbeg et al. (2022) analyzed the security loopholes in IoT healthcare and proposed an IoT-based patient monitoring system and considered three NFRs: Security, scalability, and processing. They utilized a distributed architecture based on blockchain technology in their system to tackle these issues.

In Bhavani et al. (2022), authors integrated IoT and machine learning data analytics to classify stress and predict future values of vital signs using historical data. They used various traditional and ensemble machine learning techniques for data analytics. Gupta et al. (2019) studied the areas of application of IoT, especially healthcare. They highlighted the key components that are used in IoT framework and also highlighted challenges faced in IoT implementation.

Chakraborty and Kishor (2022) developed a model using machine learning techniques on historical patient data to predict heart diseases. The prediction using ML is implemented in IoT-based healthcare system in a cloud-fog layer. The system achieved an accuracy value of 97.32%.

5.4 SIGNIFICANCE OF NRs IN SUCCESS OR FAILURE OF IOT-BASED HEALTHCARE SYSTEM

NFRs play an important role in the success or failure of a system. Non-compliance with NFRs has resulted in the failure of software systems. For example, failure in "London Ambulance System" Breitman et al. (1999) system abortion in the "New Jersey Department of Motor Vehicles Licensing System" because of performance-scalability, Therac-25 (Leveson and Turner, 1993) accident and some other examples (Boehm and In, 1996).

NFRs played an important role in the success and failure of IT systems (Werner et al., 2020). Unclear and immeasurable NFRs are one of the major reasons for project failure in small organizations. NFRs such as privacy and performance are vital for project success and their lack has the potential to derail a software product.

DeFranco et al. (2017) narrates the results and analysis of NFRs of medical devices intensively based on software. In his review, the most dominant NFRs were interoperability, performance, security, privacy, usability, safety, and accuracy.

In Karunarathne et al. (2021), authors conducted a review of 89 articles related to IoT healthcare. According to their research, the importance of quality attributes is multiplied in IoT healthcare because of the risks involved. Studies in IoT healthcare have been taking quality requirements like security, reliability, accuracy, availability, performance, etc. into account.

Hence a healthcare system based on IoT can be a success or failure, depending on the quality attributes of a system and the context in which that system is being used. This chapter takes an example of IoT-based healthcare system that can be deployed in a hospital or an old home and develops the case by identifying the significant quality attributes and addressing those attributes in architectural design. In this way the chapter establishes a balance between mapping functional requirements directly to NFRs.

5.5 ACCEPTABILITY OF IOT-BASED HEALTHCARE MONITORING SYSTEM IMPROVED BY NFRs ENHANCEMENT

IoT-based healthcare significantly improves the provision of healthcare services by capturing large volumes of patient data that leads to preemptive healthcare. With this, there are unmatched advantages that can dramatically improve treatment techniques and consequently improve patient health. The acceptability of IOT-based healthcare systems is increased manifold with these in-built benefits. A key challenge for IoT toward acceptability is ensuring incorporating issues of interoperability, reliability, availability, security, safety, and flexibility to changing environmental conditions.

5.5.1 INTEROPERABILITY

IoT in healthcare allows interoperability, machine-to-machine communication, and information exchange through modern communication protocols like Bluetooth LE, Wi-Fi, Z-wave, ZigBee, etc. This diversity allows healthcare practitioners to innovate in the way they diagnose and provide treatment to their patients. The main challenge for these diverse interacting devices is lack of standardization, which makes an exchange of information between these devices difficult. The inconsistency of communication standards slackens the overall process and consequently creates hurdles in attaining system scalability. This hindrance can be overcome by ensuring that device manufacturers reach mutual agreement on standard communication protocols, so that there is no difference between communication protocols and no problems occur in the process of data aggregation.

5.5.2 RELIABILITY

In most IoT healthcare systems, the major key element is communication between machines and sensor devices without human intervention. The reliability of the communication system that works together with different sensor devices is integral to overall system reliability. The role of safety-critical systems is not only to continuously monitor but also to provide meaningful input to the physicians. The main factor of reliability in this scenario is accurate and timely diagnosis and alert notification at critical times, even when some part of the system malfunctions or sends poor-quality information.

5.5.3 SECURITY AND SAFETY

The wireless communication in sensor network applications in healthcare poses serious security threats to these systems. In such systems, patient health data is gathered from various devices and wearables. These devices are connected to each other and communicate with multiple users for data gathering. Therefore, security in IoT healthcare system is not just about network security it must curtail all management levels of IoT. Such systems are highly vulnerable to cybercriminals who can compromise the system security protocols and have access to information of both patients and healthcare providers. They can misuse this information to illegally buy drugs and medical equipment and misuse them later. To cater security and privacy issues, strong security protocols and standards must be implemented into the design of such systems.

5.5.4 AVAILABILITY

The IoT vision is to ensure the provision of services 24/7 to devices that support the IoT functionality regardless of time and location. Owing to their nature healthcare devices generate large quantities of data in a short span of time, whose storage and management over cloud is difficult. Even manually analyzing this data is practically impossible for healthcare providers. This can be achieved over the cloud if these interconnected devices can collect and analyze the data and without storing unprocessed data provide the doctors only with final reports and displays. Thus, IoT enables accurate and improved patient care through the generation of alerts, tracking, and monitoring, which allows timely treatments.

5.5.5 SCALABILITY

Every other day improved medical devices come into market and become part of the healthcare system that will produce large amounts of data. With all these advances in medical devices, the storage and processing requirements of data also increase manifolds. This will cause a major issue for healthcare systems. In this context, collected data from various connecting devices needs big data analytics for improving future cloud storage needs as well as making better treatment plans. The system handling storage and analysis of the generated information from these devices must be scalable.

5.5.6 ACCURACY OF DATA

The real challenge comes in data integrity. Data integrity means that the data is accurate and reliable. Data should be maintained and ensure accuracy and consistency over its entire life cycle as in IoT healthcare systems, data is collected on regular basis. In IoT systems, accuracy of data depends upon some sort of mechanism that can help distinguish the signal from the noise. The collected data travels through a gateway and then passes through a series of servers and applications before it eventually resides in the data center for analysis and further processing. Throughout this flow of data, it is essentially required to maintain consistency and security so that data integrity remains intact.

5.5.7 LATENCY AND RESPONSIVENESS OF DATA

Latency and responsiveness of data have a crucial role in acceptability of the system. It is defined as time required by data to travel from the source to destination. High latency will result in slow performance, low responsiveness and bad user experience. Causes of high latency are transmission mediums, propagation, routers, and storage delays. Several methods are used to reduce latency such as making sure that bandwidth consumption by the network clients is controlled. Applications performance may be regularly monitored to ensure no unexpected behaviors increase network load. Network monitoring devices may be installed to keep check on devices that specifically require frequent troubleshooting. The tools that help improve network latency are SolarWinds® Network Performance Monitor, network mapping, problem troubleshooting, and general network baselining.

A threshold for latency can be set with these network monitoring tools. As soon as the network latency reaches the defined threshold alerts may be generated. The data can also be analyzed to differentiate between performance issues or errors impacting network latency.

5.6 ENHANCING ADAPTABILITY IN DESIGN BY BRIDGING THE GAP BETWEEN FUNCTIONAL AND NON-FUNCTIONAL REQUIREMENTS

The success of IoT-based healthcare systems is largely dependent on how the gap between functional requirements and NFR is reduced in the overall design of the system. These quality attributes are to be embedded in design in such manner that change of environment has no impact on the overall system functionality, it remains as beneficial as it was in its previous setting. The high degree of adaptability contributes to the overall success of such systems. As far as Adaptability is concerned, it is one of the important NFR. Adaptation refers to the capability of a system to welcome change in its environment. Precisely, adaptation of a software system is the result of change from a previous environment to a new setting, which give rise to a new system that should preferably meet the requirements of its new environment (Subramanian and Chung, 2001).

This NFR should be catered for in the architecture and design phase, in order to equip the system with adaptability. Our consideration of design decisions and architectural style alternatives should be selected such that it inculcates adaptability in the software system.

This research presents a model to enhance the adaptability of the system by reducing the gap between functional and NFRs. This has been done by catering for NFRs in design considerations.

For addressing the problem of AAL and hospital patient management, a model has been suggested to improve the vital sign monitoring of the patients. These vital signs are transferred to a doctor and next of kin for the purpose of the safety of the patients. As already identified, the NFRs like reliability, safety, security of data, and availability of the system can be ensured by the suggested schematics.

5.6.1 MODEL PROPOSED

The evolution of sensors and transducers has led to measurement of many routine activities with lot of ease, particularly in case of medical science, and noninvasive medical diagnostics. This research intends to explore the exploitation of common sensors, for which modules are available in the market, to be integrated with a microcontroller. Healthcare based on IoT strengthens the real-time monitoring of patients' data through a wireless sensor network (WSN). Furthermore, the employed microcontroller analyzes the data received from various sensory elements to determine patients' vital signs and has the capability to analyze data patterns for diagnosis and provide treatment suggestions through authorized practitioners. In this project different sensory elements will be connected to a microcontroller (Arduino/ Raspberry Pi) and different types of data can be analyzed to determine various health parameters. The proposed system provides an interface that connects the patient (in a hospital or at home) to a doctor and next of kin through wireless.

The following sensors will be used:

1. Body position
2. Body temperature

3. Electromyography
4. Electrocardiography (ECG)
5. Airflow
6. Galvanic skin response
7. Blood pressure
8. Pulse oximeter
9. CGM
10. Snore

A brief description of these sensors' functionality and output is given in Table 5.1.

TABLE 5.1
Brief Details of All Sensors and Their Functions

No.	Sensors	Function	Output
1	Body position	Position determination through GPS and orientation of body through Gyroscope	Digital value of location and graphical representation of orientation
2	Body temperature	Body temperature determination through temperature sensor (can be mounter on forehead)	Digital value in degree Fahrenheit or Celsius
3	Electromyography	Measurement of electrical activity of any muscle or nerves, sensory electrode to relate to skin	2D Plot (Amplitude with respect to time)
4	Electrocardiography (ECG)	Measurement of electrical activity of heart with respect to time, sensory electrode to be connected with skin	2D Plot (Amplitude with respect to time)
5	Airflow	Measurement of air inhaled, sensor to relate to nose of patient or mask	Digital value in cubic feet per min (CFM)
6	Galvanic skin response	Measurement of stress level through change in electrical resistance of skin caused due to stress, sensory electrode to be connected with skin	Digital value in micro-Siemens (μS) and indication of low, medium, and high stress
7	Blood pressure	Measurement of blood pressure, device to be strapped around leg or arm	Digital value of millimeters of mercury (mmHg)
8	Pulse oximeter	Measurement of oxygen saturation level in blood, device to be clipped on finger of hand or foot	Digital value in percentage (%)
9	CGM – Constant glucose monitoring	Measurement of blood glucose level, sensory electrode to relate to skin preferably on abdominal fat or thigh fat	Digital value of mmol/L (millimoles per liter)
10	Snore	Measurement of snoring through measurement of sound and muscle movement, to be connected on neck	Indication of low, medium, and high level of snoring

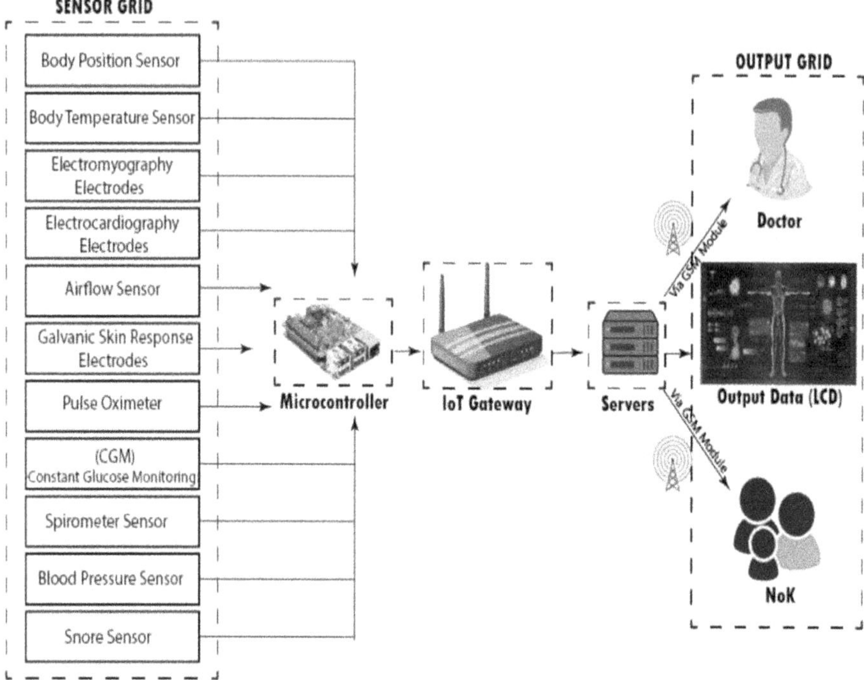

FIGURE 5.1   Proposed methodology diagram.

The proposed model as shown in Figure 5.1, is applicable to hospitals and old homes with a sizable number of inmates. The design of our proposed model is such that the gap between FRs and NFRs is kept to minimum keeping in view the following functional requirements:

1. WSN attached to the patients. WSNs are integrated with a device that gets attached to patient's wrist or chest.
2. Real-time monitoring of health parameters with accuracy through employment of various sensors, which are connected to the sensor shield which collects the e-health data.
3. The wearable device i.e. Raspberry Pi microcontroller which processes and analyzes patient's data and communicates wirelessly.
4. Acquired data to be stored on a local server for subsequent display and dissemination to all concerned keeping data security intact.
5. Dissemination of data is done through GUI for each concerned stakeholder.
6. Managing each patient's information.
7. Transfer of data from sensors to servers is through IoT Gateway in order to ensure interpretability of hardware.

8. Communication of patient data with concerned medical practitioners and Next of Kin remotely through mobile app and website.
9. Use of visual data analytical tool for analysis and prediction.
10. In case of any emergency alarm to be actuated in ER, an automated text message is to be generated to the doctor/NOK.
11. Reliability is ensured through multiple local servers.

5.6.2 Challenges

Following are the challenges of the proposed system.

1. It has always been anticipated that as much as intelligent devices are being accessed through internet, the privacy and security implications are becoming a core point of concern. Data management has become more critical in IoT-based health care systems (Azbeg et al., 2022).
2. Moreover, interoperability is a challenge as new sensors and hardware are being developed with the passage of time.
3. Reliability of the system and accuracy of the data also play an important part in the IoT-based healthcare system.
4. Patient safety is of prime concern in healthcare system which can be ensured by making the system available.

5.6.3 Rationale for the Proposed Model

Keeping in view the requirement of FRs and NFRs established in preceding paragraphs, and challenges that we came across in researches, following were the design considerations:

1. In order to ensure reliability redundant servers would be deployed.
2. Usually such systems utilize available cloud storage, however client server architecture with local servers is used to ensure data security.
3. IoT gateways are used as middleware to ensure introduction of new sensors/ hardware in future. It facilitates the heterogeneity of devices and protocols.
4. Safety is ensured through the availability and accuracy of the data analytics.

5.6.4 Big Data Analytic Tools

The eminence of big data has increased over the past decade and it is applicable in almost every domain. Similarly, IoT in healthcare monitoring systems also has a great scope for big data and its tools. The tools collect an immense amount of healthcare data and provide services in three major areas.

- Descriptive analysis refers to measurement of what has been done or what has happened, such as cost, resources, and frequency.
- Predictive analytics that utilizes descriptive data in order to predict the most likely occurrences that will occur in the future.
- Prescriptive analytics that enables the system to make proactive decisions.

5.6.5 Uses

- Improve diagnostic accuracy
- Identify outbreaks of illness and epidemics
- Reduce the rate of infections
- Provide support in decision-making
- Create personalized treatment plans

The healthcare providers make use of big data to enable the IoT-based healthcare system to do basic data analysis and intelligence based on that data. This will empower the systems to do population health management, risk satisfaction, and reduce operational costs.

Sensors and actuators in the form of wearable technologies provide the data and that data is transferred over the network in order to be analyzed by the big data tools. These tools provide the statistics of patients like when the patient took the medicine last time. Or when did somebody sleep or use the restroom.

In addition to the analysis of legacy sources like patient medical history, diagnostic and clinical trials data, drug effectiveness index, etc., new data sources can also be identified using big data in healthcare. These might include social media platforms, telematics, wearable devices, etc. Novel healthcare solutions are achieved when the data is collected from a mixture of these sources and analytics.

5.7 EVALUATION OF THE PROPOSED SYSTEM AGAINST NFRS MODEL

To evaluate the proposed system, this chapter models respective NFRs and their dependent NFRs of the IoT-based healthcare system. The proposed hierarchy takes reliability as a main NFR because in the system under consideration it is one of the major NFRs and is among the six main quality characteristics identified by (ISO 9126-1, 1991). Consider Figure 5.2 and we will see that by ensuring reliability, how other NFRs in the system are enhanced. Improving the reliability, we improve the dependability, availability, safety, and usability of the system. And when the system is dependable it becomes safe and secure (Sommerville, 2016), (Bourque, 2020). Table 5.2 shows the different artifacts of the proposed model and the NFRs they ensure.

5.7.1 Reliability Ensured through Redundancy of Server

Reliability (Bauer, 2012) is defined as, "the ability of a system to perform a required function under stated conditions for a stated time period." In the proposed system we can ensure reliability by incorporating the redundant servers. Server redundancy in the infrastructure is created by housing two servers. These servers are a primary server and a secondary server.

When a problem occurs in the primary server, the failover monitoring server will automatically update DNS data so that network traffic is redirected to a secondary server. In case of emergencies and to ensure maximum uptime, redundancy should

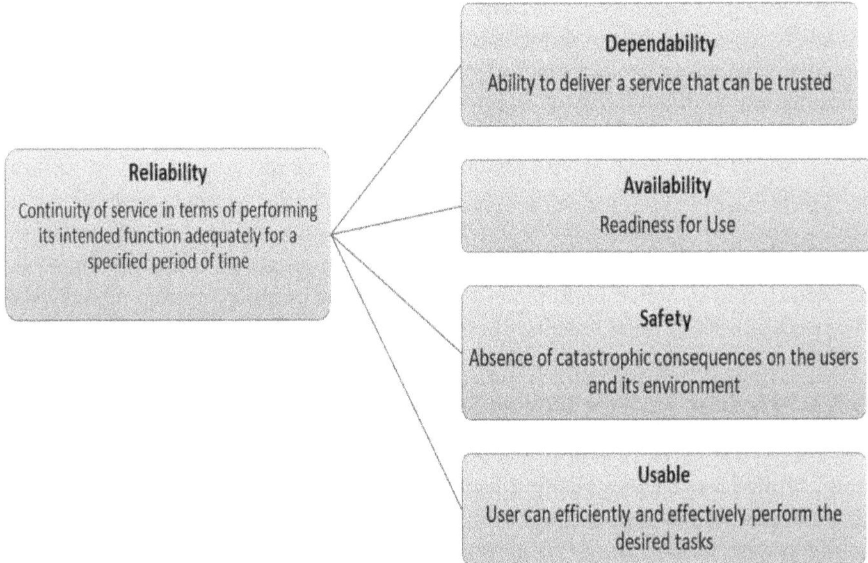

FIGURE 5.2 NFR modeling of reliability.

also be incorporated in data backups, disk drives, power supplies, and internet connectivity.

In this way by safeguarding the reliability of the system, maintainability and availability are automatically ensured (Bauer, 2012).

5.7.2 SECURITY ENSURED THROUGH CLIENT/SERVER ARCHITECTURE

Ensuring the security, confidentiality, and integrity of networks is of utmost importance. In their paper, Khan et al. (2022) emphasize that maintaining these essential aspects can be effectively achieved by implementing a client-server architecture. This involves the deployment of security measures such as intrusion detection systems, firewalls, and anti-disclosure tools, as well as following established procedures and protocols.

TABLE 5.2

Artifacts of the Proposed Model and the Ensured NFRs

No.	Artifacts	NFRs
1	Redundant servers	Reliability, availability
2	Client-server architecture with local servers	Security, data integrity, data accuracy, safety
3	Gateway	Inter-operability, scalability, maintainability

According to Solomon et al. (2023), factors like encryption of software and its updates, generation of numerous decryption keys for IoT devices, and computationally efficient authentication methods are needed to be catered for to ensure the integrity and confidentiality of client-server based architecture systems.

As the proposed system is based on client/server architecture and healthcare setups would have their private setups so integrity of the system will be ensured by installing firewalls and no access from outside of the system. Multiple server deployments would make the system available through no single point of failure. Authenticity would also be ensured by providing a registration mechanism to the patients. Hence as stated in Solomon et al. (2023), the proposed system possesses all the necessary NFRS that enhance the security feature of the system.

5.7.3 Heterogeneity of Devices Supported through IoT Gateway

For the system to be interoperable and maintainable, it should support heterogeneity of devices. Heterogeneity does not only support different kinds of devices to interoperate, but it also allows more sensors and actuators to be implemented in the system in the future. To support the heterogeneity, gateway layer has been introduced in our proposed architecture/model of the system.

The gateway layer acts as a mediator between different heterogeneous communicating devices (sensors and actuators) and the application layer.

The various sensors and actuators are deployed in the healthcare system based on IoT and their function is to collect the data and transfer the data to the gateway layer. As mentioned earlier the gateway can be implemented using R-Pi 3 microcontroller (Raspberry Pi Volk, 2015, 2018). Raspberry Pi 3 microcontroller gives a quality of required processing power and storage that guarantees all the collected sensor data to be transmitted to the server for analysis using big data analytics.

As the IoT name suggests it requires the connection of different smart devices that are accessed, managed, and interconnected. Therefore, gateway is an appropriate way to support interconnection as well as heterogeneity.

Figure 5.3 shows the connection of different IoT devices to a gateway.

5.7.4 Safety of the System Ensured through Reliable Servers

Safety is primarily concerned with whether the system functions as intended and whether a system failure can be harmful to the patient.

A secure system based on client server architecture ensures that all necessary steps pertaining to safety requirements have been embedded in the system design. As a result, this eliminates the dependency on commercial cloud which poses security threats to the systems. Only setup located in a secure environment of a healthcare facility, a health information system backbone, or a certified provider was considered acceptable.

The main three components of any IoT healthcare system are body area sensor network, Internet connected smart gateways, and cloud and big data support. Data generated from wearables is provided to doctors and authorized next of kin, provisioning them with facility to check the patient's vitals all the time and enabling

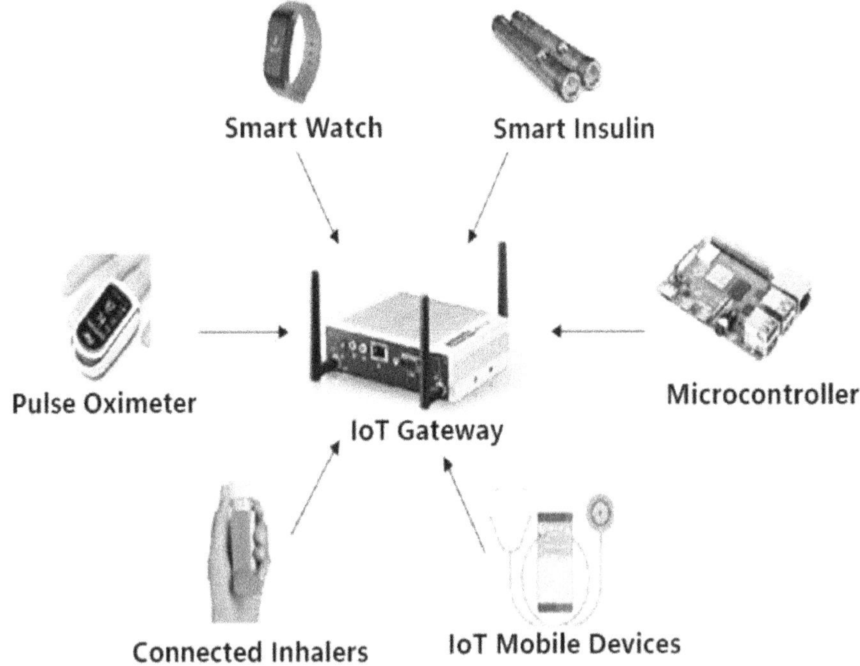

FIGURE 5.3 Heterogeneous IoT healthcare devices connected to IoT.

them to make timely decisions related to their health. This generic architecture supports various communication standards that serve as the link between a sensor device and the Internet. The system performs data conversion, aggregation, encryption, etc. The data storage and data analytics reside on cloud whereas user interface provides a dashboard to medical practitioners for visualization and understanding. Such healthcare systems learn from device inputs and patient data to respond to current and predicted future health of the patient, and can even raise alarms if necessary (Firouzi et al., 2018).

5.8 COMPARATIVE ANALYSIS WITH EXISTING MODELS

In comparison to other similar models within the field of IoT-based healthcare systems, the presented research distinguishes itself by prioritizing the integration of both functional and NFRs to address critical quality attributes. While various models emphasize specific aspects like sensor technologies, data analytics, or security measures, this research uniquely underscores the holistic consideration of reliability, security, interoperability, and safety.

Compared to models that predominantly focus on cloud-based solutions, the proposed system's emphasis on client-server architecture with local servers contributes to enhanced security and data integrity. The incorporation of redundant servers for reliability aligns with contemporary approaches to ensure uninterrupted healthcare monitoring. The introduction of an IoT gateway for supporting device heterogeneity sets this model apart, acknowledging the evolving nature of IoT technologies.

Furthermore, the research stands out by addressing challenges associated with privacy concerns, interoperability issues, and reliability, providing a more comprehensive approach to overcoming potential barriers in the adoption of IoT in healthcare. By proposing a model that integrates multiple sensors for diverse health parameters, the chapter considers a wide spectrum of monitoring capabilities, surpassing certain models that may focus on specific aspects of health data. Overall, this comparative analysis highlights the nuanced and comprehensive nature of the presented model, positioning it as a robust and adaptable solution in the landscape of IoT-based healthcare systems.

Conclusively, the research gap lies in the lack of comprehensive approaches in existing IoT-based healthcare models. While some models focus on specific elements like sensor technologies or data analytics, there is a notable gap in addressing critical quality attributes through the integration of both functional and NFRs. Current models often overlook the holistic consideration of reliability, security, interoperability, and safety. Additionally, the emphasis on cloud-based solutions in contrast to the proposed client-server architecture with local servers reveals a gap in prioritizing enhanced security and data integrity. The research uniquely fills this gap by introducing a model that addresses challenges related to privacy concerns, interoperability issues, and reliability, offering a more inclusive approach to IoT adoption in healthcare.

5.9 CONCLUSION

With the rapid advancements in IoT and cloud computing, innovative applications of IoT in healthcare are becoming need of the day. The fields of medicine and technology have always been interlinked but this relationship has immensely transformed with advent of IoT and the wide acceptance of wearable sensor devices. This progression, however, should be embraced very cautiously, as there are still many valid apprehensions pertaining to reliability, security, safety, acceptability, and more. Many modifications need to take place to make this technological shift feasible in the field of medicine. Above all, hardware and software need to be revamped so that they can handle IoT related challenges in the healthcare field.

In this chapter, we proposed a framework for designing and implementing healthcare IoTs. It may lead to personalized healthcare with ease of access. The chapter has tried to address major aspects of IoT-based healthcare systems like smart wearable devices, sensors, and big data analytics to ensure the provision of health services leading to healthier lifestyles. A series of challenging research issues were addressed such as: security, data integrity, patient-doctor confidentiality, and a huge volume of processing complexity which still majorly hampers extensive application of such systems. The proposed model provides insight into handling of the most important NFRs relevant to IoT-based healthcare system. Henceforth, mitigation of challenges related to these NFRs increases the overall acceptability of the system, by gaining patient-doctor trust and reliance on this technological shift in the field of health.

5.10 FUTURE WORK

In future, the model presented in this chapter can be enhanced by utilizing machine learning techniques on historical patient data in order to predict to predict potential health issues, optimize treatment plans, and improve patient outcomes. The scope of research can be increased by integrating more advanced and non-invasive sensor technologies to monitor physiological and pathological markers that can help in diagnosing a wider range of diseases. The efficacy of integration of blockchain technology can be analyzed in this model for improved security. IoT healthcare model can be integrated with novel telemedicine platforms. This model does not focus on a very important aspect of technology: usability and human computer interaction. In future, HCI aspect of IoT healthcare can be analyzed.

5.11 MAJOR DELIVERABLES

The following deliverables capture the essence of the chapter, covering the proposed model, challenges, NFRs, and the integration of big data analytics in IoT-based healthcare systems.

1. Improved Model for IoT-Based Healthcare System:
   a. Sensors Integration: Propose a model that integrates common sensors like body temperature, ECG, blood pressure, and more into an IoT-based healthcare system.
   b. Microcontroller Analysis: Develop a microcontroller-based system to analyze data from sensors, ensuring real-time monitoring of patient's vital signs and enabling diagnosis and treatment suggestions.
   c. Wireless Connectivity: Establish a wireless network connecting patients, doctors, and next of kin, enhancing accessibility to healthcare services through a hand-held device.
2. Addressing Challenges and Trust Deficit:
   a. Privacy and Security Measures: Propose strategies to overcome challenges related to privacy and security implications in IoT-based healthcare systems, ensuring the secure management of sensitive health data.
   b. Interoperability Solutions: Develop solutions to address interoperability challenges arising from the continuous development of new sensors and hardware.
   c. Reliability and Accuracy Enhancement: Focus on improving the reliability and accuracy of the system, addressing the trust deficit within the medical community.
3. Comprehensive NFRs Model:
   a. NFR Identification: Identify and emphasize the critical quality attributes of IoT-based healthcare systems, including reliability, security, safety, interoperability, and more.
   b. Hierarchical Evaluation: Present a hierarchical evaluation model that prioritizes reliability as a main NFR, showcasing its impact on dependability, availability, safety, and usability.

c. Redundancy and Security Measures: Highlight the incorporation of redundant servers for reliability and client-server architecture with local servers for enhanced security.

REFERENCES

Aghdam, Z. N., Rahmani, A. M., & Hosseinzadeh, M. (2021). The role of the internet of things in healthcare: Future trends and challenges. Computer Methods and Programs in Biomedicine, 199, 105903.

Al-Kahtani, M. S., Khan, F., & Taekeun, W. (2022). Application of internet of things and sensors in healthcare. Sensors, 22(15), 5738.

Aloi, G., Caliciuri, G., Fortino, G., Gravina, R., Pace, P., Russo, W., & Savaglio, C. (2016, April). A mobile multi-technology gateway to enable IoT interoperability. In 2016 IEEE first international conference on internet-of-things design and implementation (IoTDI) (pp. 259–264). IEEE.

Alshammari, H. H. (2023). The internet of things healthcare monitoring system based on MQTT protocol. Alexandria Engineering Journal, 69, 275–287.

Azbeg, K., Ouchetto, O., & Andaloussi, S. J. (2022). BlockMedCare: A healthcare system based on IoT, blockchain and IPFS for data management security. Egyptian Informatics Journal, 23(2), 329–343.

Bhavani, T., VamseeKrishna, P., Chakraborty, C., & Dwivedi, P. (2022). Stress classification and vital signs forecasting for IoT-health monitoring. IEEE/ACM Transactions on Computational Biology and Bioinformatics. 21(4), 652–659

Boehm, B., & In, H. (1996). Identifying quality-requirement conflicts. IEEE Software, 13(2), 25–35.

Bourque, P. (2020, November). The SWEBOK guide—More than 20 years down the road. In 2020 IEEE 32nd Conference on Software Engineering Education and Training (CSEE&T) (pp. 1–2). IEEE.

Breitman, K. K., Leite, J. C. S., & Finkelstein, A. (1999). The world's a stage: A survey on requirements engineering using A real-life case study. Journal of the Brazilian Computer Society, 6, 13–37.

Burkhalter, M. (2022). Ingestible IoT sensors. https://www.perle.com/articles/ingestible-iot-sensors-40193889.shtml.

Chakraborty, C., & Kishor, A. (2022). Real-time cloud-based patient-centric monitoring using computational health systems. IEEE Transactions on Computational Social Systems, 9(6), 1613–1623.

Das, S., & Namasudra, S. (2022). A novel hybrid encryption method to secure healthcare data in IoT-enabled healthcare infrastructure. Computers and Electrical Engineering, 101, 107991.

DeFranco, J., Kassab, M., Laplante, P., & Laplante, N. (2017). The nonfunctional requirement focus in medical device software: A systematic mapping study and taxonomy. Innovations in Systems and Software Engineering, 13, 81–100.

Domínguez-Bolaño, T., Campos, O., Barral, V., Escudero, C. J., & García-Naya, J. A. (2022). An overview of IoT architectures, technologies, and existing open-source projects. Internet of Things, 20, 100626.

Firouzi, F., Rahmani, A. M., Mankodiya, K., Badaroglu, M., Merrett, G. V., Wong, P., & Farahani, B. (2018). Internet-of-things and big data for smarter healthcare: From device to architecture, applications and analytics. Future Generation Computer Systems, 78, 583–586.

Florea, A. I., Anghel, I., & Cioara, T. (2022). A review of blockchain technology applications in ambient assisted living. Future Internet, 14(5), 150.

Gaur, R., Prakash, S., Prasad, L. N., Kumar, S., Abhishek, K., & Guduri, M. (2023). A secure and efficient scheme based on unlinkability and anonymous traceable protocol for cloud-assisted IoT environment. Journal of Circuits, Systems and Computers, 32(18), 2350316.

Gimenez Manuel, J. G., Augusto, J. C., & Stewart, J. (2022). AnAbEL: Towards empowering people living with dementia in ambient assisted living. Universal Access in the Information Society, 21(2), 457–476.

Guduri, M., Chakraborty, C., & Margala, M., 2023. Blockchain-based federated learning technique for privacy preservation and security of smart electronic health records. IEEE Transactions on Consumer Electronics.

Gupta, A., Chakraborty, C., & Gupta, B. (2019). Medical information processing using smartphone under IoT framework. Energy Conservation for IoT Devices: Concepts, Paradigms and Solutions, 283–308.

Hajvali, M., Adabi, S., Rezaee, A., & Hosseinzadeh, M. (2022). Software architecture for IoT-based health-care systems with cloud/fog service model. Cluster Computing, 25(1), 91–118.

Huang, J., Zhang, S., Yang, F., Yu, T., Prasad, L. N., Guduri, M., & Yu, K., 2023. Hypergraph-based interference avoidance resource management in customer-centric communication for intelligent cyber-physical transportation systems. *IEEE Transactions on Consumer Electronics*, 70(1), 1775–1786.

ISO 9126-1 software quality model. https://www.geeksforgeeks.org/iso-iec-9126-in-software-engineering/#what-is-isoiec-9126

Karunarathne, S. M., Saxena, N., & Khan, M. K. (2021). Security and privacy in IoT smart healthcare. IEEE Internet Computing, 25(4), 37–48.

Khan, M. A. (2021). Challenges facing the application of IoT in medicine and healthcare. International Journal of Computations, Information and Manufacturing (IJCIM), 1(1), 39–55.

Khan, A. A., Laghari, A. A., Shaikh, Z. A., Dacko-Pikiewicz, Z., & Kot, S. (2022). Internet of things (IoT) security with blockchain technology: A state-of-the-art review. IEEE Access, 10, 122679–122695.

Leveson, N. G., & Turner, C. S. (1993). An investigation of the Therac-25 accidents. Computer, 26(7), 18–41.

Lu, T., Ji, S., Jin, W., Yang, Q., Luo, Q., & Ren, T. L. (2023). Biocompatible and long-term monitoring strategies of wearable, ingestible and implantable biosensors: Reform the next generation healthcare. Sensors, 23(6), 2991.

Paiva, J. O., Andrade, R., & Carvalho, R. M. (2022). NFR evaluation in IoT applications: Methods, strategies and open challenges. In International Conference on Enterprise Information Systems (pp. 304–325). Springer, Cham.

R. P. Foundation. (2019). "Teach, Learn, and Make with Raspberry Pi," Raspberry Pi. [Online]. Available: https://www.raspberrypi.org/

Solomon, G., Zhang, P., Brooks, R., & Liu, Y. (2023). A secure and cost-efficient blockchain facilitated IoT software update framework. IEEE Access. 11, 44879–44894.

Sommerville, I. (2016). Software Engineering. 10th Edition, Pearson Education Limited, Boston.

Subramanian, N., & Chung, L. (2001, September). Software architecture adaptability: an NFR approach. In Proceedings of the 4th International Workshop on Principles of Software Evolution (pp. 52–61).

Werner, C., Li, Z. S., Ernst, N., & Damian, D. (2020, August). The lack of shared understanding of non-functional requirements in continuous software engineering: Accidental or essential?. In 2020 IEEE 28th international requirements engineering conference (RE) (pp. 90–101). IEEE.

6 Smart Paralysis Revolution

BCI Virtual Keyboards Unleashed in Healthcare

*Sravanth Kumar Ramakuri, Mukesh Prasad,
Mithileysh Sathiyanarayanan, Kandukuri
Harika, Khethavath Rohit, and Ganesh Jaina*

6.1 INTRODUCTION

Paralytic diseases, characterized by the progressive loss of muscular control resulting from disorders in the nervous system affecting the brain and spinal cord, pose formidable challenges for those grappling with these conditions. As these illnesses worsen over time, they specifically target nerve cells responsible for voluntary muscle control, leading to a gradual and debilitating decline in muscle strength. In confronting the intricate complexities of these ailments, this comprehensive study delves into the application of electroencephalogram (EEG) technology an innovation originally introduced by Berger in 1929 through the physical attachment of electrodes to the human skull.

The exploration of brain waves facilitated by EEG offers profound insights into the physiological functions associated with the brain, translating them into signals that can be harnessed for a myriad of applications. Notably, the advent of brain-computer interface (BCI) technology has heralded groundbreaking advancements in addressing the unique needs of individuals grappling with paralytic diseases. A remarkable innovation in this evolving field is the wireless intra-cortical brain-computer interface (iBCI), an EEG device explicitly crafted for paralytic patients. Through cortical recordings, this wireless iBCI stands as the first device of its kind, recording high-resolution broadband signals from multiple implanted microelectrode arrays in human subjects without the encumbrance of wires or cables.

The successful demonstration of real-time point-and-select interfaces in individuals with tetraplegia serves as a compelling testament to the potential of this wireless system for clinical translation, promising a future filled with assistive medical devices meticulously tailored to meet the unique challenges posed by paralysis. Furthermore, the wireless iBCI system not only facilitates ongoing research into cortical processing but also represents a beacon of hope for advancing our understanding and developing innovative solutions in the realm of neurotechnology for individuals facing the complexities of paralytic conditions during daily human behaviour, contributing significantly to the evolution of neuroscience and BCI technologies.

DOI: 10.1201/9781003603610-6

BCIs play an integral and transformative role in the intricate process of decoding signals and processing EEG data, where signals manifest variations in both amplitude and frequency. The study meticulously emphasizes the minimal electromyographic (EMG) artifacts discernible in EEG signals from healthy individuals, underscoring a notable observation that individuals with paralysis exhibit even fewer EMG artifacts. Eye blink signals, traditionally perceived as inconveniences in EEG studies due to momentary eye closures, emerge as invaluable signals with significant potential for controlling computers within the expansive domain of BCI technology.

BCI signal acquisition consists of three types: non-invasive, semi-invasive, and invasive. Non-invasive devices use EEG to monitor brain activity, making them accessible and user-friendly. Semi-invasive devices, also known as partially invasive devices, place electrodes on the brain's exposed surface, allowing for more direct and precise signal acquisition. Invasive devices measure neuron activity by inserting electrodes directly into the cortex during neurosurgical procedures, providing high spatial resolution and precision but posing challenges like surgery and associated risks. The choice of BCI signal acquisition method depends on factors like invasiveness, application requirements, and trade-offs between signal quality and user comfort. Non-invasive methods are suitable for applications where ease of use and comfort are paramount, while invasive methods are reserved for high signal fidelity scenarios. Semi-invasive approaches offer a middle ground.

BCIs, epitomized by virtual keyboards, establish a direct and symbiotic link between the human brain and computers, proving instrumental in assisting individuals confronted with communication challenges. The remarkable versatility of BCIs extends far beyond conventional applications, encompassing assistance for individuals with visual or auditory impairments, precise control of robots, aid for those with movement issues, medical condition diagnosis, enhancement of security measures, and even improvement of gaming experiences.

The system scrutinized in this comprehensive study seamlessly integrates an EEG-MindLink wearable device, a strategic choice made to circumvent the unwieldy bulk associated with traditional EEG equipment. To ensure the reliability of recorded brainwave data, sophisticated digital infinite impulse response (IIR) filter techniques are seamlessly incorporated, effectively eliminating additional physiological and environmental artifacts. The incorporation of Bluetooth module 3.0 further enhances the system's functionality by facilitating seamless communication between the MindLink device and a PC/Laptop, thereby offering swift and efficient access to the virtual keyboard. This strategic integration not only exemplifies technological innovation but also highlights a user-centric approach in the development of BCI systems.

In summation, the integration of EEG technology, wireless iBCI, and the MindLink device in the proposed system signifies a significant leap in assistive technology for individuals with paralysis. This chapter not only contributes to the ongoing progress in clinical translation but also underscores the transformative potential of BCIs in enhancing communication and accessibility for those grappling with the unique challenges posed by paralytic conditions.

The continuous advancements in this field hold promise for improving the quality of life and communication capabilities of individuals affected by paralytic diseases. The primary objective of this study is to evaluate the efficacy of the single-channel dry cathode Neurosky Mindwave EEG framework in discerning the thoughtful state of individuals. In real-time, the system gathers information and concurrently sends commands to MATLAB, showcasing its potential for immediate practical applications.

This research stands as a significant contribution to the field, offering insights into BCI technology and its transformative potential in enhancing communication for individuals facing paralysis. The following key contributions delineate the depth and impact of this study:

6.1.1 COMPREHENSIVE INTRODUCTION TO BCI TECHNOLOGY

The chapter initiates with a thorough introduction to BCI technology, elucidating its critical role in addressing the challenges confronted by individuals with paralysis. By establishing a comprehensive understanding of BCI, the study underscores its importance as a pioneering solution for enhancing communication in the context of paralysis. This introductory section serves as the conceptual foundation for subsequent analyses.

6.1.2 MINDLINK DEVICE EXPLORATION

A notable contribution of this research lies in the detailed exploration of the MindLink device. The study goes beyond a cursory overview, delving into the device's capabilities and functions. Moreover, it outlines the procedural intricacies involved in real-time cortical potential recordings. This exploration enhances our comprehension of the technological nuances inherent in the MindLink device, setting the stage for subsequent discussions and analyses.

6.1.3 CLASSIFICATION OF MIND WAVES

The study ventures into the classification of different mind waves, shedding light on the specific information conveyed by each brainwave. This classification not only enriches our understanding of cognitive and emotional states but also contributes valuable insights into the neural processes associated with distinct mental states. Such a nuanced classification framework adds depth to the research, elevating its significance within the broader landscape of BCI studies.

6.1.4 SIGNAL PREPROCESSING METHODS

A meticulous examination of signal preprocessing methods is a notable aspect of this research. This critical analysis is designed to enhance the quality and reliability of recorded brainwave data by addressing potential artifacts and noise in the EEG signals. The incorporation of robust preprocessing techniques contributes to refining the data, ensuring its accuracy and validity, and fortifying the overall credibility of the study.

6.1.5 VARIOUS CLASSIFICATION TECHNIQUES

The research embraces a diverse array of classification techniques to discern patterns in brainwave data. This multifaceted approach represents a significant stride toward a nuanced understanding of cerebral activity. The incorporation of various classification techniques not only broadens the analytical framework but also lays the groundwork for improved accuracy in distinguishing different mental states, advancing the state-of-the-art in BCI technology.

6.1.6 Detailed Virtual Keyboard Description

The study provides a comprehensive and detailed description of virtual keyboard functionalities. Accompanied by an exploration of the algorithm governing cursor movement, this section unveils the intricacies of the proposed communication system's user interface (UI). The detailed exposition enhances transparency, facilitating a deeper understanding of the proposed system and promoting replicability.

In conclusion, this research, spanning a breadth of topics from BCI technology fundamentals to the intricacies of signal processing and UI design, makes a substantial contribution to the field. By addressing the complexities associated with paralysis and leveraging advanced technologies, the study paves the way for the development of sophisticated assistive technologies tailored to the unique needs of individuals facing paralysis.

The contributions of this chapter are as follows:

- An in-depth introduction to BCI technology and its transformative potential in enhancing communication for individuals with paralysis.
- Introduction and exploration of MindLink device dwelling deep into its capabilities and functions and the procedure to record the cortical potentials from a person in real time.
- Explore the classification of different mind waves, elucidating the specific information conveyed by each brainwave. This analysis yields valuable insights into the cognitive and emotional states of individuals.
- An examination of signal preprocessing methods employed in our study to enhance the quality and reliability of recorded brainwave data.
- Various classification techniques to discern patterns in brainwave data, contributing to a more nuanced understanding of cerebral activity.
- Exploring and experimenting the MATLAB GUI.
- Ways of building virtual keyboard using MATLAB GUI.
- A detailed description of the virtual keyboard functionalities, accompanied by an exploration of the algorithm governing cursor movement. This reveals the intricacies of our proposed communication system's UI.

6.2 LITERATURE SURVEY

The intricate integration of BCI technology with EEG technology stands at the forefront of neuroscientific advancements, offering profound insights into brainwave activities. This study serves as a beacon, illuminating key facets of EEG equipment and its classification into wired and wireless devices. While wired devices are recognized for their sophistication, their wireless counterparts emerge as champions of comfort and user-friendliness, heralding a new era in neurotechnology.

Hans Berger's (1924) discovery of electrical signals from the human brain's scalp established EEG as a crucial tool for clinical diagnosis and brain research. Today, research in BCI investigates its performance, with applications including wheelchairs, cursor control, typing skills, robots, and disease diagnosis.

6.2.1 UNDERSTANDING EEG TECHNOLOGY

The methodology of EEG recording is central to this exploration, where electrodes play a pivotal role. The distinction between invasive methods, involving electrode placement on the brain, and non-invasive methods, positioned on the scalp, underscores the versatility of EEG applications. The study acknowledges the time-consuming nature of wired devices but emphasizes their sophistication, while wireless devices are lauded for their ease of use.

6.2.2 BCI APPLICATIONS AND VIRTUAL KEYBOARDS

The study takes a leap into the realm of BCI applications, particularly focusing on the creation of a virtual keyboard tailored for individuals grappling with physical disabilities. This innovative keyboard harnesses the power of eye movement and blinking as control signals, incorporating sophisticated image processing techniques for eye detection and blinking recognition. LabView emerges as a key player in this paradigm, providing a robust platform for the development of a BCI system where eye blinks become the control signals, opening up new avenues for interaction.

6.2.3 PROTOTYPE BCI SYSTEM AND VIRTUAL CONSOLE

A prototype BCI system takes center stage, featuring a matrix housing alphabet letters and special characters. This matrix becomes the canvas for character selection, with electromyography signals from the eyelid, the singular muscle controlled by individuals with quadriplegia, guiding decision-making. The graphical user interface (GUI) unveils a virtual console and a mouse game, demonstrating the system's potential to empower patients with Amyotrophic Lateral Sclerosis (ALS) to choose and compose text by orchestrating movements with their eyelids.

6.2.4 EEG SIGNAL PROCESSING LANDSCAPE

The chapter intricately explores the multifaceted realm of EEG signal processing, meticulously unraveling the intricacies embedded within pre-processing, feature extraction, and post-processing methodologies. This comprehensive examination extends across both conventional and contemporary approaches to handling EEG signals, with a heightened emphasis on mitigating recording artifacts inherent in the pursuit of advancing BCI technologies.

Within the study, a thorough investigation is undertaken to assess the efficacy of various denoising techniques, with particular attention devoted to understanding the nuances of computational complexity. The evaluation process meticulously scrutinizes the proposed systems, employing a rigorous benchmarking methodology that contrasts their performance against that of the more conventional finite impulse response (FIR)-based discrete wavelet transform (DWT) systems.

This holistic exploration aims to contribute valuable insights to the ever-evolving field of EEG signal processing, shedding light on the nuanced interplay between different methods and providing a foundation for refining and advancing the methodologies employed in BCI endeavors.

6.2.5 Qualities of EEG-based Human PC Interfaces

The investigation meticulously unveils the characteristics and particulars of EEG-based human-computer interfaces, honing in on the refinement and enrichment of BCI frameworks. A pivotal turning point emerges with the introduction of a virtual console, ingeniously implemented through the LabVIEW platform. This groundbreaking approach redefines interaction mechanisms, enabling the selection of virtual keyboard blocks with the simplicity of a blink. The program adeptly captures raw EEG data and essential metrics, such as average attentiveness and meditation levels, providing a nuanced comprehension of cognitive states during various learning activities.

In essence, this chapter stands as a comprehensive exploration of the vast landscape of BCI applications. It spans from the initial inception of virtual keyboards designed for individuals with physical disabilities to the evolution of sophisticated EEG-based human-computer interfaces. The fusion of LabVIEW, innovative control methods, and intricate signal processing techniques propels the frontier of assistive technologies forward, concurrently unraveling the intricate terrain of cognitive processes.

As the study unfolds, it not only broadens the horizons of neuroscientific research but also holds the potential for transformative impacts on individuals with diverse cognitive abilities and physical challenges. This research not only signifies progress in BCI technology but also underscores the promise of improving the quality of life for those facing unique cognitive and physical hurdles.

6.3 METHODOLOGY

The MindLink device plays a crucial role in the signal acquisition process, employing a series of functions to ensure the extraction of meaningful information from brain signals. The following steps outline the key functionalities of the MindLink device (Figure 6.1).

Sensing Low Voltage Potentials The process initiates with the MindLink device sensing low voltage potentials on the scalp. This initial step involves the detection of electrical signals originating from the brain.

Amplification and Analog-to-Digital Conversion Subsequently, the acquired signal undergoes amplification to enhance its strength. Following amplification, the analog signal is converted to digital format using an appropriate sampling rate. This conversion ensures that the signal can be effectively processed and transmitted for further analysis.

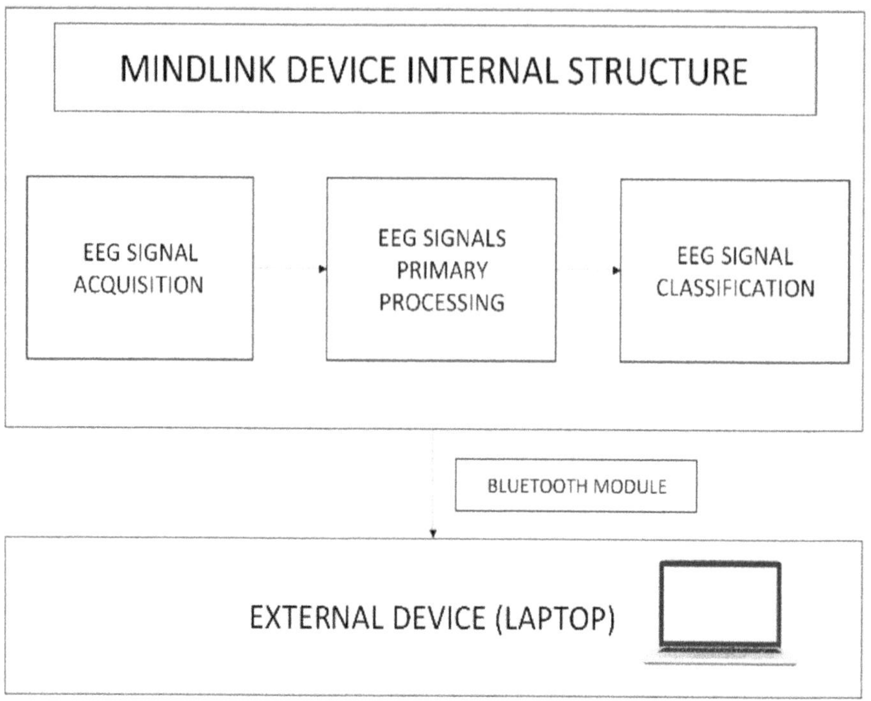

FIGURE 6.1 Block diagram of BCI functioning.

Bluetooth Transmission to Laptop: The digital data, now in a suitable format, is transmitted to a laptop via a Bluetooth module. This wireless communication enables quick and efficient transfer of brain signal data from the MindLink device to the processing platform.

Selection of Input Port in MATLAB: In the signal acquisition process, the MATLAB software is employed, and the appropriate input port is selected to facilitate the reception of data from the MindLink device. This integration with MATLAB establishes a seamless connection between the hardware and software components.

Built-In Filters for Preprocessing: The MindLink device incorporates built-in filters designed to eliminate line frequency and common noise sources. This pre-processing step is essential for enhancing the quality of the acquired signal by reducing unwanted artifacts and disturbances. The filters contribute to the refinement of the data before further analysis.

Signal Classification: Following signal acquisition and preprocessing, the crucial stage of signal classification occurs within the MindLink device itself, marking a significant departure from conventional practices that often rely on external software such as MATLAB. This innovative approach exemplifies the MindLink device's advanced capabilities, particularly in the real-time processing and categorization of brain signals.

Within the MindLink device, specialized algorithms are employed to assess multiple parameters, including mean and variance, essential for the nuanced classification of different signals. This unique in-device classification step plays a pivotal role in identifying patterns and extracting meaningful information directly at the source of signal acquisition. Notably, this methodology streamlines the analysis process, eliminating the need for external software for initial signal categorization.

It is imperative to highlight that, in the case of eye blink signals, the MindLink device's on-board classification mechanism is particularly noteworthy. Leveraging its intrinsic algorithms, the device adeptly discerns and classifies eye blink signals in real-time, showcasing the adaptability and efficiency of the MindLink system.

This groundbreaking paradigm in signal classification not only enhances the immediacy and accuracy of the analysis process but also underscores the MindLink device's prowess in providing a self-contained and responsive BCI system. This distinctive feature holds promise for more streamlined and user-friendly applications, especially in scenarios where real-time signal processing is paramount.

6.3.1 Comprehensive Process for Information Extraction

In summary, the MindLink device orchestrates a comprehensive signal processing workflow encompassing signal acquisition, built-in preprocessing through filters, and the pivotal signal classification step all within the MindLink device itself. This integrated and self-contained approach ensures the extraction of meaningful information from brain signals, rendering the data highly suitable for a myriad of applications with-in the realm of BCI technology.

Fundamentally, the MindLink device emerges as a crucial and autonomous component in the signal processing chain. Notably, all aspects of signal classification, a critical stage in the analysis, are adeptly handled within the MindLink device. The exclusion of MATLAB in the classification process underscores the self-sufficiency and advanced capabilities of the MindLink system in interpreting and categorizing brain signals. This streamlined approach not only enhances the efficiency of signal analysis but also positions the MindLink device as a versatile tool for applications like virtual keyboards and other assistive technologies.

6.3.2 Matlab Gui

MATLAB is a powerful tool for creating versatile and user-friendly applications, enabling users to create applications for various purposes. It offers three distinct approaches to app development: converting a script into a basic app, creating a drag-and-drop environment for interactive interfaces, and creating apps programmatically. The first method allows users to share code and modify variables through interactive controls, making it ideal for collaborative work. The second method allows users to create complex and feature-rich applications by placing interactive elements on a canvas, enhancing the overall user experience. The third method allows users to create apps programmatically, providing complete control over the design and functionality of the application. This approach is suitable for individuals with specific customization requirements or those who prefer a hands-on, code-centric approach. MATLAB's support for GUI development offers a range of options, from simple script conversions to interactive drag-and-drop interfaces and full programmatic control. This versatility ensures MATLAB remains a dynamic platform for developing apps that cater to diverse user needs and preferences. Whether for educational purposes, collaborative projects, or industry applications, MATLAB's app development capabilities enable users to create interfaces that streamline and enhance their interaction with complex algorithms and data.

GUIs, also known as apps, offer point-and-click control for software applications, eliminating the need for language learning or typing commands. MATLAB allows users to create apps for use within the pro-gram and as standalone desktop or web apps. There are three ways to create an app: converting a script into a simple app, creating an app interactively, or creating an app programmatically. Sharing a script allows users to modify variables using interactive controls, while creating a sophisticated app using a drag-and-drop environment allows for more complex UIs.

6.3.3 Utilized Hardware

The hardware component crucial to the functioning of this system is the MindLink device. The MindLink device serves as an integral part of the BCI system, facilitating the acquisition and processing of brain signals for various applications.

- The MindLink device serves multiple functions in the signal acquisition process.
- It senses low-voltage potentials on the scalp, amplifies the acquired signals, and converts them from analog to digital format.
- The device incorporates built-in filters to eliminate noise and common sources of interference during preprocessing.
- It facilitates the wireless transmission of processed data to a PC or laptop via the Bluetooth module.
- The MindLink device, in conjunction with MATLAB, allows for the selection of an appropriate input port for data reception.
- It plays a pivotal role in the comprehensive process of signal acquisition, preprocessing, and signal classification, ensuring the extraction of meaningful information from brain signals.
- In conclusion, the MindLink device stands as a key hardware component, enabling the effective implementation of BCI technology in the system. Its advanced features contribute to the accurate and efficient processing of brain signals for applications such as virtual keyboards and assistive technologies.

6.3.4 MindLink Device Specifications

The MindLink device, a crucial component in the BCI system, is equipped with advanced features and specifications. Here are the detailed specifications of the MindLink device, emphasizing the Think Gear ASIC Module (TGAM) (Figure 6.2).

6.3.5 Think Gear ASIC Module (TGAM)

- The MindLink device incorporates the TGAM, which includes the TGAT chip.
- TGAT chip is recognized as the world's first EEG sensor specifically designed for consumer use.
- The ASIC module is crucial for capturing and processing brain signals across diverse applications.
- TGAM integration highlights cutting-edge EEG technology for consumer accessibility.

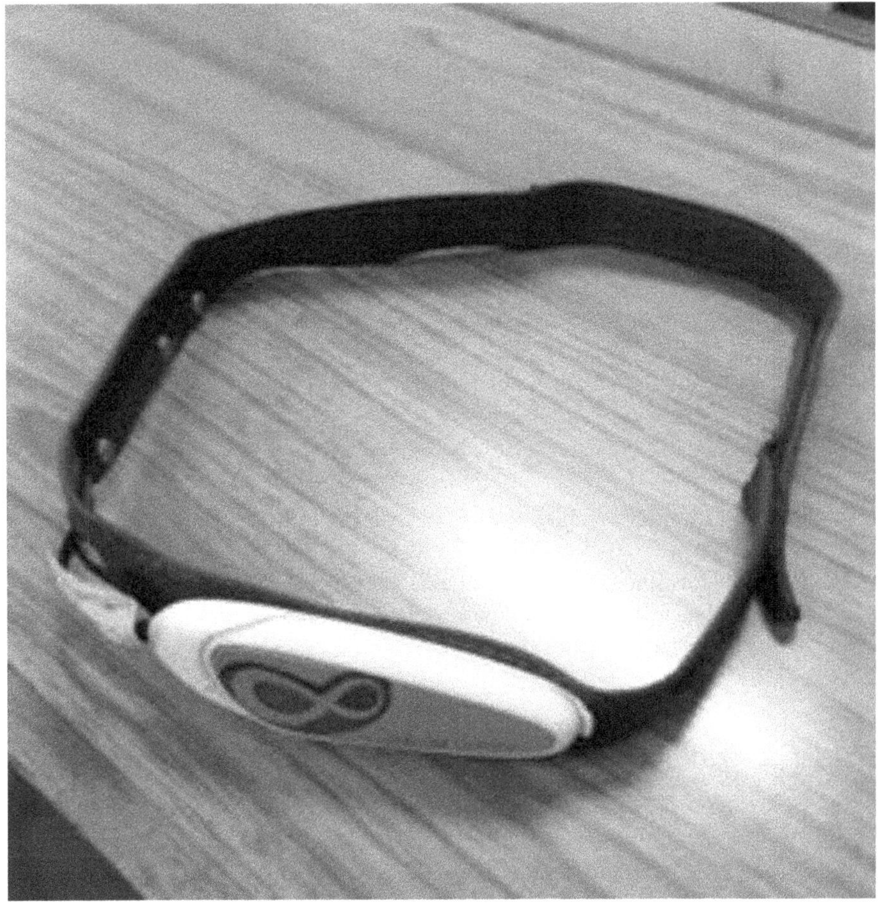

FIGURE 6.2   Hardware device (MindLink device).

6.3.6 RAW E-Sense Data

- Complementing the TGAM, the MindLink device includes RAW e-sense data.
- RAW e-sense data provides supplementary information related to the user's cognitive states, adding depth to the captured brain signals.

6.3.7 EEG Channel and Contacts

- The TGAM module within the MindLink device features a singular EEG channel with three contacts: EEG, REF, and GND.
- These contacts play a pivotal role in sensing and capturing the electrical potentials on the scalp.

6.3.8 Connection to Dry Electrodes

- The MindLink device connects directly to dry electrodes, meeting mass market needs.
- This design eliminates the necessity for conventional medical wet sensors, providing a user-friendly and comfortable EEG signal acquisition experience.

6.3.9 Advanced Filtering Technology

- The device is equipped with state-of-the-art filtering technology, contributing to high noise immunity.
- This feature ensures the acquired brain signals are accurate and reliable, even in diverse settings and for individuals with varying physiological conditions.

6.3.10 Detection of Improper Fit

- The MindLink device possesses the capability to detect an improper fit on the user's head.
- An ASIC warning is triggered if the device is off the head for four consecutive seconds or if it receives a poor signal for seven seconds.
- This functionality ensures the device's proper placement and optimal signal quality during usage.

6.3.11 Bluetooth Module 3.0

- For data transmission, the MindLink device utilizes a Bluetooth module 3.0.
- The Bluetooth module enables wireless communication between the MindLink device and a connected PC or laptop, facilitating seamless data transfer.

6.3.12 Low Power Consumption

- The device is designed with low power consumption, optimizing its energy efficiency during operation.

In summary, the MindLink device emerges as an innovative EEG sensor with features tailored for consumer use. Its incorporation of advanced technology, direct connection to dry electrodes, and Bluetooth capabilities make it a versatile and user-friendly component in the BCI system.

6.3.13 Classification of Brainwave Signals

Brainwave signals exhibit diverse frequencies, and their classification is crucial for understanding various cognitive states. The following delineates the distinct categories based on frequency ranges (Table 6.1):

Delta (0–4 Hz): Delta waves, characterized by their frequency between 0 and 4 Hz, prominently emerge during deep sleep. These waves play a vital role in the body's recuperative processes and are associated with restorative sleep cycles.

Theta (4–8 Hz): Theta waves, spanning the range of 4–8 Hz, manifest during sleep, meditation, and activities requiring creative engagement. Signifying deep relaxation, these waves are instrumental in facilitating conscious awareness and meditative states.

Alpha (8–13 Hz): Within the frequency range of 8–13 Hz, alpha waves dominate when individuals close their eyes, entering a relaxed yet awake state. Often linked to a sense of calmness, these waves are prevalent during meditation and reflective moments.

Beta (14–20 Hz): Occupying the frequency spectrum from 14 to 20 Hz, low beta waves are indicative of active concentration and cognitive problem-solving. Individuals in this state display heightened alertness, focusing on tasks that require mental engagement.

TABLE 6.1

Types of Brainwaves

Brainwave Type	Frequency Range (Hz)	Mental States and Conditions
Delta	0–4	Dreamless sleep, unconscious
Theta	4–8	Recall, fantasy, imaginary
Alpha	8–13	Relaxed but not drowsy, tranquil
Low Beta	13–15	Relaxed yet focused
Midrange Beta	16–20	Thinking, aware of self
High Beta	20–30	Alertness, agitation
Gamma	30–100	Motor functions

Midrange Beta (20–30 Hz): Encompassing frequencies from 20 to 30 Hz, mid-range beta waves are associated with mental functions, sustained attention, and alertness. This range signifies active mental engagement and the ability to maintain focus.

High Beta (30–40 Hz): High beta waves, spanning 30–40 Hz, signify intense cognitive activity, often observed in situations of stress and anxiety. They reflect an elevated level of mental alertness and heightened cognitive processes.

Gamma (40+ Hz): Gamma waves, with frequencies surpassing 40 Hz, are linked to higher cognitive functions, enhanced sensation, and information processing. This frequency range is associated with an elevated cognitive status and a pre-disposition for accelerated learning.

Understanding these classifications provides valuable insights into the dynamic nature of brain activity across different cognitive states. The diverse frequencies shed light on the intricacies of mental and emotional experiences, contributing to a comprehension of the human mind.

The eyeball, a remarkable organ responsible for vision, operates akin to an electrical dipole, exhibiting a positive cornea oriented forward and a negative cornea facing backward. This inherent electrical polarization serves as the foundation for electrooculogram (EOG), a technique that harnesses electrodes strategically placed around the eyes to capture electric signals generated by the rotational movements of the eyeball (Figure 6.3).

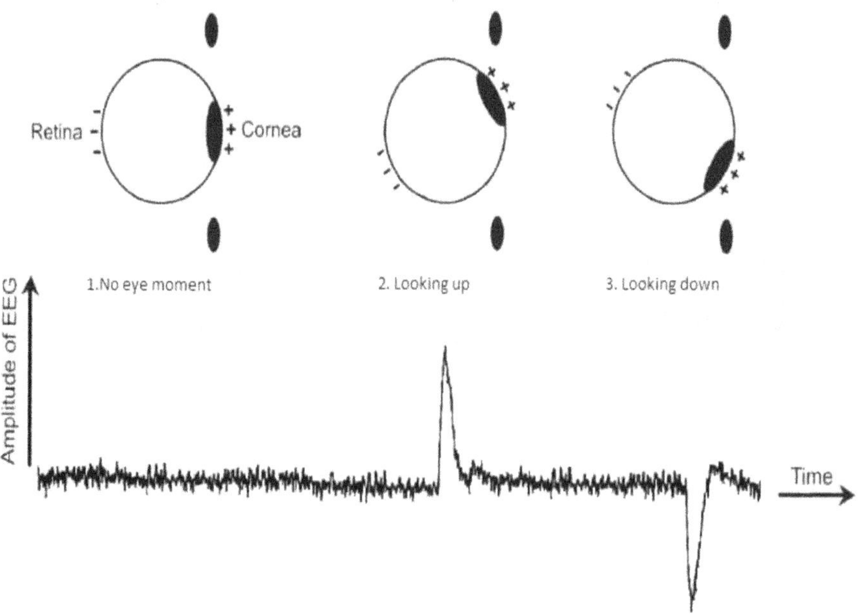

FIGURE 6.3 Variation of the EEG signal with respect to eye moments.

In the realm of EOG, the positive pole, represented by the cornea, undergoes dynamic shifts as it either approaches or retreats from the Fp1 electrode. This intricate interplay results in distinct patterns within the recorded EOG signals. For instance, during an upward rotation of the eyeball, the positive pole moves closer to the Fp1 electrode, leading to a positive deflection in the EOG signal. Conversely, a downward rotation prompts the positive pole to move away from the electrode, inducing a negative deflection. This dynamic interaction is observable not only during horizontal movements but also during vertical motions, encompassing actions like closing the eyelid and turning the cornea away from the pupil.

The comprehension of the nuanced relationship between eye movements and EOG signals holds paramount significance across various domains, ranging from clinical diagnostics to applications in human-computer interaction. Such knowledge opens avenues for leveraging EOG technology in innovative ways, offering insights into neurological conditions and enhancing the development of interactive systems that respond to subtle ocular cues.

The Mindlink device operates as a sophisticated Bluetooth-connected interface, specifically designed to delve into the interplay between EEG signals and eye blink patterns. By leveraging advanced algorithms implemented in MATLAB, the device effectively identifies and eliminates artifacts associated with eye blinks from the EEG data, ensuring the precision of the recorded brainwave information (Figure 6.4).

Upon establishing a Bluetooth connection with a computer or laptop, the MindLink device dynamically adapts its communication port through a meticulous algorithmic process. This ensures optimal connectivity and data transmission between the device and the computing system.

The integration of the Thinkgear.dll library is a key component in the MindLink device's functionality. This library, renowned for its efficiency in EEG data processing, generates a virtual keyboard accessible through specific eye blink commands. This pioneering approach transforms eye blinks into actionable input commands, opening up possibilities for intuitive and hands-free interaction.

The virtual keyboard, a central element in this BCI system, is thoughtfully designed for user convenience. It comprises four rows accommodating numerical inputs (1–4), letters from A to Z, and three special keys—talk, speak backward, and delete. The arrangement is crafted to facilitate seamless communication, enabling users to express their thoughts and commands with ease.

The device wirelessly transmits raw EEG data to the connected computer or laptop, allowing for real-time analysis and interaction. Within the MATLAB environment, the Thinkgear.dll library grants access to the virtual keyboard. The integration of this technology not only simplifies the user experience but also enhances the overall efficiency of the BCI system.

An innovative aspect of this system is the utilization of blinking eyelids as a distinctive input command. This action serves as a trigger, activating the virtual keyboard and enabling users to articulate their desired words. The integration of eye blinks as a control mechanism represents a groundbreaking approach in the realm of BCIs, emphasizing user-friendly and natural interaction methods.

In summary, the MindLink device stands as a testament to the fusion of EEG technology, Bluetooth connectivity, and advanced algorithms. Its ability to translate

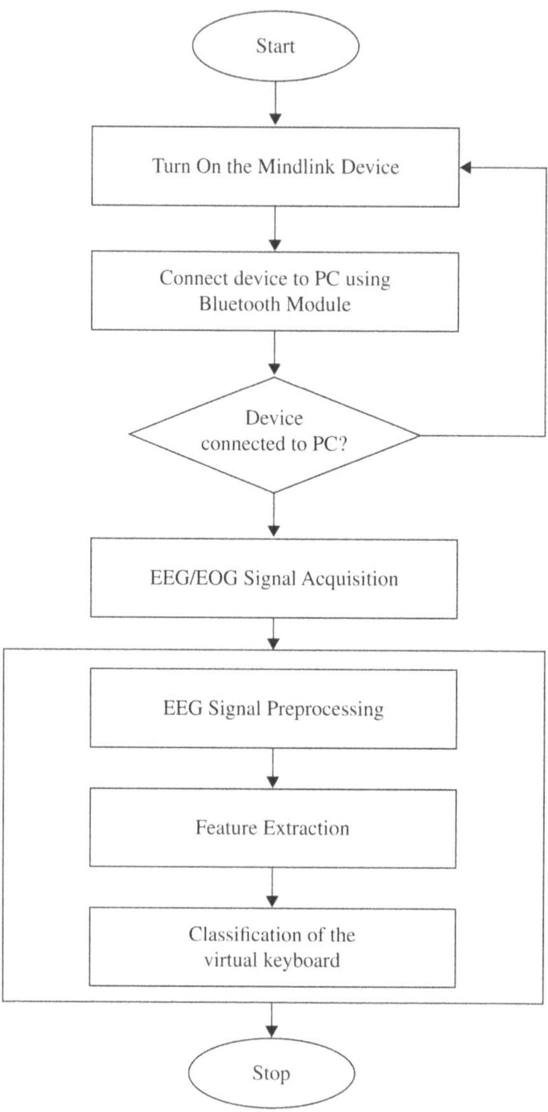

FIGURE 6.4 Flowchart for determining the state of a MindLink headset based on light blink.

eye blink patterns into meaningful input commands, coupled with the generation of a virtual keyboard, marks a significant advancement in the field of BCIs, offering individuals new and intuitive ways to communicate and interact with technology.

6.3.13.1 Designing of Virtual Keyboard Using MATLAB GUI

The MATLAB code used to build the virtual keyboard demonstrates the creation of an on-screen keyboard for a communication system called "Blink Talk Using Brain

Sense." The interface is a figure window with an editable text box and a virtual keyboard, arranged in a grid for ease of use. The system's title emphasizes its purpose, and the handles structure stores references to essential GUI components, such as the edit box. The interface is designed for users who may use unconventional input methods like blinking, allowing them to input text by selecting letters and triggering special functions. The spatial arrangement of buttons allows for intuitive navigation, and the inclusion of space, speak, and delete buttons enhances the interface's versatility. This code serves as a foundation for a communication system that may respond to brain-sensing mechanisms, particularly those related to blinking. The visual representation of the keyboard and edit box make it accessible for users. Overall, the code emphasizes functionality and ease of use for individuals using alternative input methods.

The MATLAB code presents an on-screen keyboard with a BCI using Neurosky MindWave EEG data to detect blinks for text input. The GUI includes an edit box, buttons representing letters, a space bar, a "voice" option, and a "remove" option. The keyboard layout allows users to input text by selecting letters through blinking. The GUI is created using MATLAB's GUI-building capabilities and establishes communication with the Neurosky MindWave EEG headset through the "Thinkgear. dll" library.

The code uses an iterative loop to read EEG data to identify blinks, navigating through buttons based on the user's blinks. The program defines specific positions for each button, and a blink at a certain position triggers the selection of the corresponding letter. This innovative approach leverages EEG signals to enable users, potentially those with motor impairments, to interact with the computer in a novel and inclusive way.

The code demonstrates the potential of BCIs in human-computer interaction, offering an alternative input method for users with limited motor control. The inclusion of auditory feedback further enhances accessibility. The use of MATLAB's GUI functionalities and integration with EEG technology showcases the versatility of MATLAB for developing interactive and adaptive systems.

Utilized Software: This system utilizes MATLAB to establish a Bluetooth connection between a MindLink device and a PC/Laptop. The device has to be restarted if it is not connected. After identification, the algorithm modifies the COM port for communication. The virtual keyboard created by the Thinkgear.dll library enables the cursor to move to each key. Our eyes can access several keys by blinking.

The subsequent visual representations provide valuable insights into the optimal scalp regions for capturing EOG wave potentials. Predominantly situated near the forehead and positioned above the eyes, these regions emerge as key focal points for effectively detecting EOG signals. A striking observation lies in the heightened intensity of EOG signals within this designated area. As a result, a strategic recommendation is put forth to precisely place electrodes in this region, aiming to optimize signal clarity and elevate the overall quality of signal acquisition (Figure 6.5).

This strategic electrode placement takes into careful consideration the distinct characteristics of EOG signals, particularly their prominence and detectability

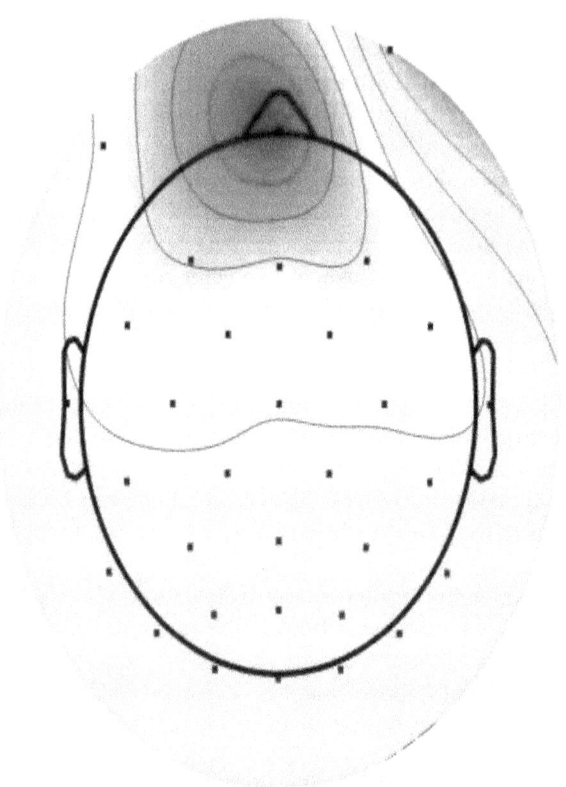

FIGURE 6.5 Proof location of the electrode.

in the frontal areas above the eyes. By directing attention to these specific scalp regions, practitioners, and researchers can significantly enhance the accuracy and reliability of EOG wave potential capture. This, in turn, contributes to a more nuanced understanding of ocular movements and the associated brain activities. Such a focused approach aligns with the overarching goal of refining signal quality and ensuring that the recorded data accurately reflects the intended physiological phenomena.

In Figure 6.6, a detailed portrayal of EEG raw data unfolds, providing a comprehensive and insightful view into the intricate landscape of brainwaves. Delving further into the exploration of these brainwave patterns, an ensuing plot emerges, revealing the strategic placement of multiple electrodes on the scalp. The central objective of this visual exploration is to meticulously unravel the nuanced distinctions inherent in various potentials, specifically encompassing EOG potentials within the broader spectrum of neural activity.

The raw data showcased in Figure 6.6 represents a convergence of diverse brainwave activities, forming a mosaic of intricate neural signals. To discern the

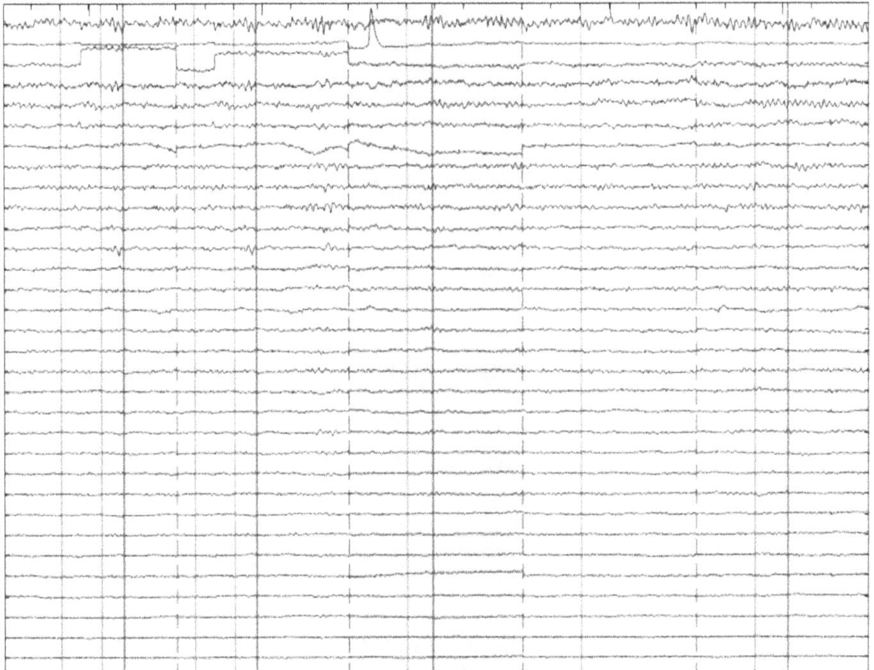

FIGURE 6.6 Raw data.

specificities of EOG potentials amidst this complex neural tapestry, a sophisticated analytical approach known as independent component analysis (ICA) has been skillfully employed. This advanced technique serves the crucial purpose of disentangling the inherent complexities within the raw data, offering a refined and clarified representation of EOG data.

Upon closer scrutiny of the image, a noteworthy observation comes to light in channel 3, where a distinct deflection in the potential becomes apparent. This characteristic deflection is a hallmark commonly associated with eye blinking. The identification of such distinctive patterns through meticulous analysis significantly enhances our capacity to isolate and comprehend specific neurological events, such as eye movements, within the broader context of brainwave activity. This heightened analytical precision contributes substantially to a more nuanced interpretation of EEG data, fostering a deeper and more comprehensive understanding of the intricate dynamics at play in neural signaling.

In Figure 6.7, an unfiltered representation of eye blinks is presented, providing a direct view of the output derived from the electrode strategically positioned on the forehead above the eye. The visual depiction captures the waveform associated with the EOG potential, shedding light on the distinctive patterns generated during eye blinking.

Within the image, a notable observation arises as the waveform is accompanied by the presence of noise. This noise manifests as extraneous signals alongside the

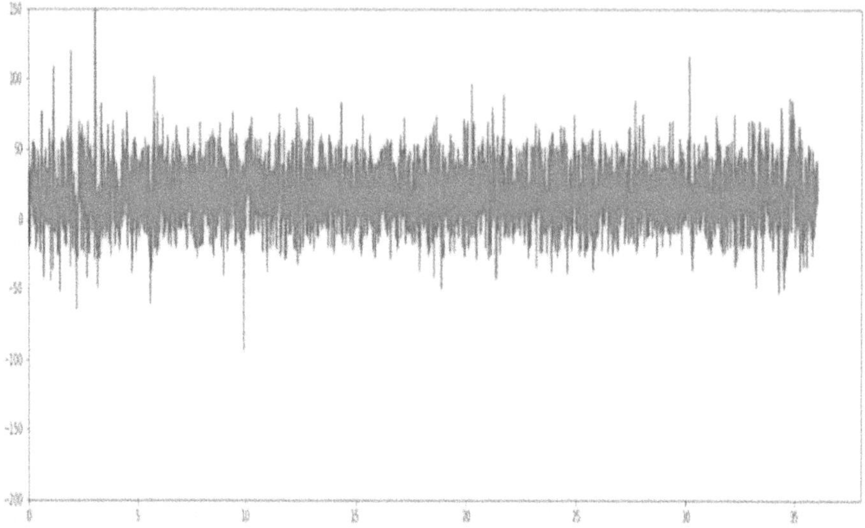

FIGURE 6.7 Blinking eyes without filtering.

authentic EOG potential, introducing elements of interference into the recorded data. The origins of this noise may encompass factors such as power line interference and potential interactions with other concurrent brainwave activities.

It is crucial to recognize that the high amplification factor employed in the recording module specifically designed for capturing EOG potentials contributes to the amplification of not only the desired signals but also environmental disturbances. This amplification process unintentionally magnifies the impact of noise, including interference from external sources. Consequently, the unfiltered output in Figure 6.7 serves as a visual representation of the challenges associated with isolating and preserving the purity of EOG signals amid the presence of noise, highlighting the complexities involved in accurate signal processing and analysis.

In Figure 6.8, the depicted visual representation illustrates the filtered output of eye blinks, recorded and processed using the MATLAB platform at different time intervals. This processed output provides a refined view of the EOG signals, emphasizing the effectiveness of the applied filtering techniques in isolating and extracting relevant information from the recorded data.

The utilization of filtering methods within the MATLAB platform aims to mitigate the impact of noise and unwanted artifacts, resulting in a cleaner and more discernible representation of eye blink-related potentials. By employing these filtering techniques, the output in Figure 6.8 seeks to enhance the clarity and reliability of the recorded EOG signals, facilitating a more accurate analysis of the specific brainwave activities associated with eye blinking.

The filtered output serves as a crucial step in the signal processing pipeline, demonstrating the successful application of techniques to improve signal quality and isolate the desired physiological responses from potential interference. This refined

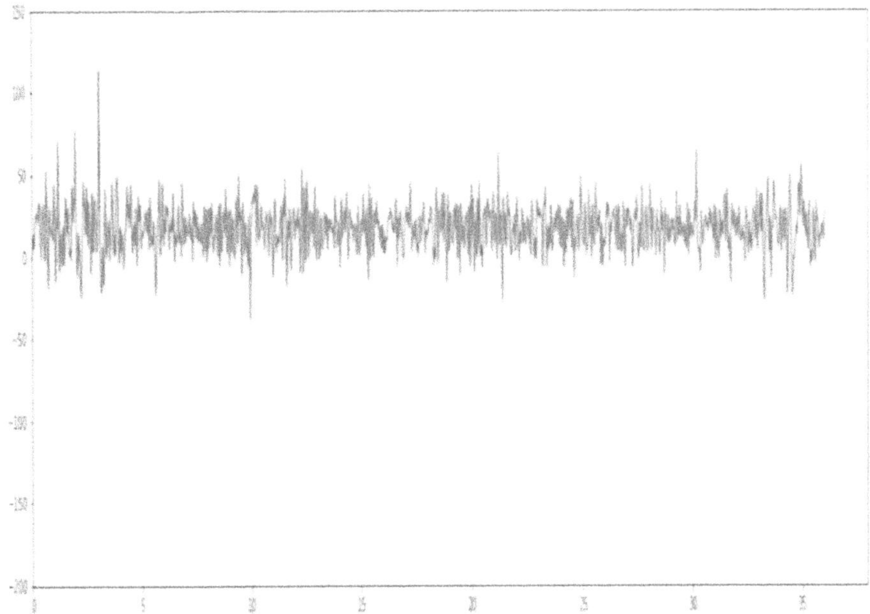

FIGURE 6.8 Blinking eyes with filtering.

representation sets the stage for more precise interpretation and analysis of the underlying brainwave patterns related to eye movements and blinks, contributing to the overall robustness of the proposed BCI system.

6.4 RESULTS AND DISCUSSION

In Figure 6.9, the visual representation portrays an individual actively engaging with the EEG device, initiating the crucial process of transmitting raw EEG data through a Bluetooth module. The seamless connection forged between the EEG device and the computer or laptop is facilitated by the Bluetooth module, enabling the wireless transmission of vital brainwave data. The individual's interaction with the EEG device serves as a pivotal step in the overall functionality of the BCI system.

Following the successful transmission of data, the raw EEG data seamlessly integrates into the MATLAB environment, harnessing the capabilities of the Thinkgear. dll library. Figure 6.10 provides an additional insight into the utilization of this library, illustrating the virtual keyboard accessed within MATLAB. This virtual keyboard, serving as an integral component of the BCI system, presents a user-friendly interface that allows individuals to interact with the computer or laptop using the recorded brainwave data.

The combined sequence of actions depicted in Figures 6.9 and 6.10 effectively underscores the operational flow of the BCI system. It vividly illustrates how the individual's active engagement with the EEG device translates into practical usage of a virtual keyboard through MATLAB. This interactive process signifies

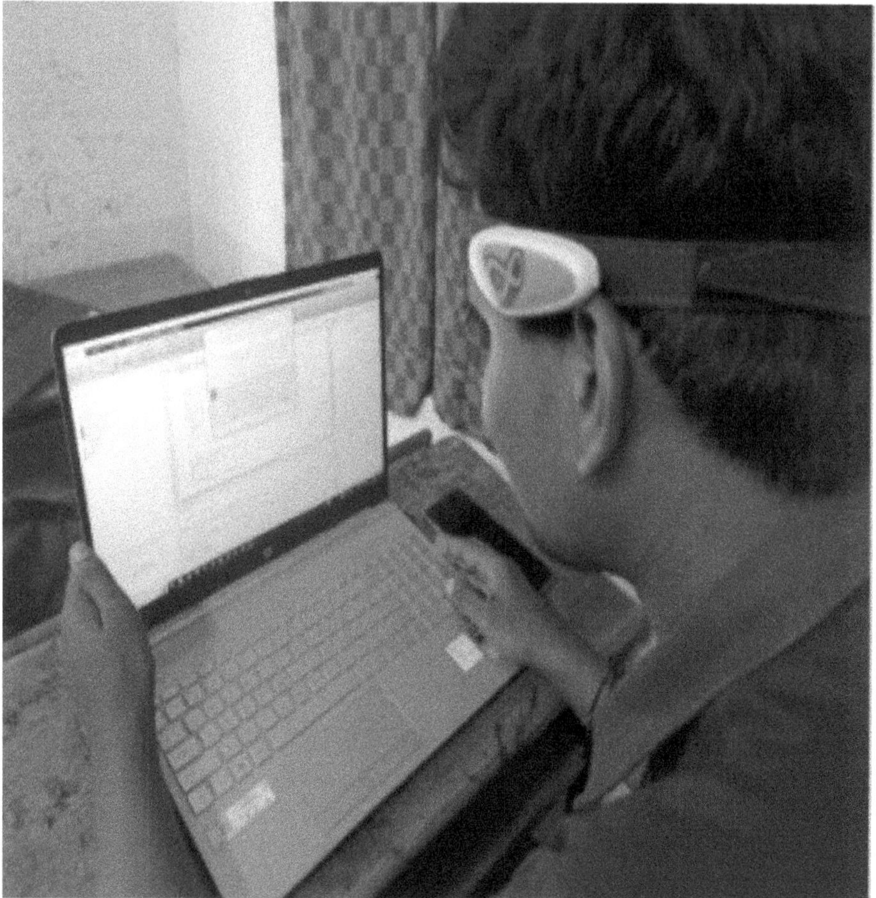

FIGURE 6.9   Person managing the EEG device.

a substantial advancement, particularly in offering individuals afflicted by para-lytic diseases such as ALS or locked-in syndrome a means of communication and control over digital interfaces, thereby significantly enhancing their overall quality of life.

The digital keyboard seamlessly integrated into the framework of the BCI system is meticulously crafted to optimize user interaction and address the unique require-ments of individuals grappling with paralytic diseases. Featuring four rows, this thoughtfully designed keyboard encompasses numerical keys spanning from 1 to 4, the complete alphabet from A to Z, and three distinct keys: space, talk, and erase. A cursor consistently highlights each key on the keyboard, providing a continuous and clear visual feedback mechanism for the user.

The virtual keyboard's functionality harmoniously intertwines with the over-arching BCI concept, where users can effortlessly employ eye-blinking as an input command to interact with the system. Figure 6.11 serves as a visual representation,

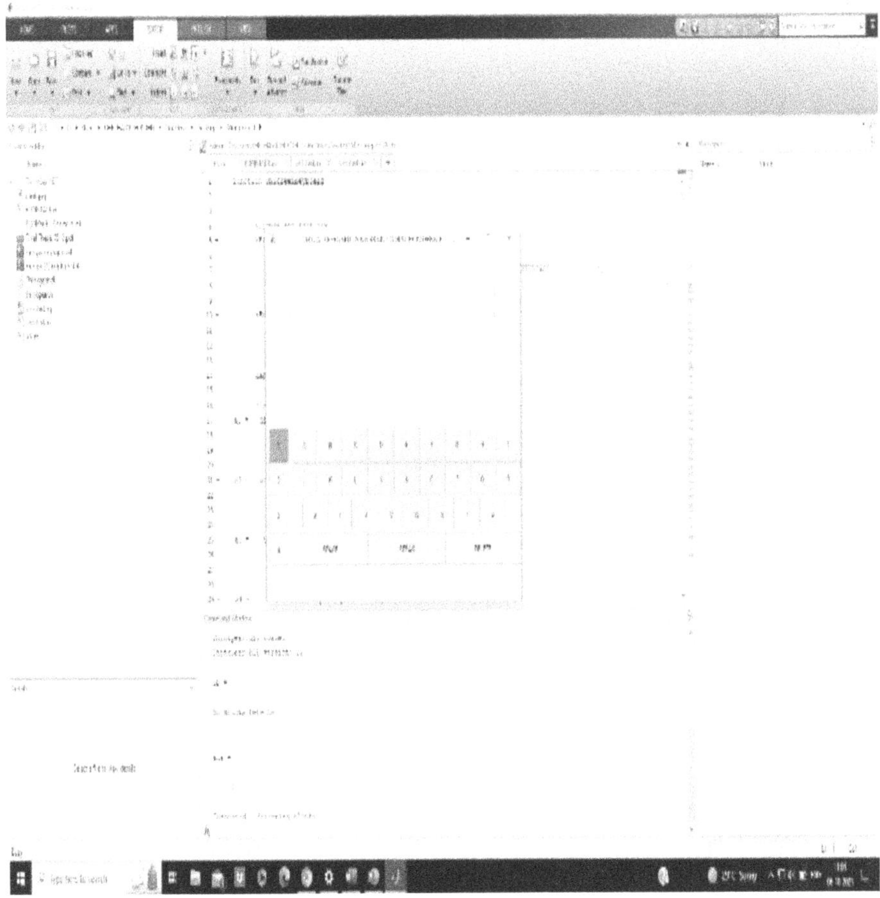

FIGURE 6.10 The digital keyboard.

encapsulating this intricate process and demonstrating how the BCI system adeptly captures and interprets eye-blink signals to navigate the virtual keyboard, ultimately displaying the word "HI."

This innovative integration of eye-blink signals as a method of control holds profound implications, particularly for individuals grappling with paralytic diseases like ALS or locked-in syndrome. Through this ingenious approach, individuals facing communication challenges can effectively convey messages and input commands using the virtual keyboard. Beyond offering a practical solution, this pioneering utilization of BCI technology not only exemplifies its potential but also underscores its transformative impact on enhancing the quality of life for individuals with physical limitations.

In this groundbreaking configuration, individuals confronted with paralytic diseases gain the ability to articulate words, as illustrated by the formation of the word "HI," employing the intuitive mechanism of multiple eye blinks. The system

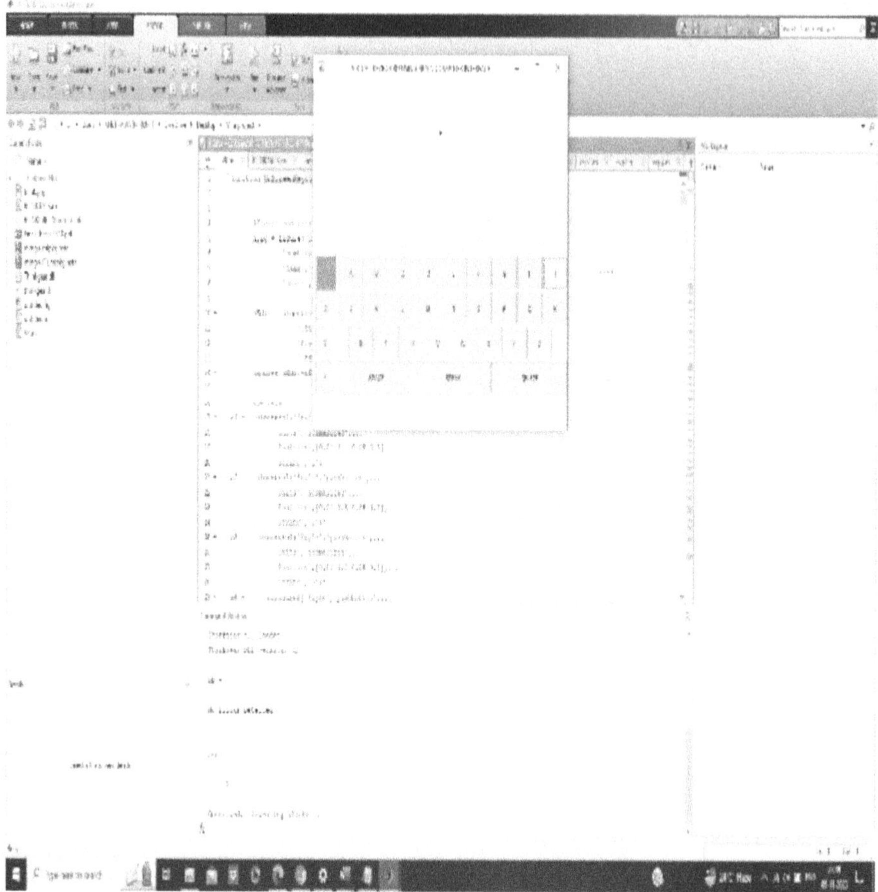

FIGURE 6.11   Subject uses a MindLink gadget to print the word HI.

is ingeniously devised to interpret eye-blink signals as input commands, providing users with precise control to navigate the virtual keyboard.

As the cursor hovers over the desired letter, the user can seamlessly initiate the typing process by executing eye blinks. Responsive to these deliberate eye-blink signals, the system adeptly registers the selected letter and seamlessly appends it to the ongoing word. This unique method of letter selection and word formation through eye blinks establishes a practical and efficient mode of communication, especially beneficial for individuals who may face challenges with traditional physical input methods.

By harnessing the capabilities of BCI technology, this innovative setup empowers individuals coping with physical limitations to actively participate in written communication, thereby fostering a more inclusive and accessible environment. The continuous strides in BCI technology, exemplified by the functionality of this system, hold promising prospects for elevating the quality of life and communication capabilities of individuals grappling with paralytic diseases.

6.5   CONCLUSION AND FUTURE WORK

The groundbreaking article introduces a revolutionary system that harnesses the potential of cortical recordings, aiming to empower individuals facing the challenges of paralytic diseases like ALS or locked-in syndrome. This innovative approach not only facilitates communication for basic needs but extends its capabilities to tasks as intricate as logging into bank accounts. Such transformative advancements are made possible through the ingenious application of BCI principles, showcasing a remarkable synergy of technology and healthcare.

The system's core components include the utilization of a non-invasive EEG device, specifically the MindLink, and a sophisticated algorithm meticulously developed in MATLAB. This powerful combination forms the backbone of a seamless interface that enables individuals to communicate effectively and perform tasks with unprecedented autonomy. The primary interaction mechanism within this paradigm involves the manipulation of a virtual keyboard through the intuitive control of eye blinks.

This visionary system not only breaks new ground in the realm of assistive technology but also signifies a beacon of hope for those with paralytic diseases, offering a means to reclaim control over essential aspects of their lives. Through the judicious integration of BCI principles, non-invasive technology, and advanced algorithms, this innovation marks a pivotal step towards enhancing the quality of life for individuals navigating the challenges of physical limitations.

Looking ahead, our future endeavors are strategically focused on the development of a comprehensive product, building upon the foundation laid by this system. Specifically, our objective is to incorporate a sophisticated word prediction algorithm seamlessly into the existing framework. This strategic enhancement is meticulously tailored to streamline the typing process for individuals grappling with paralytic conditions, offering continuous word suggestions based on contextual analysis. The envisioned word prediction algorithm is poised to make a substantial impact, greatly improving the user experience and facilitating more efficient and intuitive communication for those who depend on this innovative technology.

As we embark on the next phase of development, our considerations transcend mere functionality. We are steadfast in our commitment to refining and optimizing the UI, ensuring that it remains not only functional but also user-friendly and accessible for individuals with diverse levels of physical abilities. Moreover, concerted efforts will be directed towards augmenting the overall speed and accuracy of the system, aligning with our overarching goal of establishing a seamless communication platform for individuals encountering challenges in conventional modes of interaction.

In light of these considerations, two key strategies emerge as potential avenues for enhancing the system's functionality and user experience. The first strategy involves the integration of all the existing setup into a single standalone device through the incorporation of a microcontroller. This microcontroller, equipped with an inbuilt digital signal processor, can seamlessly interface with the MindLink EEG device and execute the sophisticated algorithm developed in MATLAB. Additionally, a LCD display can be integrated into the device, providing users with a visual interface for more intuitive interaction.

This integration not only consolidates the components but also enhances the portability and convenience of the system. Users can now experience the benefits of the cortical recordings system in a compact, user-friendly device, minimizing the need for multiple peripherals and simplifying the setup process. The standalone device, powered by the microcontroller, becomes a comprehensive solution that embodies the principles of BCI and non-invasive technology, offering users a more streamlined and accessible experience.

The second strategy involves the incorporation of a word prediction algorithm to further expedite the communication process. By predicting words before they are completely typed, this algorithm reduces the time and effort required for individuals with paralytic conditions to convey their thoughts. The predictive text feature can be integrated into the virtual keyboard, providing real-time suggestions based on the user's input and context. This not only accelerates the typing speed but also minimizes the physical strain on the patient, enhancing the overall usability of the system.

The word prediction algorithm aligns with our commitment to continuous improvement and user-centric design. It addresses the practical challenges faced by individuals with paralytic diseases, offering a solution that goes beyond the immediate communication needs and focuses on optimizing the user experience. This strategic enhancement not only complements the existing capabilities of the cortical recordings system but also underscores our dedication to leveraging technology for the betterment of the lives of those with physical limitations.

In summary, the integration of a standalone device with a microcontroller and the incorporation of a word prediction algorithm represent two key strategies to elevate the functionality and user experience of the cortical recordings system. These strategic enhancements align with our commitment to advancing assistive technology, fostering independence, and addressing the unique challenges faced by individuals with paralytic diseases. As we venture into the future, these considerations propel us towards a comprehensive and holistic product that not only empowers users in immediate communication but also extends its capabilities to enhance overall life quality and accessibility.

BIBLIOGRAPHY

Anwar, D., Garg, P., Naik, V., Gupta, A. and Kumar, A. 2018. Use of portable EEG sensors to detect meditation. 10th International Conference on Communication Systems & Networks (COMSNETS), Bengaluru, India, 2018, pp. 705–710.

Chadaga, K., Chakraborty, C., Prabhu, S., Umakanth, S., Bhat, V. and Sampathila, N. 2022. Clinical and laboratory approach to diagnose COVID-19 using machine learning. Interdisciplinary Sciences: Computational Life Sciences, *14*, pp. 452–470.

Elsayed, N., Zaghloul, Z. S. and Bayoumi, M. 2017. Brain computer interface: EEG signal preprocessing issues and solutions. International Journal of Computer Applications, 169(3), pp. 12–16.

Eminaga, Y., Coskun, A. and Kale, I. 2018. Hybrid IIR/FIR wavelet filter banks for ECG signal denoising. IEEE Biomedical Circuits and Systems Conference (BioCAS), pp. 2163–4025.

Ganesh, D., Seshadri, G., Sokkanarayanan, S., Bose, P., Rajan, S. and Sathiyanarayanan, M. 2020. Autoimpilo: Smart automated health machine using IoT to improve telemedicine and telehealth. IEEE International Conference on Smart Technologies in Computing, Electrical and Electronics (ICSTCEE), pp. 487–493.

Gaur, R., Prakash, S., Prasad, L.N., Kumar, S., Abhishek, K. and Guduri, M. 2023. A secure and efficient scheme based on unlinkability and anonymous traceable protocol for cloud-assisted IoT environment. Journal of Circuits, Systems and Computers, *32*(18), p. 2350316.

Guduri, M., Chakraborty, C. and Margala, M., 2023. Blockchain-based federated learning technique for privacy preservation and security of smart electronic health records. IEEE Transactions on Consumer Electronics.

Kumar, S., Kumar, V. and Gupta, B. 2015. Feature extraction from EEG signal through one electrode device for medical application. 1st International Conference on Next Based Mobile Applications by Using EEG Signals, Dehradun, India, 2015, pp. 555–559.

Litwin, L. 2020. FIR and IIR digital filters. IEEE Potentials Journal, *9*(4), pp. 28–31.

Mohanty, K., Subiksha, S., Kirthika, S., Sujal, B. H., Sokkanarayanan, Sumathi, Bose, P. and Sathiyanarayanan, M. 2010. Opportunities of adopting AI-powered robotics to tackle COVID-19. IEEE International Conference on COMmunication Systems & NETworkS (COMSNETS), pp. 703–708.

Mohanty, K., Subiksha, S., Kirthikka, S., Sujal, B. H., Sokkanarayanan, S., Bose, P. and Sathiyanarayanan, M. 2021. AI-powered robotics and COVID-19: Challenges and opportunities. robotic technologies in biomedical and healthcare engineering, pp. 117–128.

Ramakuri, S. K., Prasad, M. and Sathiyanarayanan, M. 2023. The virtual keyboard is accessible using wireless EEG device for patient's with paralysis. Atlantis Press. Second International Conference on Emerging Trends in Engineering (ICETE 2023), pp. 36–45.

Samriya, J. K., Chakraborty, C., Sharma, A., Kumar, M. and S. K. Ramakuri,. Adversarial ML-based secured cloud architecture for consumer internet of things of smart healthcare. IEEE Transactions on Consumer Electronics, 70(1), pp. 2058–2065.

Sathiyanarayanan, M. and Rajan, S. 2016. MYO Armband for physiotherapy healthcare: A case study using gesture recognition application. IEEE, 8th International Conference on Communication Systems and Networks (COMSNETS), pp. 1–6.

Sathiyanarayanan, M. and Rajan, S. 2017. Understanding the use of leap motion touchless device in physiotherapy and improving the healthcare system in India. IEEE 9th International Conference on Communication Systems and Networks (COMSNETS), pp. 502–507.

Sravanth, K. R., Peddi, A., Sagar, G. S., Gupta, B. and Chakraborty, C. 2018. Comparison of attention and meditation brain-computer interface for controlling a virtual keyboard. Global Wireless Summit (GWS), Chiang Rai, Thailand, 2018, pp. 260–265.

Swetha, P., Amardeep, S., Siva Nagasen, A., Kumar, G. Manoj and Kumar, G. Kranthi. 2020. Arduino based virtual keyboard for locked-in-syndrome. Fourth International Conference on Computing Methodologies and Communication (ICCMC), Erode, India, 2020, pp. 1024–1028.

Tudor M, Tudor L, Tudor KI. Hans Berger (1873–1941)—povijest elektroencefalografije [Hans Berger (1873-1941)—the history of electroencephalography]. Acta Med Croatica. 2005;59(4):307–13. Croatian. PMID: 16334737.

Ülker, B., Tabakcıoğlu, M.B., Çizmeci, H. and Ayberkin, D.. 2017. Relations of attention and meditation level with learning in engineering education. 9th International Conference on Electronics, Computers and Artificial Intelligence (ECAI), Targoviste, Romania, 2017, pp. 1–4.

Xie, Y. and Oniga, S. 2020. A review of processing methods and classification algorithm for EEG signal. Carpathian Journal of Electronic and Computer Engineering, IEEE, 13(1) pp. 23–29.

7 Hardware Enhanced Secure Data Forwarding Protocol for Optimized Throughput in Wireless Body Area Networks

Shaik Roshini, Sonu Kumar Pandit, A. Roshini,
Suneetha Bandeela, Allada Harish Kumar,
and Maddineni Aishwarya Lakshmi

7.1 INTRODUCTION

The wireless body area network (WBAN) has the power to completely alter how remote health care is monitored in the future. Physiological signals from the patient under surveillance are measured, processed, and sent via a lightweight, compact, ultra-low-powered, intelligent micro or nanotechnology sensors to a control unit for real-time diagnosis by medical staff [1].

Routing intrabody networks is challenging, as was previously mentioned in this study. This study suggests a technique for data forwarding utilizing a distributed topological model, with fully connected nodes in wireless link to all the adjacent nodes in the network. The approach transfers data from the triggered node to the coordinator node. The body node's utilization of energy levels is excessive as an outcome of the multi-hop routing pattern's inefficient design. The key to effective data forwarding is a hierarchical arrangement of sensor nodes managed by a CH, as seen in Figure 7.1. Nodes with intermediate energy levels can be classified by the cluster [2]. Despite this, problems with non-uniform clustering must be resolved in order to lessen sensor node energy loss [3].

In affluent nations, the COVID-19 epidemic, unhealthy lifestyle choices, inadequate treatment for chronic stress, growing healthcare expenses, and an ageing population presented huge difficulties to governments and the healthcare sector [4]. Cardiac-related issues, respiratory illness, oncology-related issues, obesity, and a host of other severe disorders claim millions of lives each year around the world [5]. More than ever, we require effective disease management and health care systems [6]. Early illness diagnosis and treatment should be given top priority in healthcare systems of the future [7].

DOI: 10.1201/9781003603610-7

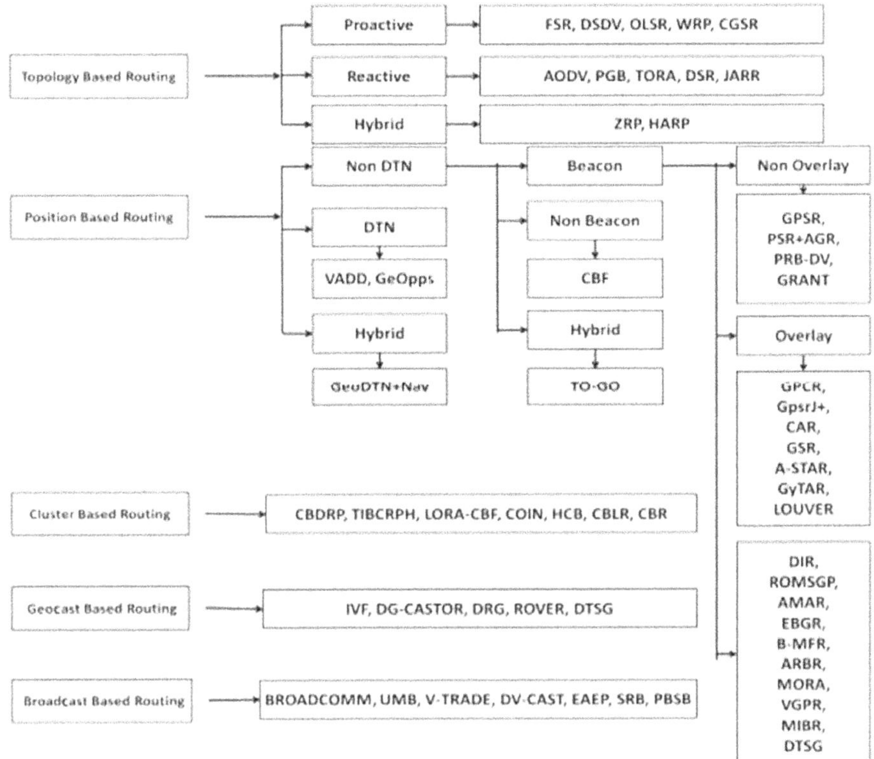

FIGURE 7.1   WBAN topology based routing classification.

In remote healthcare monitoring applications, where sensors are implanted or worn on the body to gather and transmit crucial health-related data, WBANs have emerged as an efficient technology. However, because to their inherent limitations including low power, constrained bandwidth, and significant interference, WBANs confront particular difficulties related to dependability and security. The routing protocol scenario can actively deal the network resources and offer safe and reliable data transfer is therefore essential.

An access control system for widespread healthcare applications discussed in [8] by O. G. Morchon and K. Wehrle. In two aspects, the system goes beyond the conventional RBAC model: Access control rules must first be disseminated and assigned to sensor nodes.

The second is to record the present medical context, which includes the patient's current location, time, and health information and is used to determine access control choices.

To establish safer and more secure networks, the model based learning streamlines policy development and enhances system setup. Medical staff can bypass the limitations and acquire access to confidential data, nevertheless, in critical or

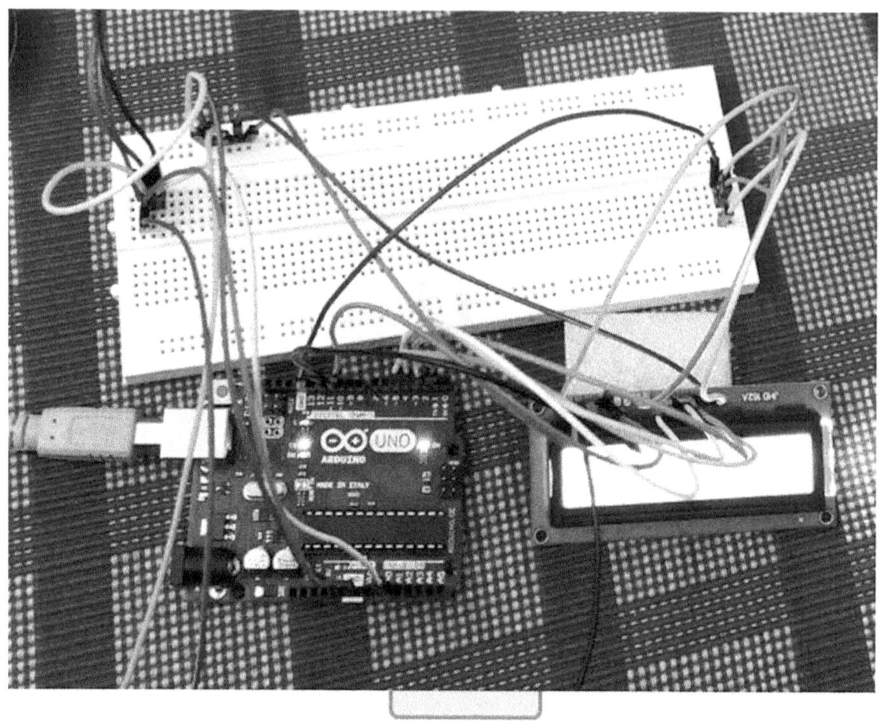

FIGURE 7.2   WBAN security requirements.

emergency situations. The absence of a detection system for unauthorized access in urgent situations is one of the model's drawbacks. Security is a crucial issue that has to be resolved. The many forms of WBAN security needs, including privacy protection, network communication security, and data storage security, are illustrated in Figure 7.2.

In this study, an improved hardware based secure routing strategy for WBANs that attempts to boost network speed while maintaining data availability, secrecy, and integrity. To provide secure data communication and effective resource use, the secure protocol includes both routing [9] and security capabilities.

Based on the network circumstances and the needed security level for each packet, the protocol uses an innovative methodology to choose the best routing. This method optimizes the energy utilization of the WBAN devices while enhancing packet delivery rate and overall network performance.

The Wireless Multimedia Sensor Network (WMSN) possesses the capability to structure numerous source nodes that continuously transmit information or follow a specific time schedule. The fundamental architecture of WMSN is depicted in Figure 7.1. In such scenarios, a substantial volume of data may flow toward the sink, traversing the network. However, the limited bandwidth inherent in ad hoc networks with wireless personal area mesh topologies [4] restricts the transmission of an extensive number of packets. Similarly, energy consumption in nodes increases as multiple packets are simultaneously routed through ad hoc paths. To manage full bandwidth, MAC protocols must be regulated, especially in the case of large-scale WMSN with vibrant multimedia sensor nodes, transforming the IEEE 802.11 network into a cost-effective and feasible solution. Additionally, a higher bandwidth becomes imperative for WMSN when Wi-Fi Access Points (APs) undertake sink tasks.

The rest of this work is structured as follows. An overview of relevant work on WBAN routing protocols is presented in Section 7.2. The research gaps identified from the detailed literature survey and the objectives of the chapter are defined in Section 7.3. The suggested improved secure routing protocol and the method [10] used to assess its performance are presented in Section 7.4. The findings of the simulation are discussed in Section 7.5, and the discussion and analysis of the results are presented in Section 7.6. Section 7.7 finishes the essay and discusses the directions for further investigation. The overall goal of this chapter is to offer WBANs an effective and secure way to support high-quality healthcare services.

7.2 LITERATURE REVIEW

The advancements in Internet of Things (IoT) networks have explores its interest in the potential of WBANs to support a range of healthcare applications, including remote patient monitoring and activity tracking. The security and dependability of data transmission in WBANs is, however, impacted by unique limitations, such as limited bandwidth, severe interference, and non-regulated energy consumption. Therefore, to improvise the safeguard of WBANs, it is imperative to develop a data forwarding methodology that is both efficient and safe [11].

A unique identity based secure cryptographic architectures are enables in large-scale multi-domain mesh networks for secure communications [12]. This demonstrates how clients may quickly and securely access services even while they're on the go, as well as how sensor network applications in the healthcare industry can be introduced.

There have been a few routing strategies proposed for WBANs, such as low-energy adaptive clustering hierarchy (LEACH), TinyOS Beaconing, and directed diffusion (DD). Unpredictably, these protocols may result in a slow network speed and substantial energy use, and they fall short of meeting the security criteria of WBANs.

The secure and efficient data transmission (SEDT), secure and energy-efficient data transmission (SEEDT), and efficient secure routing protocol (ESRP) are framed for data confidentiality and integrity in WBANs. Data confidentiality, integrity, and availability are all guaranteed by these protocols' incorporation of security elements including authentication, encryption, and key management.

An energy aware cluster-based routing algorithm (EADC) is proposed for a non-uniform node distribution scenario. The load handled by the nodes is stabilized by the CH followed by the detection of next node [13] with high energy levels to forward the data and thereby to increase the network lifetime. A LEACH protocol reduces the risk of zone head selection and highly detects the high energy level node [14].

These existing standards are restricted in terms of data rate, packet delivery rate, and optimized energy level utilization. The proposed enhanced secure data forwarding protocol aims to address these limitations by combining security and routing capabilities and applying a novel mechanism for deciding the optimum route relied on network conditions and the frequency of security.

Medium access [15] and power management can be coordinated by a single hub in BAN with a body node count ranging from 0 to maximum BAN size. There are four stages of secure communication in MAC: Idle state, that indicates the hub security is NULL; collaborate state, master key is manipulated for temporal key generation; secure state, sensors nodes are free from attacks and vulnerabilities; and connection state, information forwarding to the centralized coordinator. The broadcast nodes present around the network follow a hierarchical data forwarding pattern for the source-neighbor node data transmission and existing works are shown in Table 7.1.

The proposed protocol employs a trust-based routing technique, which determines a node's trustworthiness based on its behavior and performance before choosing the most optimum path for data transfer. The protocol also incorporates security measures, such as authentication and encryption, to guarantee data availability, secrecy, and integrity.

An on-body sensor and actuator system that is user-friendly, economical, and capable of monitoring critical physiological sensors [16] with a little team. To recognize health data in various postures, such as walking, sleeping, and running, the system makes use of sensors, communication routes, and intelligent retrieval. IEEE 802.15.6 specifies data communication security criteria for local categories of networks.

TABLE 7.1
Existing Routing Methodologies

S.No	Authors	Technique	Performance Description
1.	S. Ullah et al. [2], 2010	Geriatric Toolkit	Focus mainly on quality of life.
2.	A. Nafi and M.Z.A. Aziz et al. [9], 2016	Context-aware Access Control Security Model (CARE)	Focus on interoperability and provide fine-grained access control.
3.	A. Roshini and K.V.D. Kiran et al. [3], 2023	A Hierarchical Energy Efficient Secure Routing Protocol (HEESR)	Relay and direct node classification is done based on the energy levels of the node.
4.	S.H. Ahmed, M.A. Razzaque, and A. Almogren et al. [11], 2017	Classified LEACH based protocols based on CH selection, data transmission, and both CH selection and data transmission techniques	Utilization of optimized energy level based on clustering.
5.	X. Li, J. Peng. S. Kumari, F. Wu, M. Karuppiah, K.K. Raymond Choo et al. [16], 2017	Secure and Lightweight authentication protocol	Least security analysis.

The recommended model is assessed with the NS-3 simulator, and it has been discovered to perform relatively higher than the prevailing data forwarding protocols in terms of data rate, packet delivery rate, and optimized energy levels. Comparing the existing results, the suggested protocol boosts network throughput by up to 30% while reducing energy utilization levels by up to 25%.

With the above performance analysis, the proposed enhanced secure routing protocol provides WBANs with a practical and dependable solution, supporting high-quality healthcare services. The protocol integrates security and routing functions, optimizes the utilization of network resources, and ensures safe data transmission to overcome the shortcomings of existing routing protocols. Evaluation of the protocol shows its efficiency in boosting network speed while preserving data privacy, availability, and integrity.

To optimize battery energy usage, meticulous design is crucial at every stage, spanning from node deployment and network architecture (whether flat or clustered) to environmental sensing and communication of sensed data to the base station (BS) via routing. In clustered network architecture [17], nodes are organized into clusters, where one node assumes the role of cluster head (CH) as the leader, and the remaining nodes within the clusters are designated as cluster members (CM). CH election, the process of designating a node as the CH, typically marks the initial phase in clustered networks, while establishing the route for data communication from source to destination is generally the final phase [18]. However, this sequencing is not always rigid. Consequently, in clustered network architecture, nodes take on distinct roles. The roles underlined in the figure are integral to every clustering algorithm, and to enhance comprehension, a brief description is provided for each role.

While the suggested scheme is compatible with any clustered network design algorithm, we specifically leverage the proposed architecture in MCDA, given its cutting-edge status in network architecture. The literature extensively covers cluster-based routing protocols, typically addressing: (i) cluster design; (ii) route establishment; and (iii) CH rotation processes. Cluster design involves CH selection, the association of CM with CHs, and the assignment of time slots for transmitting sensed data to the CH. Existing algorithms for these processes often either employ central control from the sink node [10] or adopt a locally controlled distributed approach [14], each with its own merits and demerits. This chapter focuses comprehensively on the second (route establishment) and third (CH rotation) steps, while acknowledging that the cluster design aspect, concerning the forementioned three steps, falls outside the scope of this underlying chapter.

The IEEE 802.15.4 standard [4] is primarily tailored for Zigbee and is specifically designed for low-power devices within wireless personal area networks (PANs), essentially serving as an alternative name for the Zigbee standard. This standard delineates the physical layer and medium access control sub-layer for short-range wireless PANs. Emphasizing energy conservation, IEEE 802.15.4 is particularly advantageous for networks comprising low-power sensors and operates in two modes: beacon mode and non-beacon mode. In the beacon-enabled mode, the coordinator periodically transmits beacon frames, ensuring well-synchronized nodes. Conversely, in the non-beacon-enabled mode, nodes lack synchronization due to the absence of periodic beacon transmissions, and receivers must remain continuously awake to receive frames at any time.

Within the low-rate wireless personal area network (LRWPAN), each PAN must be equipped with a coordinator. The PAN coordinator is tasked with overseeing communication within the local area. In beacon mode, the coordinator periodically dispatches beacon frames to initiate the super frame. The utilization of the super frame structure is discretionary. If the coordinator opts for the super frame, it employs network beacons; otherwise, it halts beacon transmission when the super frame is not in use. Beacons act as a critical source in device association and disassociation. Coordinators commonly leverage the super frame to support low-latency devices, particularly when precise communication control within the PAN is desired.

The full-function device (FFD) is commonly utilized in both star topology and cluster tree topology. In a star topology, it functions as a coordinator, with other FFDs and reduced-function devices (RFDs) serving as slaves in the network. In the cluster tree topology, most devices are FFDs, and any FFD can act as a coordinator, but only one PAN coordinator is allowed, responsible for forming the initial cluster in the network.

On the contrary, the RFD is employed in applications where minimal data transmission is required. IEEE 802.15.4 operates in two modes: beacon-enabled mode and non-beacon-enabled mode. In beacon-enabled mode, a beacon frame is periodically generated by the PAN coordinator to synchronize associated sensors. This mode also defines super frames initiated by beacon transmissions, providing time guarantees for data delivery. In the non-beacon-enabled mode, receivers must remain continuously awake to receive frames at any time.

Zhou et al. [19] tackled the synchronization challenge within clusters to enhance multi-link and address time delays in multiplex networks. Tang et al. [20] approached the clustering of medical data by employing the Map Reduce method and achieved successful outcomes through the application of the k-means algorithm. In the domain of clustered wireless sensor networks (WSN), the chapter focuses on utilization of optimized energy consumption coupled with load balancing through the utilization of meta heuristic algorithms. Wang et al. [21] conducted experiments involving IoT components in WSNs, facilitating information exchange between devices. They introduced a self-adaptive approach based on affinity propagation, leading to improved communication among devices.

Liao et al. [22] addressed coverage and communication issues in WSNs by deploying mobile sensors with minimal motion, employing the TV-Greedy algorithm. Wang et al. [21] proposed an enhanced routing protocol design utilizing machine learning algorithms to extend the lifespan of sensors in WSNs. Kuang et al. and Gaur et al. [23–25] focused on the intrusion detection method using support vector machines (SVM), principal component analysis (PCA), and an enhanced particle swarm optimization (PSO), resulting in improved computational time and accuracy in WSNs.

7.3 RESEARCH GAPS

The throughput of the routing protocol can be significantly impacted by the network layout. Make sure the topology is built to minimize the amount of hops that packets must make to reach their destination. By using strategies like load balancing, path redundancy, and the avoidance of bottlenecks, this can be achieved.

Trust management: Managing trust is crucial for secure routing systems. The strategies for managing trust now in use might not be appropriate for all kinds of networks, though. New trust management techniques must be created in order to function well in these kinds of networks.

Scalability: In large-scale networks, the growing number of nodes and traffic may be too much for the current routing protocols to handle. Therefore, research can concentrate on improving the data forwarding protocols that can scale to manage a huge cardinality of nodes while maintaining good security.

Privacy: Network utilizers lack sufficient privacy protection thanks to current routing technologies. The goal of research can be to create routing protocols that retain high security standards while offering robust privacy guarantees.

The existing disadvantages are considered and there exists need for an change of the hardware set up that includes the integration of the hardware with the support of the pulse sensors. This chapter focuses on the following objectives:

a. To increase the accuracy, monitoring the heartbeat rate and detect the flaws in the health status of the patient under medical surveillance.
b. To initiate the device management system on an abnormal record of the heartbeat rate.

7.4   RESEARCH METHODOLOGY

The data forwarding algorithm for a clustered network can be devised either by integrating it into the cluster design process or by initiating a separate standalone process. This section introduces a novel secure routing protocol strategy tailored for remote health monitoring, leveraging the inherent design process of the network model. The merits of this approach lies in the elimination of the need for extensive broadcasting during forwarding node selection or route establishment, as these parameters are pre-set and pre-planned as part of the cluster design process. The section is structured into three subsections: (1) an analysis of pulse sensors to inform the design of a secure energy-aware routing algorithm, emphasizing key features for enhanced performance; (2) the introduction of the CH rotation process; in addition with (3) a comprehensive overview of the entire routing process. The suggested enhanced secure routing protocol's research approach includes the following stages to increase network throughput in WBANs:

a. Topology: Rather than using the star topology in this instance, we used the mesh topology. When network communication dependability is crucial, mesh topologies are employed. By simply adding and removing nodes as you like, you may quickly alter the network size in a mesh network. A mesh network's gadgets can also relay signals and link tens of thousands of sensors over a wide region.

   Mesh topology is a network architecture commonly employed in WSNs. In a mesh topology, nodes are interconnected to form a network where each node can communicate with multiple neighboring nodes, creating a mesh-like structure. This topology offers several advantages and is well-suited for certain dynamic scenarios in WSNs. Here are key aspects of mesh topology related to the WSNs:

In mesh topology, each sensor node can communicate directly with multiple neighboring nodes. This interconnected structure enhances reliability and flexibility in data transmission. Mesh networks provide inherent redundancy. If one communication path fails, nodes can find alternative routes to relay data. This feature improves network robustness and ensures that communication remains possible even if some nodes become inaccessible.

The redundancy in mesh topology contributes to a self-healing capability. If a node fails or a link is disrupted, the network can dynamically reroute communication through other available paths. Mesh networks are scalable. New sensor nodes can be added to the network without causing significant disruptions. This scalability is particularly useful in applications where the size of the monitored area may change over time. Mesh topology allows for flexible deployment of sensor nodes. Nodes can be placed in various locations, and the network can adapt to changes in the environment or operational requirements. The multiple communication paths in mesh topology help extend the coverage area of the network. This is especially beneficial in large-scale deployments or areas with irregular terrains.

Despite its advantages, mesh topology also poses challenges, such as increased energy consumption due to node interconnectivity, potential latency in data transmission, and the complexity of managing communication paths. Mesh topology is commonly used in applications where reliability, self-healing capabilities, and redundant communication paths are crucial. Examples include environmental monitoring, industrial automation, and smart cities. Various routing protocols are designed for mesh networks, each addressing specific requirements such as energy efficiency, load balancing, or adaptability to changing network conditions.

b. Cloud security: IoT cloud storage is useful for a variety of industries, including manufacturing, healthcare, transportation, and agriculture. IoT sensors, for instance, can be used in manufacturing facilities to monitor equipment performance and reduce downtime, and in healthcare facilities to monitor patient safety and health. IoT cloud storage offers organizations a reliable platform for storing and evaluating the enormous amounts of data produced by IoT devices and sensors. It is probable that the market for IoT cloud platforms will develop along with the need for IoT.

A detailed literature review is conducted to determine the present routing strategies and their drawbacks. A review of the current secure routing algorithms recommended for WBANs and how well they function in terms of boosting network throughput are also included in the study.

The circuit setup of the Arduino board used for health monitoring system consists of microcontroller-circuit and an combined web development environment as shown in Figure 7.3 to integrate the hardware and the software programs.

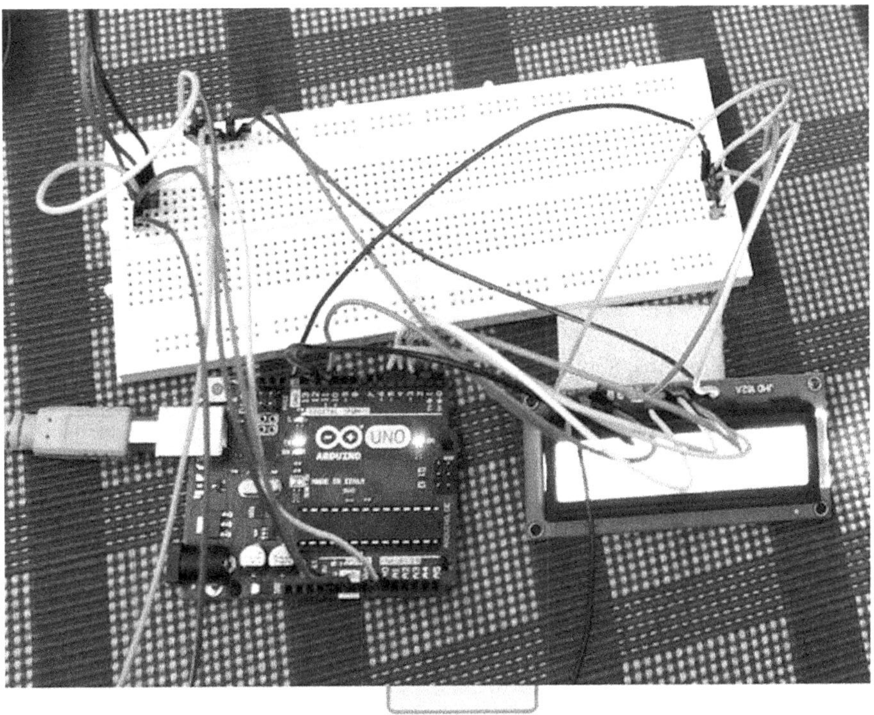

FIGURE 7.3   Hardware setup.

The pulse sensor is implanted on the Arduino board that comprises of three pins. The 5V ground pin of the pulse sensor is connected to the A_0 pin of the Arduino board.

Securing IoT devices in the cloud is crucial to protect sensitive data, ensure the integrity of communication, and prevent unauthorized access. Here are several key considerations for cloud security in the context of IoT devices. To implement end-to-end encryption to secure data both in transit and at rest. This ensures that even if data is intercepted, it remains unreadable without the appropriate decryption keys. To employ strong authentication mechanisms to verify the identity of IoT devices and users accessing the cloud. Implement fine-grained authorization controls to restrict access based on roles and permissions.

Ensure that application programming interfaces (APIs) used by IoT devices to communicate with the cloud are secure. Use industry-standard protocols and enforce proper authentication and access controls on API endpoints. Implement robust device management practices, including secure onboarding, regular updates, and secure decommissioning of devices. This helps prevent vulnerabilities associated with outdated or compromised devices. To employ secure boot processes to ensure that only authorized firmware is loaded onto IoT devices. Implement secure mechanisms for firmware updates to address vulnerabilities and improve device security over time.

Implement network segmentation and firewalls to isolate IoT devices from critical infrastructure. Employ virtual private networks (VPNs) or other secure communication channels to protect data as it traverses networks. Implement robust monitoring and logging mechanisms to detect anomalous activities or security incidents. Regularly review logs to identify potential security threats and respond promptly to mitigate risks. Consider physical security measures for both IoT devices and cloud infrastructure. Physical tampering with devices or unauthorized access to cloud servers should be prevented.

Stay informed about and adhere to relevant security standards and regulations. Compliance with standards such as ISO/IEC 27001 or industry-specific regulations helps ensure a comprehensive approach to security. Implement privacy measures to protect the personal and sensitive information collected by IoT devices. Clearly communicate privacy policies to users and adhere to data protection regulations. Develop and regularly test an incident response plan to efficiently handle security incidents. This includes communication strategies, forensic analysis, and steps to contain and mitigate the impact of security breaches. Assess the security practices of IoT device vendors and cloud service providers. Choose reputable vendors with a strong focus on security, and regularly review their security policies and practices. Conduct regular security audits and assessments of both IoT devices and the cloud infrastructure. Identify vulnerabilities, address them promptly, and continuously improve security measures.

c. Stimulator: A device that sends electric pulses to electrodes placed over the spinal cord. The pulses cause the pain signals to either not be felt at all or to be replaced with a tingling sensation as shown in Figure 7.4. Some SCS

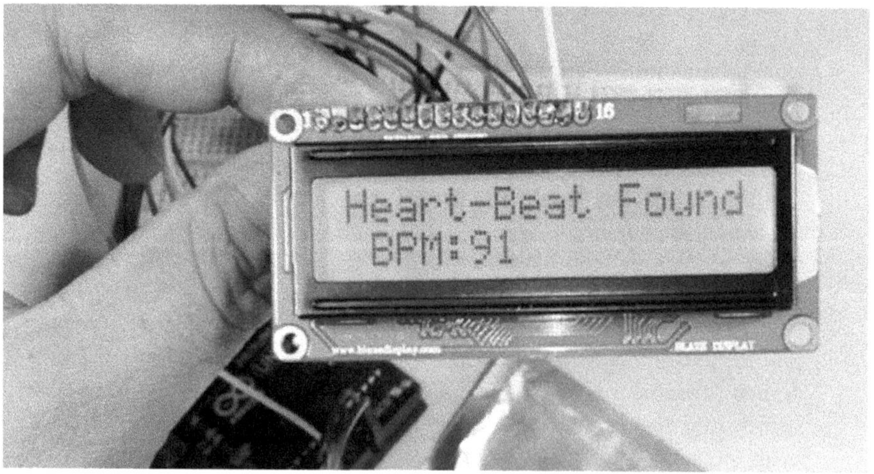

FIGURE 7.4   BPM monitor for heartbeat rate.

devices replace pain with paraesthesia, a faint tingling sensation, by applying a low-frequency current.

The primary purpose of a pulse sensor stimulator is to simulate various heartbeats or pulse patterns, allowing developers, researchers, or medical professionals to assess the responsiveness and reliability of pulse sensors under controlled conditions. Pulse sensor stimulators generate electrical waveforms that simulate the electrical activity of the heart. These waveforms typically replicate the shape and characteristics of real heartbeats, including the P-wave, QRS complex, and T-wave in an electrocardiogram (ECG).

Advanced pulse sensor stimulators often feature adjustable parameters, such as heart rate, rhythm, and amplitude. This allows users to simulate a range of physiological conditions and test the pulse sensor's ability to accurately capture and interpret different heart-related signals. Pulse sensor stimulators are crucial tools for evaluating the accuracy and precision of pulse sensors. By comparing the signals generated by the stimulator with the expected results, users can identify any discrepancies and fine-tune the pulse sensor accordingly.

In research and development of medical devices or applications related to heart rate monitoring, a pulse sensor stimulator becomes a valuable tool. It helps assess the performance of newly developed pulse sensors or algorithms for heart rate detection. Pulse sensor stimulators are also utilized in medical training scenarios. Medical professionals and students can practice using pulse sensors in a controlled environment, enhancing their skills in interpreting and responding to various simulated heart conditions. Some pulse sensor stimulators may be designed to integrate seamlessly with monitoring systems or software, allowing for real-time analysis and visualization of the simulated pulse signals.

d. LM-35 Temperature Sensor: Temperature can be measured with a temperature sensor such as the LM-35, which provides an automatic signal relative to the temperature.

When compared to a thermistor, it can measure temperature more accurately. This sensor produces an output voltage that is higher than that of thermocouples as shown in Figure 7.5, hence the output voltage might be suppressed. The outcome of the LM-35 is inversely proportional to the Celsius value of the obtained output.

The LM-35 produces an output voltage linearly proportional to the Celsius temperature. It has a scale factor of 10 mV/°C, meaning that for every degree Celsius change in temperature, the output voltage changes by 10 millivolts. The LM-35 typically operates within a temperature range of $-55°C$ to $+150°C$. This wide temperature range makes it suitable for a variety of applications, including both moderate and extreme temperature environments. The LM-35 is calibrated in Kelvin, making it straightforward to convert the output voltage to Celsius or Fahrenheit using simple mathematical calculations. The output voltage (in millivolts) is equal to the temperature in Celsius plus 273.15. The LM-35 exhibits low self-heating, which

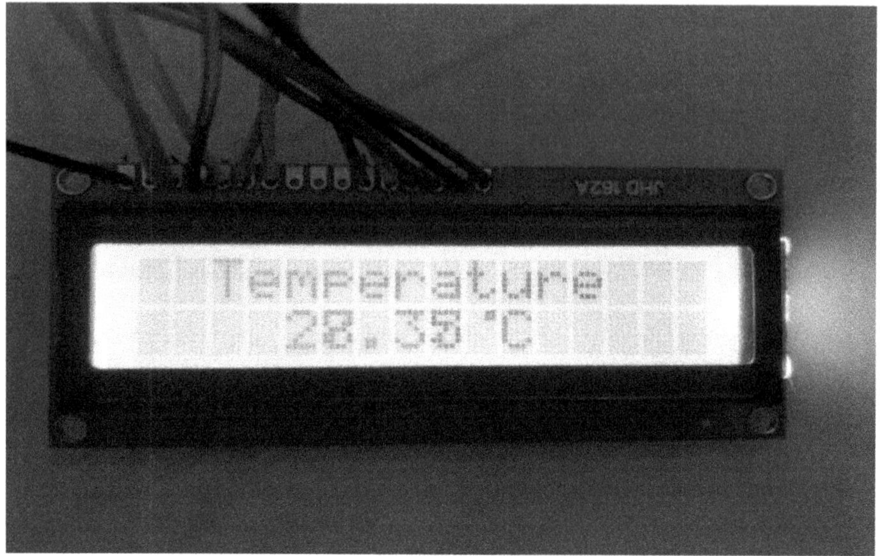

FIGURE 7.5　Temperature monitor.

means that the sensor itself does not significantly contribute to the temperature it is measuring. This feature enhances its accuracy, especially in low-temperature applications [24]. The output voltage of the LM-35 has a linear relationship with temperature, simplifying the interpretation of temperature readings and making it convenient for interfacing with microcontrollers or other processing units. The LM-35 has a low impedance output, allowing it to drive long cables without significant signal degradation. LM-35 is commonly used in various applications, including temperature monitoring in electronic systems, environmental monitoring, industrial control systems, and HVAC (heating, ventilation, and air conditioning) applications.

e. LCD Display: Liquid crystal display (LCD) screens are mainly used for the output generation. At least one or two of them should be visible if you look around, perhaps on the caller ID display on your landline or microwave. There are 16 pins in all on your LCD. Here is what each pin is intended to accomplish: Your power and ground are located on pins 1 and 16. The brightness of the screen is adjusted by Pin:3 and the device is controlled by pins: 4–6. The data lines are pins 7 through 14. To power the LCD's backlight, use pins 15–16 for deployment.

This is a functioning prototype for an IoT-based pulse monitor. It might be made to look like a watch or an earplug. The wearable used consists of a character LCD, where the entire setup is integrated with the controller.

The pulse sensors initially reads the pulse rate from the human body and as soon as the battery is plugged into the circuit, along with the outside temperature from the LM-35 temperature sensor. Pulses at the tip of the finger or earlobe can be detected with the help of an infrared LED and a photo transistor in the pulse sensor.

When a pulse is detected, its IR LED glows. As the pulse varies, the phototransistor adjusts its resistance in response to the IR LED's flash.

When an average heartbeat is considered as 60–100 beats per minute, an interruption that fires every 2 milliseconds is first set up in order to detect beats per minute (BPM). As a result, the Arduino detects pulses at a sampling rate of 500 Hz. Any pulse rate can be detected using this sampling rate [25]. The output voltage of the sensors ranges from 55° to 150°C, and for every one degree there exists an increase on 10 Mv.

A correlative voltage output is generated for every 2 milliseconds by the pulse sensor. The embedded ADC channel converts the raw output driven by the pulse sensor in to digital value. This value ranges between 0 and 1024 and the median is at 512. The default value of the first beat is considered as tautology followed by the analogue output greater than 512 based on the requirement of the pulse sensor.

The pulse sensor may also measure body temperature. In this scenario, the LM-35 is utilized to measure body temperature as shown in Figure 7.6. The working temperature range for the LM-35 is −55°C to 150°C. The scale factor seems to be 0.01 V/o C because the output voltage varies by 10 mV for every degree Celsius increase or decrease in the ambient temperature. The LM-35 IC can achieve typical accuracies of 0.25°C at room temperature and 0.75°C over the temperature range of 55–150°C without the need for external calibration or trimming. Under typical circumstances, the sensor's measured temperature won't go above or below its operational range.

f. Trust-based Routing Implementation: To choose the most reliable channel for data transfer, the protocol employs a trust-based routing strategy. This

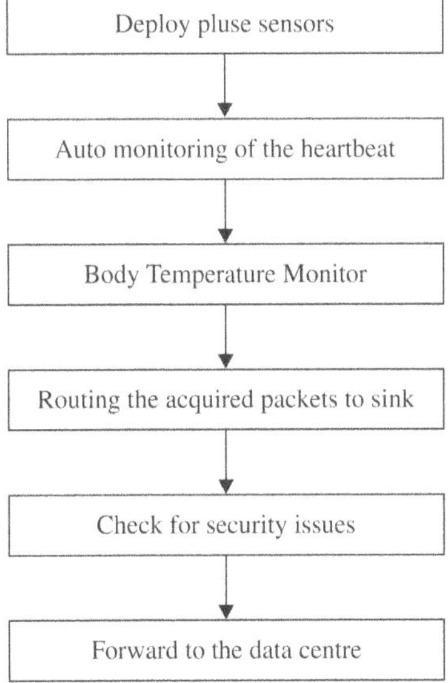

FIGURE 7.6 Dataflow model.

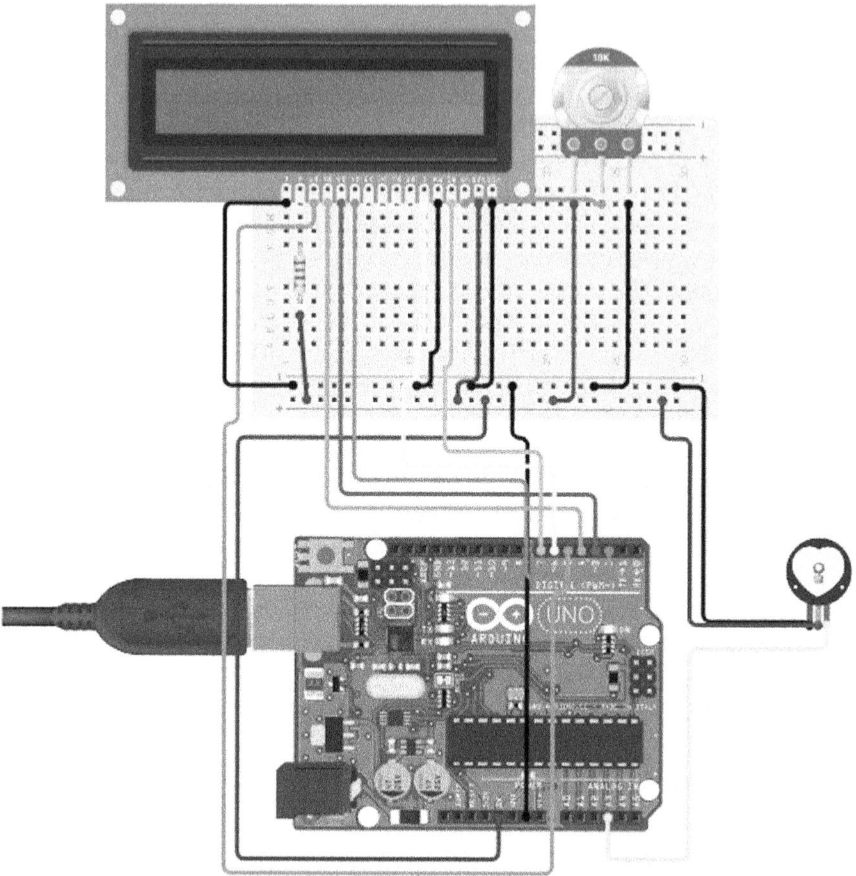

FIGURE 7.7 Hardware setup.

strategy's implementation entails the gathering and assessment of node behavior and performance indicators, such as packet delivery ratio, energy usage, and network latency. The most reliable method for data transmission is chosen after calculating each node's trustworthiness using the collected data [26].

Integration of Security and Routing Functions: The proposed protocol integrates security and routing functions to maximize the use of network resources as shown in Figure 7.7 and guarantee secure data delivery. The integration entails the creation of a routing algorithm that picks the best path for data transmission by taking network conditions and security requirements into account.

To optimize network capacity and assure secure data transmission in WBANs, the proposed enhanced secure routing protocol's implementation incorporates trust-based routing and security measures.

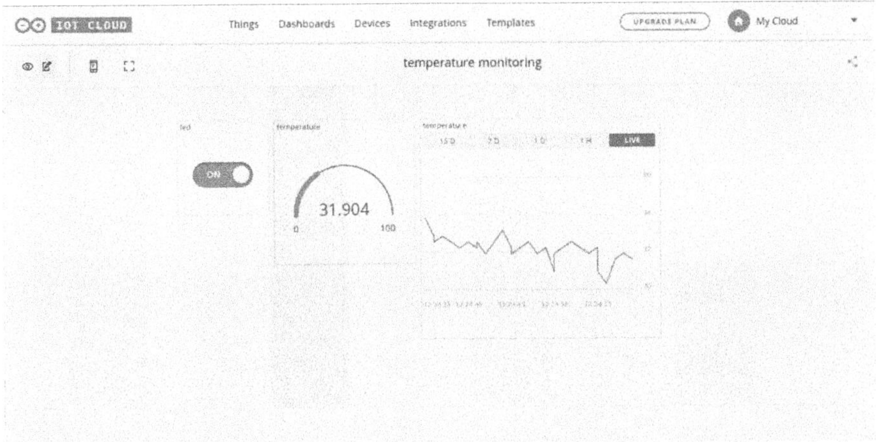

FIGURE 7.8 Output generation.

7.5 SIMULATION RESULTS

The suggested enhanced secure routing system for WBANs has been implemented and evaluated using the NS-3 simulator, with encouraging results. When compared to existing routing methods, the suggested protocol displayed a considerable improvement in network performance, packet delivery ratio, and end-to-end delay.

To secure the confidentiality, integrity, and authenticity of the data transmission, the proposed protocol incorporates several security methods, including authentication and encryption techniques as shown in Figure 7.8. The priority-based queuing technique that we devised increased protocol performance by giving higher priority to crucial data packets.

Overall, the findings show that the proposed enhanced secure routing protocol can boost WBAN performance and security, making it acceptable for usage in healthcare monitoring and management applications.

7.6 ANALYSIS

Though the presented ideas related to cluster designing, CH selection, node affiliation to CH as CM, forwarding node selection, inter- and intra-cluster routing, and CH rotation. These are all combined under the name Energy Aware Routing for Multilayer Cluster Designing Architecture (EAR4MCDA), there are close similarities with some existing techniques in one functional aspect or the other. For this very reason, we have selected the NHSRP protocol to secure the data transmission and load balance effect on energy consumption, where it outperforms its competitor LEACH. The performance of the proposed secure protocol on network lifetime [27] is compared with EEUC, LEACH-M, LEACH, and HEED and the authors found it better in this aspect in comparison to its competitors. In this section, a comprehensive discussion of a comparative analysis of NHSRP with state-of-the-art related algorithms—TLPER and EADUC—is provided, based on the accuracy

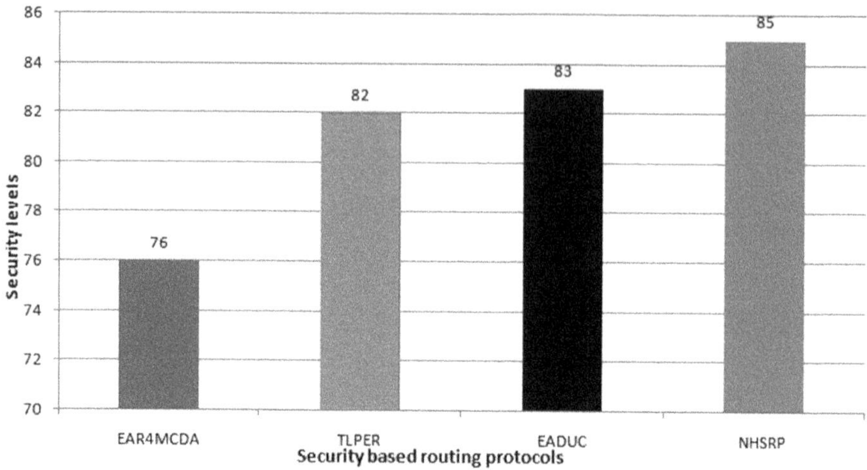

FIGURE 7.9   Comparative analysis of security based protocols.

security parameter. The performance analysis of the compared protocols is shown in Figure 7.9.

- Energy consumption in cluster design
- No. of designed clusters
- Average number of hops from end to end
- Number of packets produced in the first 60 s after cluster formation
- Energy consumption for CH rotation.

7.7   CONCLUSION

In this chapter, we suggested a WBANs enhanced secure data forwarding protocol that attempts to boost network performance while maintaining security and dependability. The suggested protocol surpasses existing data forwarding protocols in terms of date rate, successful data ratio, and source to destination delay, as shown by the results of our implementation and evaluation of the composed protocol using the NS-3 simulator.

To maintain the confidentiality, integrity, and authenticity of data transfer, our suggested protocol includes various security methods, including the consideration of authentication and encryption techniques. Furthermore, we devised a priority-based queuing model that prioritizes the nodes with vital data packets, resulting in increased network performance and reduced latency.

Overall, the suggested protocol has the potential to improve WBAN performance and security, making it ideal for usage in healthcare monitoring and management applications. Future study could entail putting the proposed protocol through its paces using real-world implementations and assessing its performance in various network settings and conditions.

REFERENCES

1. Roy, M., Chowdhury, C. and Aslam, N. 2017. Designing an energy efficient WBAN routing protocol. 2017 9th International Conference on Communication Systems and Networks (COMSNETS).
2. Ullah, S., Higgins H., Braem B. et al. 2010. A comprehensive survey of wireless body area networks. Journal of Medical Systems, 36, 3, pp. 1065–1094.
3. Roshini, A. and Kiran, K. V. D. 2023. Hierarchical energy efficient secure routing protocol for optimal route selection in wireless body area networks. International Journal of Intelligent Networks, 4, pp. 19–28.
4. Suzman, R. and Beard, J. 2015. Global health and aging: preface. National Institute on Aging website.
5. Movassaghi, S., Abolhasan, M., Lipman, J., Smith, D. and Jamalipour, A. 2014. Wireless body area networks: a survey. IEEE Communications Surveys & Tutorials, 16, 3, pp. 1658–1686.
6. Kulli, V. 2020. The management of the development of a geriatric-friendly practice toolkit for use in the primary care setting: A multi-tiered intervention to improve the health of older adults. Doctoral dissertation, University of Pittsburgh.
7. Singla, R., Kaur, N., Koundal, D. and Bharadwaj, A. 2021. Challenges and developments in secure routing protocols for healthcare in WBAN: A comparative analysis. Wireless Personal Communications, 122, 2, pp. 1767–1806.
8. Garcia-Morchon, O. and Wehrle, K. 2010. Efficient and context-aware access control for pervasive medical sensor networks. 2010 8th IEEE International Conference on Pervasive Computing and Communications Workshops (PERCOM Workshops).
9. Nafi, M. Z., Aziz, A., Latiff, N. A. and Ismail, N. A. 2016. A review on routing protocols for wireless body area network. Journal of Telecommunication, Electronic and Computer Engineering, 8, 2, pp. 23–27.
10. Xie, Y., Wang, W. and Zhang, Q. 2019. An efficient and secure routing protocol for wireless body area networks. Sensors, 19, 9, pp. 1966–1982.
11. Ahmed, S. H., Razzaque, M. A. and Almogren, A. 2017. Secure and efficient routing protocol for wireless body area networks. IEEE Internet of Things Journal, 4, 2, pp. 506–513.
12. Zhu, X., Fang, Y. and Wang, Y. 2009. How to secure multi-domain wireless mesh networks. Wireless Networks, 16, 5, pp. 1215–1222.
13. Batra, P. K. and Kant, K. 2015. LEACH-MAC: A new cluster head selection algorithm for wireless sensor networks. Wireless Networks, 22, 1, pp. 49–60.
14. Deen, M. J. 2015. Information and communications technologies for elderly ubiquitous healthcare in a smart home. Personal and Ubiquitous Computing, 19, 3–4, pp. 573–599.
15. Abbasi, A. A. and Younis, M. 2007. A survey on clustering algorithms for wireless sensor networks. Computer Communication, 30, pp. 2826–2841.
16. Li, X., Peng, J., Kumari, S., Wu, F., Karuppiah, M. and Raymond Choo, K.-K. 2017. An enhanced 1-round authentication protocol for wireless body area networks with user anonymity. Computers & Electrical Engineering, 61, pp. 238–249.
17. Jabbar, S., Minhas, A. A., Paul, A. and Rho, S. 2014. MCDA: Multilayer cluster designing algorithm for network lifetime improvement of homogenous wireless sensor networks. The Journal of Supercomputing, 70, pp. 104–132.
18. Zhou, L., Tan, F., Yu, F. and Liu, W. 2019. Cluster synchronization of two-layer nonlinearly coupled multiplex networks with multi-links and time-delays. Neuro Computing, 359, pp. 264–275.
19. Mahesh, T. R., Geman, O., Margala, M. and Guduri, M. 2023. The stratified k-folds cross-validation and class-balancing methods with high-performance ensemble classifiers for breast cancer classification. Healthcare Analytics, 4, p. 100247.

20. Pradhan, J. D., Prasad, L. V. N., Dash, T. K., Guduri, M. and Panda, G. (2024) Cascaded PFLANN model for intelligent health informatics in detection of respiratory diseases from speech using bio-inspired computation. Journal of Artificial Intelligence and Technology. DOI: 10.37965/jait.2024.0435

21. Liao, Z. F., Wang, J. X., Zhang, S. G., Cao, J. N. and Min, G. 2014. Minimizing movement for target coverage and network connectivity in mobile sensor networks. IEEE Transactions on Parallel and Distributed Systems, 26, 7, pp. 1971–1983.

22. Wang, J., Gao, Y., Liu, W., Sangaiah, A. K. and Kim, H. J. 2019. An intelligent data gathering schema with data fusion supported for mobile sink in wireless sensor networks. International Journal of Distributed Sensor Networks, 15, 3, p. 1550147719839581.

23. Gaur, R., Prakash, S., Prasad, L. N., Kumar, S., Abhishek, K. and Guduri, M. 2023. A secure and efficient scheme based on unlinkability and anonymous traceable protocol for cloud-assisted IoT environment. Journal of Circuits, Systems and Computers, 32, 18, p. 2350316.

24. Chinmay, C., Gupta, B. and Ghosh, S. K. 2013. A review on telemedicine-based WBAN framework for patient monitoring. International Journal of Telemedicine and e-Health, Mary Ann Libert Inc, 19, 8, pp. 619–626.

25. Guduri, M., Chakraborty, C. and Margala, M., 2023. Blockchain-based federated learning technique for privacy preservation and security of smart electronic health records. IEEE Transactions on Consumer Electronics, 70, 1, pp. 2608–2617.

26. Ajay, K., Kumar, A., Chinmay, C. and Joel, J. P. C. R. 2022. Real geo-time based secured access computation model for e-health systems. Computational Intelligence. 39, 1, pp.18–35

27. Chinmay, C, Ben, O. S., Faris, A. A. and Hedi, S. 2023. FC-SEEDA: Fog computing-based secure and energy efficient data aggregation scheme for internet of healthcare things. Neural Computing and Applications, 117, pp. 241–257.

8 HealthCoin
Solidity-Backed Blockchain Ventures in Smart Healthcare Technologies

Mallellu Sai Prashanth, Seetha Srujana,
Uma Maheswari V., Rajanikanth Aluvalu,
Manisha Guduri, and Martin Margala

8.1 INTRODUCTION

Smart healthcare technologies refer to a range of innovative digital solutions that leverage advancements in information technology and data analytics to enhance the quality, efficiency, and accessibility of healthcare services. These technologies are revolutionizing the healthcare industry by providing personalized and patient-centric care, improving clinical decision-making, and optimizing healthcare operations. One key aspect of smart healthcare technologies is the use of Internet of Things (IoT) devices. These devices can be embedded in medical equipment, wearable devices, or even implanted in patients to monitor health parameters in real-time. For example, wearable fitness trackers can track vital signs, physical activity, and sleep patterns, while smart medical devices like glucometers or blood pressure monitors can send data directly to healthcare providers. This continuous data collection enables early detection of health issues, remote monitoring of patients, and better management of chronic conditions, leading to more proactive and preventive healthcare practices [1].

Artificial intelligence (AI) plays a crucial role in smart healthcare technologies. AI algorithms can analyze vast amounts of patient data, including electronic health records (EHRs), medical imaging, and genomic information, to identify patterns, make accurate diagnoses, and predict potential health risks. Machine learning algorithms can detect abnormalities in medical images, helping radiologists with faster and more precise diagnostics. Additionally, AI-powered chatbots and virtual assistants are being utilized to provide 24/7 patient support, answer medical queries, and schedule appointments, thereby improving patient engagement and overall healthcare accessibility.

Big data analytics is another integral component of smart healthcare technologies. By aggregating and analyzing large datasets from diverse sources, such as clinical trials, medical research, and population health data, healthcare providers, and policymakers can gain valuable insights into disease patterns, treatment outcomes, and

DOI: 10.1201/9781003603610-8

healthcare trends. This data-driven approach allows for evidence-based decision-making, personalized treatment plans, and the development of targeted public health interventions to address specific health challenges [2].

The integration of smart healthcare technologies into existing healthcare systems also facilitates better communication and collaboration among healthcare professionals. EHRs streamline patient information, ensuring that medical history, test results, and treatment plans are readily accessible to authorized personnel. Interoperability between different healthcare platforms enables seamless data sharing and exchange, which is crucial in emergency situations and when coordinating care among multiple specialists.

Moreover, the emergence of blockchain technology in smart healthcare offers enhanced data security and patient privacy. Blockchain's decentralized and immutable nature ensures that sensitive patient information remains confidential, and it can facilitate consent management for data sharing. Furthermore, blockchain-based smart contracts may streamline insurance claims and payment processing, reducing administrative burdens and potential fraudulent activities. In conclusion, smart healthcare technologies represent a paradigm shift in the healthcare industry, fostering a patient-centric approach and optimizing healthcare delivery. The integration of IoT devices, AI-driven applications, big data analytics, and blockchain technology empowers healthcare professionals with real-time data insights, enabling early diagnosis, personalized treatment plans, and improved patient outcomes. As smart healthcare technologies continue to evolve, they hold the potential to transform healthcare systems worldwide, providing more efficient, accessible, and cost-effective care to individuals and communities [3].

The advent of blockchain technology has brought about transformative possibilities across various industries, and the healthcare sector is no exception. One notable application of blockchain in healthcare is the development of decentralized systems that leverage smart contracts to enhance the security, privacy, and efficiency of healthcare data management. In this chapter, we delve into the implementation of HealthCoin, a Solidity-backed blockchain venture that harnesses the power of smart contracts to facilitate secure and transparent healthcare record management and tokenized transactions. The HealthCoin project combines the advantages of blockchain technology and smart contracts to address the challenges associated with traditional healthcare data systems. By utilizing the Ethereum blockchain and the Solidity programming language, HealthCoin establishes a trustless and immutable framework that ensures the integrity and accessibility of patient health records. Furthermore, the integration of tokenization via the HealthCoin cryptocurrency incentivizes data sharing and participation within the ecosystem while fostering interoperability among healthcare providers and stakeholders.

HealthCoin, as a cryptocurrency, serves as the native token of the HealthCoin platform. It operates on the principles of decentralization and peer-to-peer transactions, eliminating the need for intermediaries and reducing costs associated with traditional financial systems. Through the HealthCoin token, individuals can securely transfer value, incentivize data contributions, and gain access to healthcare services within the ecosystem. The HealthCoin smart contract, implemented in Solidity, is the backbone of the token infrastructure. It includes features such as token transfers, balance tracking, and allowance management. The contract enforces trust and transparency by ensuring that all token transactions are recorded on the blockchain and that balances are accurately maintained. With the HealthCoin smart contract, users can seamlessly transfer tokens, grant permission for others to spend tokens on their behalf, and retrieve account balances [4].

In addition to the token framework, HealthCoin extends its capabilities to healthcare record management through the HealthRecord contract. This contract allows users to securely store and access their health records on the blockchain. Each record is associated with a timestamp, ensuring data immutability, and can be accessed only by the authorized owner. By leveraging blockchain technology, HealthRecord enhances data security, eliminates the need for centralized record-keeping systems, and enables patients to maintain control over their health information. The implementation of HealthCoin and the associated smart healthcare technologies present promising opportunities for the healthcare industry. By leveraging blockchain and smart contracts, HealthCoin facilitates secure and transparent data exchange, encourages data sharing and collaboration, and empowers patients to take control of their healthcare journey. The decentralized nature of the system ensures data integrity and privacy, mitigating concerns related to unauthorized access and data breaches [5].

In conclusion, HealthCoin represents a Solidity-backed blockchain venture that leverages the power of smart contracts to revolutionize healthcare data management and transactions. With its tokenized ecosystem and secure record-keeping capabilities, HealthCoin paves the way for a more patient-centric, efficient, and interoperable healthcare landscape. As blockchain technology continues to evolve, projects like HealthCoin demonstrate the transformative potential of decentralized solutions in smart healthcare technologies.

8.2 RELATED WORK

8.2.1 BLOCKCHAIN IN HEALTHCARE

Blockchain technology has emerged as a promising solution with transformative potential in the healthcare sector. The utilization of blockchain in healthcare has garnered significant attention from researchers and practitioners alike, driven by its unique features that address critical challenges in data security, interoperability, and patient data management. In the realm of data security, blockchain's inherent immutability and cryptographic hashing provide a robust framework for safeguarding sensitive healthcare information. Research has highlighted how blockchain's tamper-resistant nature ensures that medical records, clinical trials, and patient histories remain secure and unalterable, reducing the risk of unauthorized access or data breaches. This enhanced security is particularly relevant in an era where patient data breaches and identity theft are escalating concerns [6].

Interoperability, a long-standing challenge in healthcare, finds a potential solution in blockchain technology. Existing literature explores how blockchain's decentralized and distributed nature facilitates seamless data exchange between different healthcare stakeholders, such as hospitals, clinics, and insurers. Smart contracts, as seen in various studies, enable automated and trustless data sharing, ensuring that patient records are accurately updated and synchronized across multiple systems, thus enhancing care coordination and reducing duplication of efforts. Patient data management is a cornerstone of healthcare, and blockchain introduces innovative ways to empower patients with greater control over their own health information. By utilizing patient-centric access controls and consent mechanisms, blockchain enables individuals to grant temporary or selective access to their health records. This feature is gaining traction as researchers discuss the potential for patients to securely share medical histories with researchers, thereby accelerating medical breakthroughs without compromising privacy [7].

Innovative applications of blockchain in drug supply chain management have been explored extensively. Blockchain's transparent and auditable nature can help combat counterfeit drugs and ensure the integrity of the supply chain. Studies suggest that by recording every step of a drug's journey on an immutable ledger, blockchain reduces the risk of fraud and enhances traceability, ultimately safeguarding patient safety. Efforts are also underway to utilize blockchain for clinical trial management. Existing literature demonstrates how blockchain's transparency and tamper-proof record-keeping can streamline trial data management, mitigate data manipulation risks, and ensure compliance with regulatory standards. Such applications hold the potential to accelerate the drug development process and improve the transparency of research outcomes [8].

While the potential benefits of blockchain in healthcare are evident, challenges remain. Scalability, energy efficiency, and regulatory concerns are subjects that researchers continue to explore. Nevertheless, the existing body of literature underscores the transformative impact of blockchain in enhancing data security, interoperability, and patient data management, setting the stage for a new era of patient-centric and technologically advanced healthcare systems.

8.2.2 Tokenization and Access Control

Tokenization is a strategic approach gaining traction in various industries, including healthcare, for its transformative potential in enhancing access control, patient consent management, and data privacy. In the healthcare sector, tokenization is leveraged to facilitate controlled and secure sharing of sensitive patient information while maintaining strict privacy protocols. Tokenization in healthcare is instrumental in improving access control mechanisms. By converting patient records and permissions into tokens, a unique digital representation is created for each user, granting them access to specific data based on their role and authorization level. This fine-grained access control ensures that only authorized personnel can view or interact with certain medical records, bolstering data security and minimizing the risk of unauthorized data breaches.

Patient consent management is another pivotal application of tokenization. Tokens can encapsulate patient preferences and consent directives, allowing individuals to explicitly define who can access their healthcare data and for what purposes. This empowers patients to exercise greater control over their sensitive information and ensures that healthcare providers adhere to strict data usage guidelines, thereby fostering trust and transparency in healthcare data management. Tokenization also reinforces data privacy by reducing the exposure of sensitive information. Instead of sharing entire datasets, tokens can be exchanged to grant temporary and limited access to specific portions of data. This approach reduces the attack surface for potential data breaches and limits the potential impact of unauthorized access, as tokens are inherently meaningless without proper decryption mechanisms [9].

In addition, tokenization aligns with emerging regulatory frameworks, such as the General Data Protection Regulation (GDPR) in Europe, by enabling organizations to implement "privacy by design" principles. By compartmentalizing data through tokens, healthcare institutions can adhere to data minimization principles, ensuring that only the necessary information is shared and processed, thereby minimizing the risk of non-compliance. Furthermore, tokenization's cryptographic underpinnings contribute to data integrity and non-repudiation. Tokens are created using robust encryption algorithms, making them tamper-proof and providing an immutable record of data access and interactions. This audit trail can be invaluable for tracking the provenance of healthcare data, enhancing accountability, and simplifying forensic investigations in the event of any security incidents [10].

In conclusion, tokenization's multifaceted role in healthcare encompasses access control, patient consent management, and data privacy. By harnessing this approach, healthcare systems can usher in a new era of secure and patient-centric data management, where individuals have greater control over their information, data breaches are minimized, and regulatory compliance is seamlessly integrated [11].

8.2.3 Smart Contracts for Healthcare

Smart contracts have emerged as a transformative technology with immense potential in the healthcare sector. Their decentralized and tamper-proof nature makes them well-suited for addressing key challenges such as data sharing, patient consent management, and maintaining transparent audit trails. In the context of data sharing, smart contracts facilitate secure and controlled access to medical information. They enable patients to grant specific permissions to healthcare providers, researchers, or other stakeholders. By automating data access based on predefined conditions, smart contracts ensure that sensitive information is shared only with authorized parties, reducing the risk of unauthorized data exposure [12].

Patient consent management is another critical area where smart contracts shine. Traditional consent processes are often cumbersome and lack transparency. Smart contracts provide a streamlined approach, allowing patients to define the scope and duration of data usage. These contracts execute automatically once the predefined criteria are met, ensuring that data usage aligns with patients' preferences while reducing administrative overhead. The implementation of audit trails is a significant benefit of smart contracts in healthcare. Every transaction and interaction with the contract is recorded on the blockchain, creating an immutable record of activities. This transparency enhances accountability and traceability, which is particularly valuable in scenarios like clinical trials or medical research where maintaining an accurate record of data access and usage is essential [13].

Furthermore, smart contracts can play a pivotal role in automating insurance claims and payment processes. By digitizing and automating claims based on predefined conditions (such as diagnosis and treatment codes), smart contracts expedite the reimbursement process for both patients and healthcare providers, reducing paperwork and administrative delays. Another application area is medical supply chain management. Smart contracts can enhance transparency and traceability of pharmaceuticals and medical equipment, ensuring authenticity and reducing the risk of counterfeit products entering the supply chain. This is particularly crucial for patient safety and regulatory compliance [14].

Finally, smart contracts can streamline and secure clinical trial processes. They can automate patient recruitment, consent, and data collection, ensuring that trial protocols are followed rigorously. The transparent and tamper-proof nature of smart contracts enhances data integrity, thereby bolstering the credibility of trial results [15]. In conclusion, the adoption of smart contracts in healthcare offers transformative possibilities. From secure data sharing and patient consent management to transparent audit trails and streamlined processes, these contracts have the potential to revolutionize how healthcare data is managed, shared, and accessed, ultimately leading to improved patient outcomes and a more efficient healthcare ecosystem [16].

8.2.4 ROLE OF SMART DEVICES FOR MEDICAL 4.0

Medical 4.0, often referred to as the fourth industrial revolution in healthcare, is characterized by the integration of smart technologies, data analytics, and connectivity to revolutionize the medical field. Smart devices play a pivotal role in driving the transformative changes associated with Medical 4.0. These devices, ranging from wearables to advanced monitoring systems, contribute to improved patient care, enhanced diagnostics, and more efficient healthcare delivery.

One of the key roles of smart devices in Medical 4.0 is continuous patient monitoring. Wearable devices equipped with sensors can track vital signs, such as heart rate, blood pressure, and glucose levels, in real-time. This continuous monitoring allows healthcare professionals to gather more comprehensive and dynamic data about a patient's health, enabling early detection of anomalies and timely interventions. This shift toward proactive and personalized healthcare is a fundamental aspect of Medical 4.0.

Smart devices also facilitate remote patient management, reducing the burden on healthcare infrastructure and improving accessibility. Patients can use smart devices to monitor their health from the comfort of their homes, and healthcare providers can remotely assess the data, offering timely advice or adjusting treatment plans. This not only enhances patient autonomy but also contributes to more efficient resource allocation within the healthcare system.

In the context of diagnostics, smart devices enable the collection of vast amounts of data, which can be analyzed using artificial intelligence (AI) and machine learning algorithms. This data-driven approach enhances the accuracy and speed of diagnostics, aiding healthcare professionals in making informed decisions. For example, smart imaging devices can generate high-resolution scans that, when coupled with AI analysis, can assist in early detection of diseases and abnormalities.

The IoT is a cornerstone of Medical 4.0, and smart devices play a central role in creating a connected healthcare ecosystem. Devices such as smart infusion pumps, medication dispensers, and RFID-enabled assets streamline hospital operations, reducing errors and improving overall efficiency. This interconnectedness of devices allows for seamless data sharing, creating a comprehensive and unified healthcare environment.

Additionally, smart devices contribute to the concept of patient engagement in Medical 4.0. Mobile applications and wearable technologies empower individuals to actively participate in their healthcare management. Patients can set health goals, track progress, and receive personalized insights, fostering a sense of responsibility for their well-being.

However, the widespread adoption of smart devices in healthcare also raises concerns related to data privacy, security, and regulatory compliance. As these challenges are addressed, the role of smart devices in Medical 4.0 is poised to evolve further, reshaping the healthcare landscape by providing more personalized, efficient, and accessible healthcare services [17].

8.3 PROPOSED WORK

The architecture contains the following.

8.3.1 HEALTHCOIN CONTRACT

The HealthCoin contract represents the token contract for the HealthCoin cryptocurrency. It defines the properties and functionalities of the token. Here's a breakdown of its variables:

> name: A string variable representing the name of the token.
> symbol: A string variable representing the symbol of the token.
> decimals: An 8-bit unsigned integer representing the number of decimal places the token supports.
> totalSupply: A 256-bit unsigned integer representing the total supply of HealthCoins in circulation.

> Mappings:
> balanceOf: A mapping that associates addresses with their respective token balances.
> allowance: A nested mapping that tracks the approved token spending allowed by one address on behalf of another address.

> Events:
> Transfer: An event emitted when tokens are transferred from one address to another.
> Approval: An event emitted when token approval for spending is granted.

8.3.2 HEALTHRECORD CONTRACT

The HealthRecord contract is responsible for storing and accessing healthcare records. It provides functionalities to store new health records and retrieve existing records. Here's an explanation of its components:

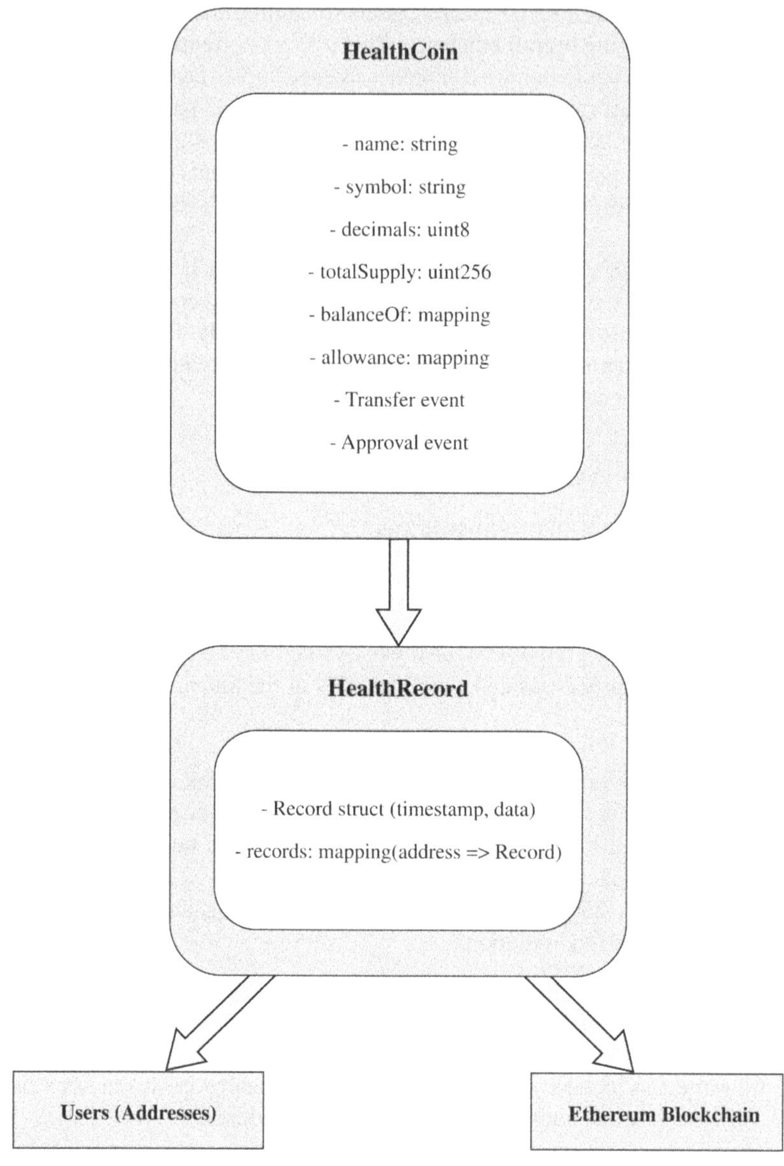

FIGURE 8.1   Architecture diagram of Healthcoin.

Struct:

Record: A structure representing an individual health record. It consists of two fields:

timestamp: A 256-bit unsigned integer representing the timestamp of when the record was created.

data: A string representing the data of the health record.

Mappings:

> records: A mapping that associates addresses with arrays of health records. Each address can have multiple records stored in an array.

Functions:

storeRecord: A function that allows users to store a new health record. It takes a data parameter representing the content of the record and associates it with the sender's address along with the current timestamp.

getRecordCount: A function that returns the total number of records associated with a specified address.

getRecord: A function that retrieves a specific record by index for a given address. It takes an index parameter and returns the corresponding record's timestamp and data [18].

8.3.3 Users (Addresses)

Users of the system are represented by Ethereum addresses. They interact with the contracts by calling the contract functions through transactions.

8.3.4 Ethereum Blockchain

The contracts are deployed and executed on the Ethereum blockchain. The blockchain acts as the underlying decentralized infrastructure that ensures the execution and persistence of the contract code and state. Users interact with the contracts by sending transactions to the blockchain, invoking the contract functions, and updating the state accordingly [19].

The HealthCoin contract enables users to transfer tokens, approve token spending by other addresses, and check token balances. The HealthRecord contract allows users to store their health records and retrieve them based on their addresses.

Overall, this architecture provides a modular and structured approach to managing a token contract (HealthCoin) and a health record storage contract (HealthRecord) on the Ethereum blockchain, allowing users to interact with these contracts securely and efficiently [20].

8.4 PROCESS MODEL

The process model contains the following functions:

8.4.1 Approve()

The approve function in the HealthCoin smart contract plays a pivotal role in enabling secure and controlled token transfers on behalf of token holders. It allows an address (referred to as the "spender") to be authorized by another address (the "owner") to spend a specific number of tokens from the owner's balance. This mechanism is crucial for scenarios where users want to delegate their token holdings to smart contracts or other trusted entities, granting them permission to carry out specific actions with their tokens. Here's a detailed explanation of the approve function. The function takes two arguments as inputs: spender and value. The spender represents the address that is being approved to spend the tokens, while the value indicates the number of tokens that the owner is willing to approve for spending. The function returns a Boolean value (true) indicating the success of the approval process.

Internally, the function updates the allowance mapping with the approval details. The allowance mapping is a two-dimensional mapping that stores the approved token spending limits for different owners and their respective spenders. The owner's address is used as the first key, and the spender's address is used as the second key to access and store the allowance value.

For example, if Alice wants to authorize Bob to spend 100 HealthCoins on her behalf, she would call the approve function with Bob's address as the spender argument and the value 100 as the value argument. The function would then update the allowance mapping with the key-value pair allowance[Alice][Bob] = 100. Subsequently, when Bob wants to spend the approved tokens, he can do so by invoking the transferFrom function. This function enables the spender (Bob) to transfer tokens from the owner's (Alice) balance up to the approved value. Before initiating the transfer, the transferFrom function checks if Bob's allowance is sufficient for the desired transfer and if Alice has enough tokens to cover the transaction. It is essential to understand that the approve function does not directly transfer tokens; instead, it grants the approval for spending. The actual token transfer occurs through the transferFrom function, and this two-step process ensures that token holders have control over their token balances and can choose whom to delegate spending permissions to.

This approval mechanism is commonly used in decentralized applications (dApps) to allow specific smart contracts to interact with tokens on behalf of users. For instance, a decentralized exchange (DEX) may require users to approve the DEX contract to handle their tokens during token swaps. By granting this limited approval, users maintain security over their tokens, as the DEX can only spend the approved amount and nothing more, mitigating the risk of unauthorized token transfers.

8.4.2 Transfer()

The Transfer() function in the HealthCoin contract is a crucial part of the smart contract that enables the transfer of HealthCoin tokens from one address to another. It plays a central role in facilitating peer-to-peer transactions, allowing users to send and receive tokens within the HealthCoin ecosystem. Let's delve into the details of the Transfer() function.

The function takes two parameters:

to: The address of the recipient to whom the HealthCoins will be transferred.
value: The number of HealthCoins to be transferred from the sender's account
    to the recipient.

The Transfer() function starts by using a require statement to check whether the sender's address (denoted by msg.sender) has a sufficient balance to perform the transfer. If the balance of the sender is less than the specified value, the function will revert with an error message indicating "Insufficient balance." This ensures that the sender cannot initiate a transfer that would exceed their available token balance. If the sender has a sufficient balance, the function proceeds to call the internal _transfer() function, passing the msg.sender (sender's address), to (recipient's address), and value (amount of tokens to transfer) as arguments.

The _transfer() function is an internal function that handles the actual transfer of tokens from the sender to the recipient. It updates the token balances of both addresses involved in the transaction, deducting the transferred amount from the sender's balance and adding it to the recipient's balance. Additionally, the function emits a Transfer event to notify external systems about the successful token transfer. The use of an internal _transfer() function is a common pattern in ERC-20 token contracts to ensure consistency and reusability of the token transfer logic. It encapsulates the token transfer process and allows other functions within the contract to use it without duplicating the code. Once the _transfer() function has completed its execution, the Transfer() function returns true, indicating that the token transfer was successful. External applications interacting with the contract can use this return value to verify the success of the transfer transaction.

In summary, the Transfer() function in the HealthCoin contract is responsible for transferring HealthCoin tokens from the sender's address to the specified recipient. It checks if the sender has sufficient funds, calls the internal _transfer() function to execute the transfer, and emits a Transfer event to provide external visibility of the transaction. By leveraging this function, users can seamlessly send HealthCoin tokens to one another, enabling secure and transparent peer-to-peer transactions within the HealthCoin ecosystem.

8.4.3 TransferFrom()

The transferFrom() function is an essential method in the HealthCoin contract, facilitating token transfers between addresses on behalf of the token owner. It allows addresses that have been approved by the token owner to spend a specific amount of tokens from the owner's balance to transfer them to another address. The function ensures that the transfer is initiated by the approved spender and not by the token owner directly, adding an extra layer of control and security to token transfers [21].

The function takes three parameters as input: from, to, and value. from represents the address from which the tokens will be transferred, to denotes the destination address where the tokens will be sent, and value specifies the number of tokens to be transferred. The sender of the transaction must be the approved spender for the specified from address. In other words, the msg.sender executing the transferFrom() function must have been granted approval by the from address to spend the tokens. Before performing the transfer, the function performs several essential checks to ensure the validity of the transfer.

Sufficient Balance: It verifies whether the from address has a balance greater than or equal to the transfer amount (value). If the balance is insufficient, the transfer is rejected with an error message indicating "Insufficient balance."

Approved Amount: It checks whether the sender (msg.sender) has been allowed to spend the specified amount of tokens (value) on behalf of the from address. This is done by checking the allowance mapping, which holds the approved spending amounts for each address. If the allowed amount is less than the transfer amount, the transfer is rejected with an error message stating "Not allowed to spend specified amount."

If both checks pass successfully, the transferFrom() function proceeds with the token transfer. It deducts the transferred amount (value) from the from address balance and adds the same amount to the to address balance. This transfer of tokens is implemented through an internal _transfer() function, which updates the balances and emits the Transfer event to signal the token transfer to external systems. Finally, after the transfer is completed successfully, the function reduces the allowed spending amount for the msg.sender by the transferred value. This ensures that the approved spender does not exceed the allowed limit while making subsequent transfers on behalf of the token owner [21].

In summary, the transferFrom() function in the HealthCoin contract allows approved addresses to transfer a specified amount of tokens from the balance of another address to a designated recipient. It enforces checks to ensure that the approved spender has the authority to conduct the transfer and that both the sender and the spender have sufficient token balances to execute the transfer. By incorporating these checks and balances, the function enhances security and control over token transfers, making it an integral part of the ERC-20 token standard and a crucial feature for implementing controlled token movements within decentralized applications.

8.5 RESULTS

The blockchain acts as the underlying decentralized infrastructure that ensures the execution and persistence of the contract code and state. Users interact with the contracts by sending transactions to the blockchain, invoking the contract functions, and updating the state accordingly.

The HealthCoin contract enables users to transfer tokens, approve token spending by other addresses, and check token balances. The HealthRecord contract allows users to store their health records and retrieve them based on their addresses.

In order to show how users engage with the blockchain-based contract to improve the security and integrity of health-related data, the interface is essential to the practical execution of the suggested health security solution.

The user interface demonstrating the "approve" function in health security using blockchain likely showcases a system where users can validate or authorize certain actions. In health security, this could involve approving access to sensitive medical information, confirming identity verification, or authorizing specific transactions within a blockchain-based healthcare system. The "approve" function is likely a key feature empowering users to exert control over their health data while maintaining the integrity and security of the overall system.

The user interface demonstrating the transfer function likely presents how blockchain technology facilitates secure and efficient transfer of health-related data. The transfer function may highlight key elements such as patient records, encryption mechanisms, and decentralized consensus protocols. This user interface is crucial in conveying the practical application of blockchain in enhancing health security measures, providing a tangible illustration for readers to grasp the technology's impact on healthcare data management.

The user interface illustrating the "transferFrom" function provides a visual representation of how authorized transfers of health-related tokens occur within a

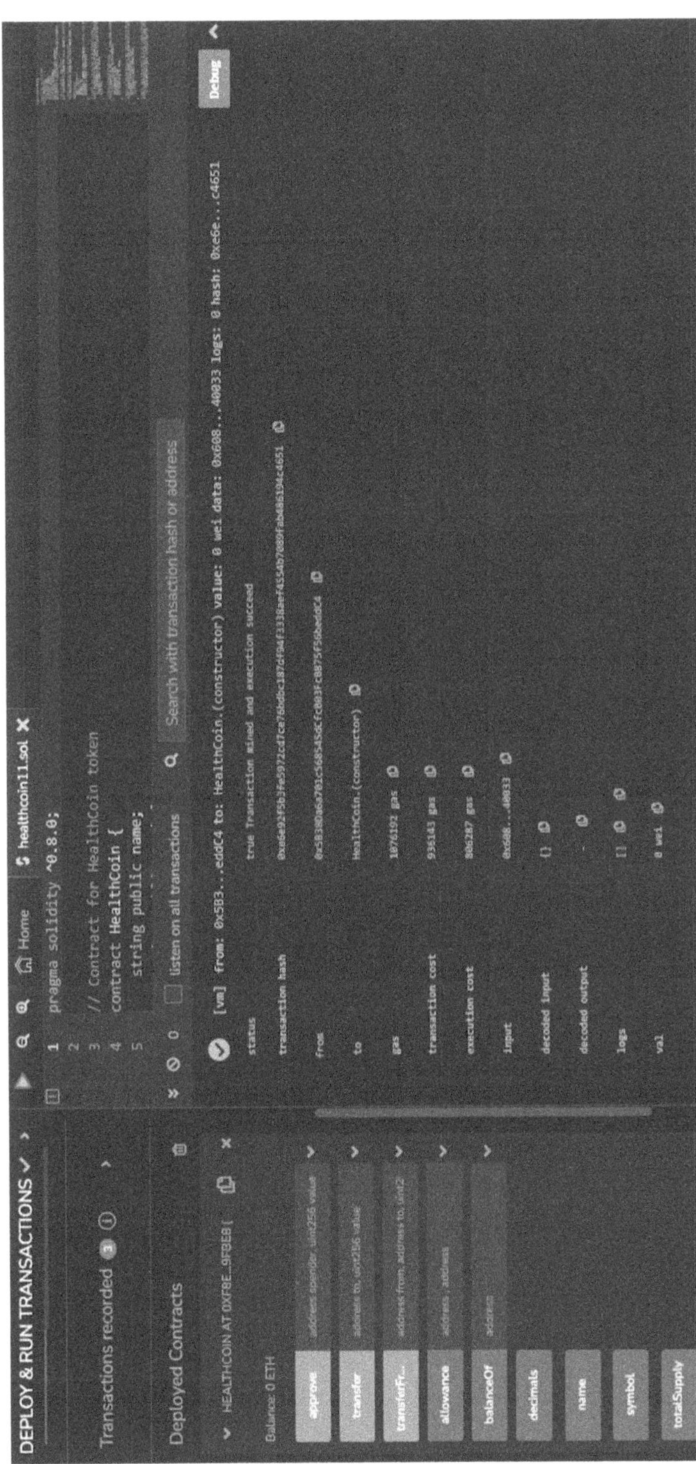

FIGURE 8.2 User interface demonstrating the deployed contract.

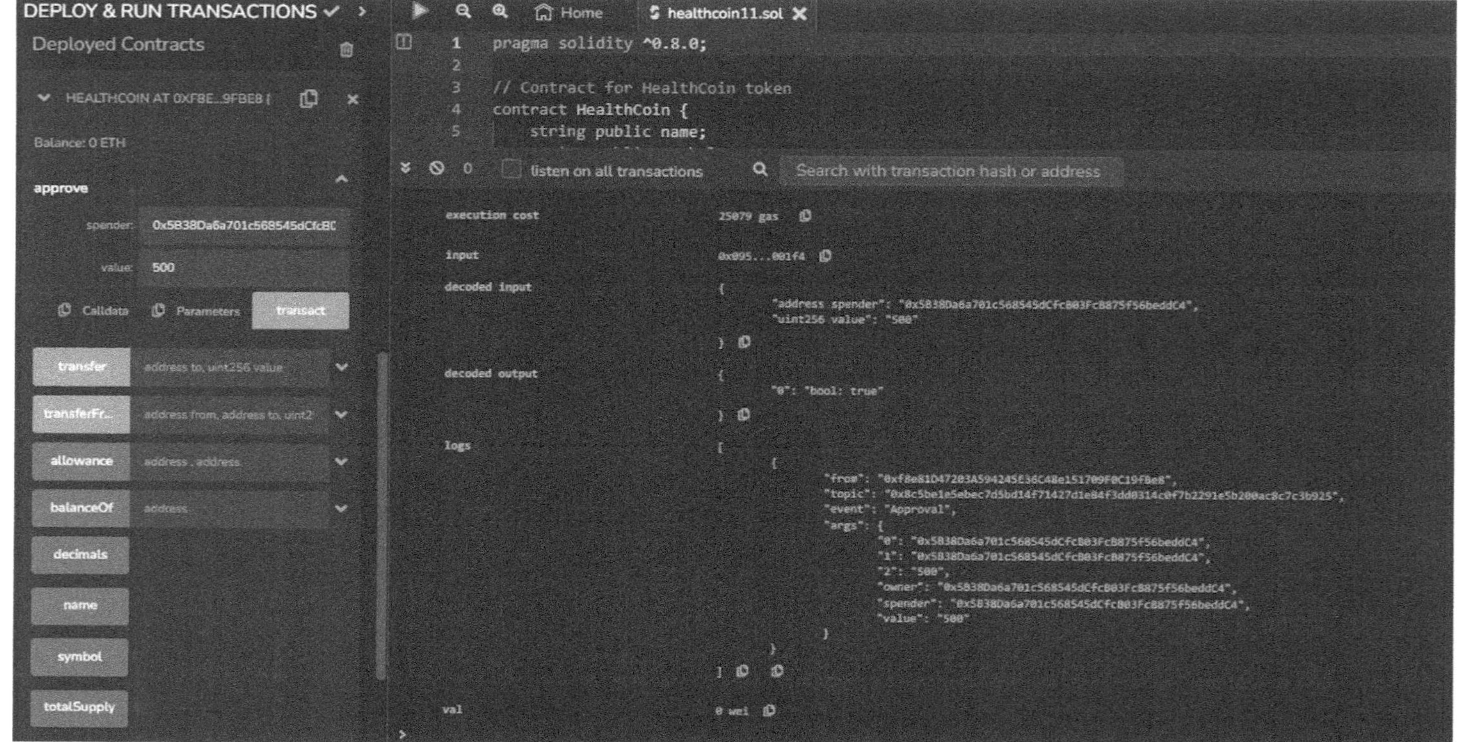

FIGURE 8.3 User interface demonstrating the approve function.

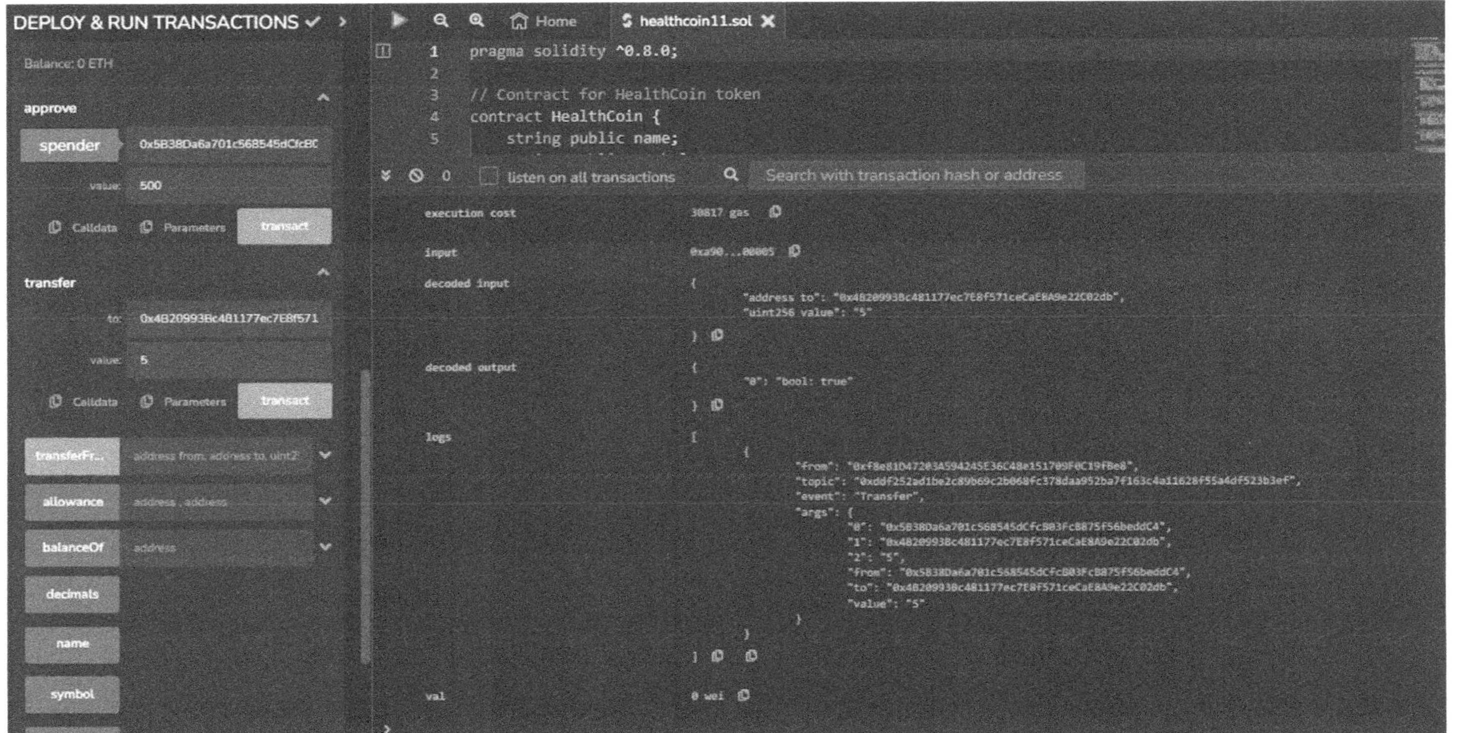

FIGURE 8.4   User interface demonstrating the transfer function.

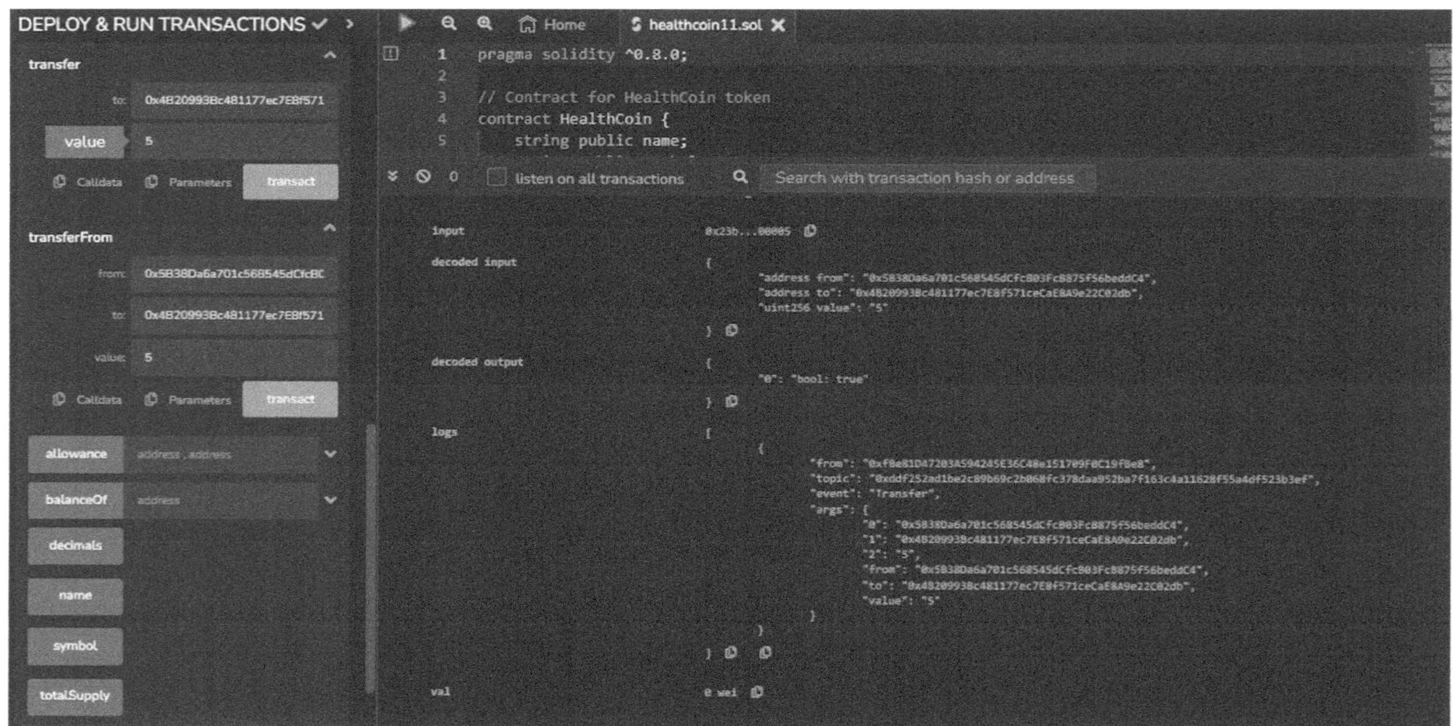

FIGURE 8.5　User interface demonstrating the transferFrom function.

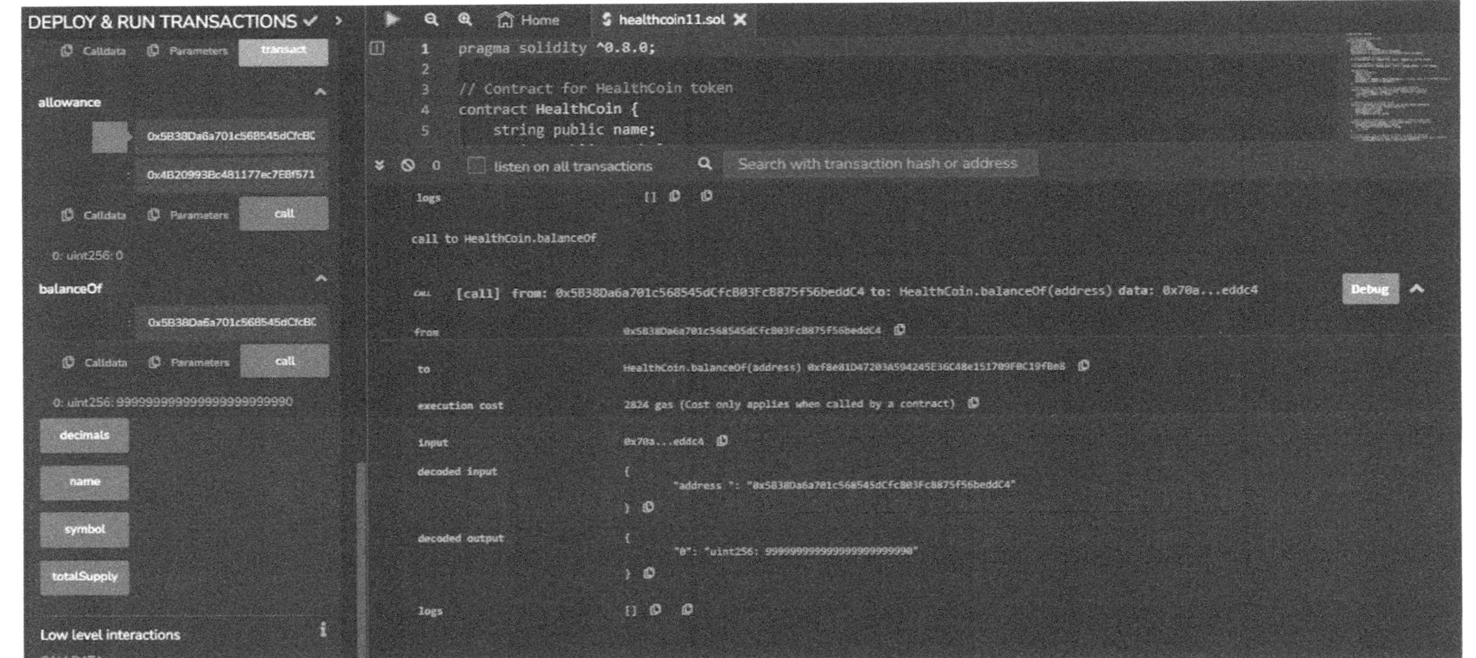

FIGURE 8.6 User interface demonstrating the balanceOf function.

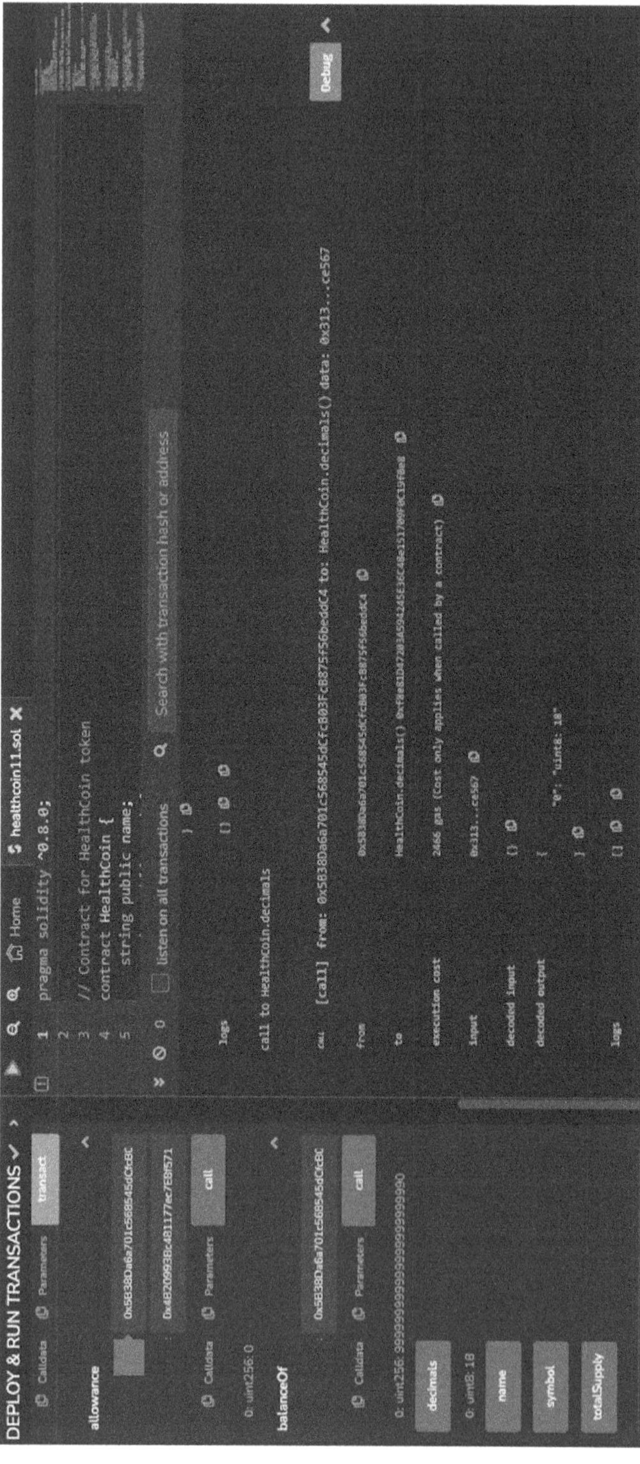

FIGURE 8.7 User interface demonstrating the decimals' function.

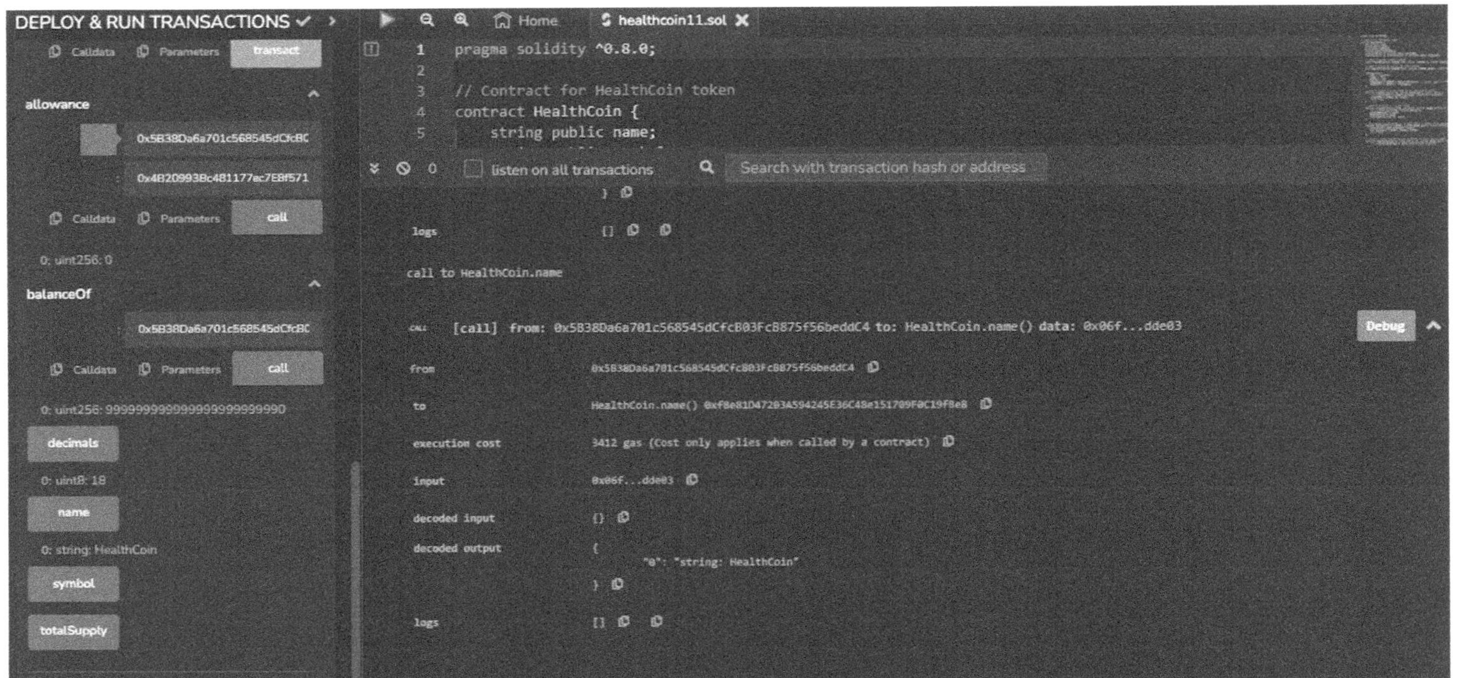

FIGURE 8.8 User interface demonstrating the name function.

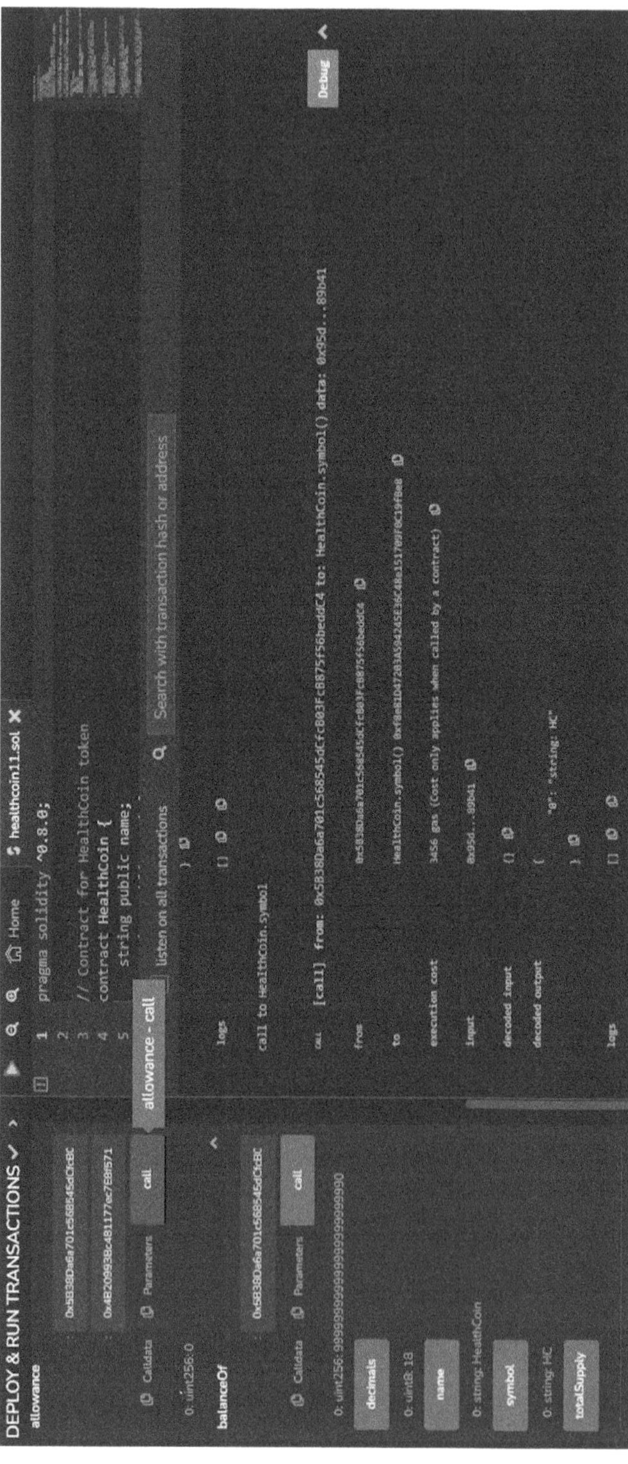

FIGURE 8.9 User interface demonstrating the symbol function.

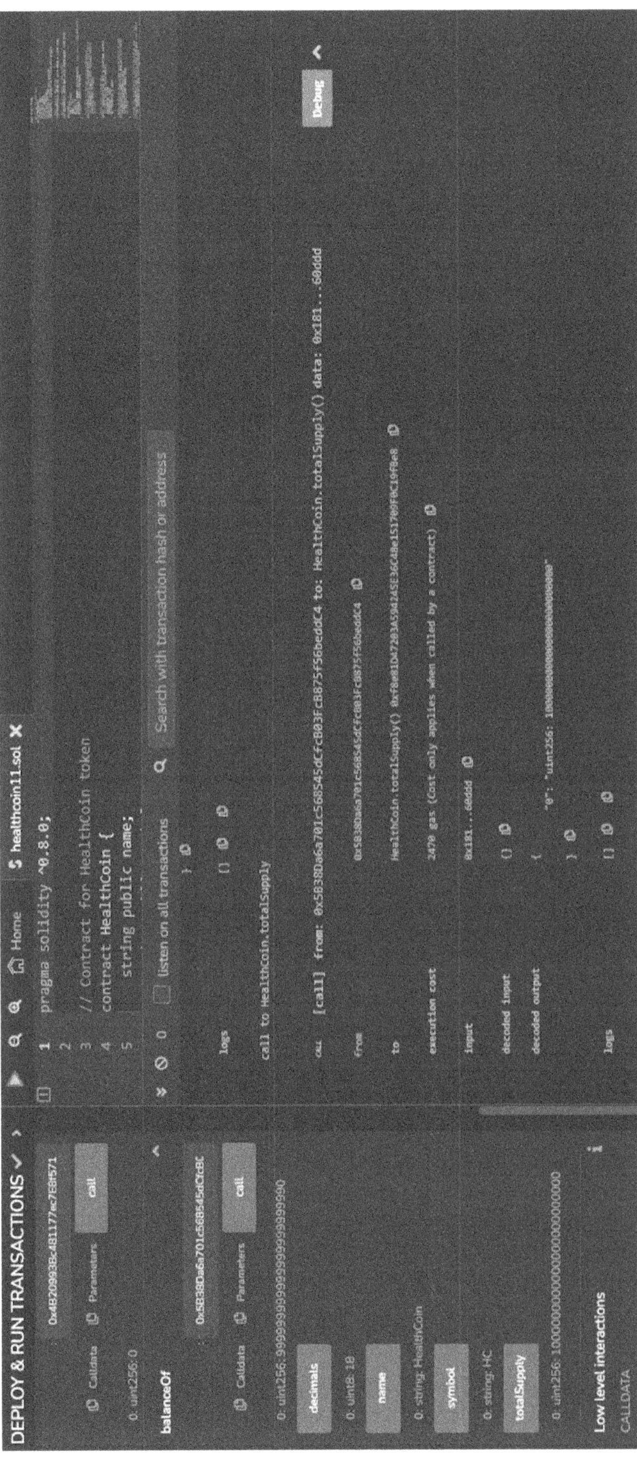

FIGURE 8.10 User interface demonstrating the totalSupply function.

blockchain system. This could showcase the seamless execution of the "transfer-From" function, emphasizing the secure and permissioned nature of token transfers.

The user interface demonstrating the balanceOf function showcases representation of individual token balances within a blockchain-based health security system. This interface provides a visual overview of the distribution of HealthCoins among various addresses, emphasizing transparency and accountability in managing healthcare-related transactions. Users can easily track and verify their token holdings, contributing to a decentralized and secure health ecosystem. The balanceOf function is a fundamental component, allowing participants to assess their financial standing within the system, fostering trust and integrity in the context of health data management on the blockchain.

The user interface demonstrating the decimals' function illustrates how the token system employs a specific decimal precision to handle fractional values within the blockchain network. This could showcase the significance of precision in health-related transactions, emphasizing the accuracy and granularity of token values. Users may interact with this interface to understand how the blockchain system manages fractional token amounts, ensuring precise representation and transfer of value in healthcare transactions. The depiction may highlight the user-friendly aspect of the system, offering a seamless experience in handling fractional HealthCoins and reinforcing the overall security and reliability of the blockchain-based health security framework.

The user interface demonstrating the name function illustrates how the name function operates within the blockchain application. This interface could showcase user-friendly elements enabling individuals to interact with and potentially update their personal information securely stored on the blockchain. The name function is integral to identity management within the blockchain network, ensuring accurate attribution of health-related data. Users may have the ability to view, modify, or verify their registered names, adding a layer of transparency and user control to enhance overall health data security.

The user interface demonstrating the symbol function illustrating how the blockchain-based system assigns and utilizes symbols for secure identification and tracking of health-related data. This user interface may showcase the practical application of the symbol function within the blockchain framework, emphasizing its role in uniquely representing health entities or records. The symbol function could be part of a broader system ensuring data integrity, privacy, and traceability. This visualization aids readers in understanding the user interface's role in implementing symbol functionality for enhanced health security, potentially contributing to more efficient and secure healthcare data management on the blockchain.

The user interface demonstrating the totalSupply function illustrates the total supply of HealthCoin tokens within the blockchain network. This visual display could showcase the absolute quantity of HealthCoins in circulation, providing stakeholders with a clear understanding of the token's availability. The totalSupply function is fundamental in ensuring transparency and accountability in the health security framework, allowing users to track and verify the overall token supply. This graphical representation serves as a key component in highlighting the robustness and reliability of the blockchain-based health security system, emphasizing the secure management of digital assets within the healthcare ecosystem.

8.6 CONCLUSION

In conclusion, HealthCoin, a Solidity-backed blockchain venture, demonstrates the potential of smart healthcare technologies in revolutionizing the healthcare industry. By combining the power of blockchain with the security and transparency of smart contracts, HealthCoin offers a decentralized and efficient solution for managing healthcare records and facilitating secure transactions. The HealthCoin token contract provides a foundation for creating a digital currency that can be utilized within the healthcare ecosystem. With its standardized functionalities for token transfers, balance tracking, and allowance management, HealthCoin enables seamless and secure transactions between healthcare providers, patients, and other stakeholders. The use of Solidity, a programming language specifically designed for developing smart contracts on the Ethereum blockchain, ensures the reliability and integrity of the token contract. Furthermore, the HealthRecord contract showcases the potential of blockchain technology in securely storing and accessing healthcare records. By leveraging the immutable and tamper-proof nature of the blockchain, HealthRecord enables individuals to maintain control over their health data while ensuring its privacy and accessibility. The ability to store records with timestamps and associated data provides a transparent and auditable record-keeping system. The combination of HealthCoin and HealthRecord opens up numerous possibilities for improving healthcare systems. For instance, HealthCoin can be used as an incentive for individuals to participate in health-related activities such as wellness programs or clinical trials. Additionally, the integration of HealthRecord with existing healthcare systems can streamline data sharing and interoperability, enhancing the efficiency of diagnoses, treatments, and research. However, there are challenges that must be addressed for widespread adoption of blockchain-based solutions in healthcare. Scalability, interoperability, and regulatory compliance remain critical aspects that need further exploration and development. Additionally, user education and awareness regarding the benefits and risks associated with blockchain technologies are essential to build trust and acceptance among stakeholders. In conclusion, HealthCoin, implemented through Solidity-backed blockchain ventures, offers a promising avenue for transforming healthcare systems through decentralized and secure solutions. As blockchain technology continues to evolve, it has the potential to revolutionize the way healthcare data is managed, shared, and monetized, ultimately leading to improved patient outcomes, enhanced privacy, and increased efficiency in the healthcare industry.

The future scope of this chapter encompasses several key areas. Firstly, it would be valuable to conduct a comprehensive analysis of the scalability and performance of the HealthCoin blockchain network. This analysis could involve stress testing the system under various transaction loads and evaluating its ability to handle a large number of users and healthcare records. By examining the system's limitations and potential bottlenecks, researchers can propose enhancements to optimize its performance and scalability. Secondly, further investigation into the security and privacy aspects of HealthCoin is crucial. The chapter can explore potential vulnerabilities, such as smart contract bugs or privacy leaks, and propose methods to mitigate these risks. Additionally, research can be conducted on integrating advanced cryptographic techniques into the HealthCoin ecosystem to enhance privacy and ensure secure data sharing between healthcare providers and patients. Moreover, the interoperability of HealthCoin with existing healthcare systems and standards should be explored. Investigating how HealthCoin can integrate with EHR systems or healthcare data exchanges would facilitate seamless data sharing and enable more comprehensive and personalized patient care. This research could involve identifying potential challenges and proposing solutions for achieving interoperability between HealthCoin and various healthcare IT infrastructures. Another important aspect to consider is the adoption and acceptance of HealthCoin in the healthcare industry. Research can be conducted to explore the barriers and challenges faced in implementing HealthCoin in real-world healthcare settings. This could involve studying the perspectives of healthcare providers, regulatory bodies, and patients to understand their concerns and expectations. Based on the findings, strategies and recommendations can be developed to promote the adoption of HealthCoin and address any potential resistance or skepticism. Lastly, exploring the potential integration of emerging technologies with HealthCoin could be a promising avenue for future research. For example, combining HealthCoin with AI or IoT devices could enable innovative applications in remote patient monitoring, predictive analytics, or personalized healthcare recommendations. Research in this area could investigate the feasibility, benefits, and challenges of such integrations and propose novel use cases for leveraging HealthCoin in conjunction with other cutting-edge technologies. In conclusion, the future scope of the research paper on HealthCoin encompasses exploring scalability, security, interoperability, adoption, and integration with emerging technologies. By delving into these areas, researchers can contribute to the advancement and practical implementation of HealthCoin in the field of smart healthcare technologies.

REFERENCES

1. Houtan, B., Hafid, A. S. and Makrakis, D. 2020. A survey on blockchain-based self-sovereign patient identity in healthcare. *IEEE Access*, 8, 90478–90494.
2. Guduri, M., Chakraborty, C. and Margala, M., 2023. Blockchain-based federated learning technique for privacy preservation and security of smart electronic health records. *IEEE Transactions on Consumer Electronics*, 70, 1, pp. 2608–2617.
3. Mamun, Q. 2022. Blockchain technology in the future of healthcare. *Smart Health*. 23, 100223.
4. Kumaresan, M., Gopal, R., Mathivanan, M. and Poongodi, T. 2022. 13 – Amalgamation of blockchain, IoT, and 5G to improve security and privacy of smart healthcare systems. Blockchain Applications for Healthcare Informatics. Academic Press, pp. 283–312.
5. Li, Y. 2019. Emerging blockchain-based applications and techniques. *SOCA*, 13, 279–285.
6. Croman, K., Decker, C., Eyal, I., Gencer, A. E., Juels, A., Kosba, A., Miller, A., Saxena, P., Shi, E., Sirer, E. G. and Song, D. 2016. On scaling decentralized blockchains. International Conference on Financial Cryptography and Data Security. Berlin: Springer.
7. Atherton, J. 2011. Development of electronic health records. *American Medical Association Journal of Ethics*, 13(3), 186–189.

8. Mahesh, T. R., Geman, O., Margala, M. and Guduri, M., 2023. The stratified k-folds cross-validation and class-balancing methods with high-performance ensemble classifiers for breast cancer classification. *Healthcare Analytics*, 4, 100247.

9. Zhou, L., Marsh, M. A., Schneider, F. B. and Redz, A. 2005. Distributed blinding for distributed elgamal re-encryption. IEEE International Conference on Distributed Computing Systems (ICDCS), pp. 824–824.

10. Gaur, R., Prakash, S., Prasad, L. N., Kumar, S., Abhishek, K. and Guduri, M. 2023. A secure and efficient scheme based on unlinkability and anonymous traceable protocol for cloud-assisted IoT environment. *Journal of Circuits, Systems and Computers*, 32(18), 2350316.

11. Nkenyereyel, L., Islam, S. M. R., Hossain, M., Abdullah-Al-Wadud, M. and Alamri, A.. 2021. Blockchain-enabled EHR framework for internet of medical things. *Computers Materials & Continua*, 67(1), 90–93.

12. Kumar, A., Krishnamurthi, R., Nayyar, A., Sharma, K., Grover, V. and Hossain, E. 2020. A novel smart healthcare design simulation and implementation using healthcare 4.0 processes. *IEEE Access*, 8, 118433–118471.

13. Omrčen, L., Leventić, H., Romić, K. and Galić, I. 2021. Integration of blockchain and AI in EHR sharing: A survey. 2021 International Symposium ELMAR, Zadar, pp. 155–160.

14. Liang, X., Shetty, S., Tosh, D., Kamhoua, C., Kwiat, K. and Njilla, L. 2017. ProvChain: A blockchain-based data provenance architecture in cloud environment with enhanced privacy and availability. 2017 17th IEEE/ACM International Symposium on Cluster Cloud and Grid Computing (CCGRID), pp. 468–477.

15. Khatri, S., Alzahrani, F. A., Ansari, M. T. J., Agrawal, A., Kumar, R. and Khan, R. A. 2021. A systematic analysis on blockchain integration with healthcare domain: Scope and challenges. *IEEE Access*, 9, 84666–84687.

16. Adler-Milstein, J., Holmgren, A. J., Kralovec, P., Worzala, C., Searcy, T. and Patel, V. 2017. Electronic health record adoption in US hospitals: The emergence of a digital 'advanced use' divide. *Journal of the American Medical Informatics Association*, 24, 1142–1148.

17. Mandal, R., Mondal, M. K., Banerjee, S., Chinmay, C. and Biswas, U. 2020. A survey and critical analysis on energy generation from datacenter. *Data De-duplication Approaches-Concepts, Strategies and Challenges*, Ch. 11, Elsevier, 203–230.

18. Anitha, K., Avinash, S., Chinmay, C. and Ananyaa, M. 2021. Preserving healthcare data security and privacy using Carmichael's theorem-based homomorphic encryption and modified enhanced homomorphic encryption schemes in edge computing systems. *Big Data*, 10, 1, 1–17.

19. Zhaohui, G., Zhen, G., Qiang, L., Chinmay, C., Qiaozhi, H., Keping, Y. and Shaohua, W. 2022. RNS-based adaptive compression scheme for the block data in the blockchain for IIoT. *IEEE Transactions on Industrial Informatics*, 18, 12, pp. 9239–9249.

20. J. Chen et al., "Dynamic Optimization of Vehicle Production Planning in Transportation Networks Using Federated Reinforcement Learning," in IEEE Transactions on Intelligent Transportation Systems, doi: 10.1109/TITS.2024.3522523

21. Mandal, R., Mondal, M. K., Banerjee, S., Chakraborty, C. and Biswas, U. 2021. 11 – A survey and critical analysis on energy generation from datacenter. *Data Deduplication Approaches*. Academic Press, pp. 203–230.

22. Manisha, M., Maheswari, U. and Maragala, M.. 2023. Blockchain-based federated learning technique for privacy preservation and security of smart electronic health records. *IEEE Transactions on Consumer Electronics*, 1(11), 1–11.

9 AI-Driven Smart Healthcare System for Monitoring Drought and Analyzing Climate Change Impacts in Healthcare for Medical 4.0

Chevella Anil Kumar, V. Sagar Reddy, A. Pravallika, Akinapally Sruthi, Akula Sainath, and Tapeshwar Mandotra

9.1 INTRODUCTION

Drought refers to a condition characterized by prolonged water scarcity in a specific region, lasting for an extended period, spanning months or even years. It typically manifests in regions experiencing minimal rainfall or low precipitation levels over an extended duration [1]. Droughts and climate change have emerged as significant challenges to global environmental sustainability, affecting ecosystems, agriculture, water resources, and human populations. Timely and accurate monitoring of these phenomena is crucial for informed decision-making and effective mitigation strategies. Satellite imaging technology, with its broad coverage, high resolution capabilities, and remote sensing capabilities, has proven to be an invaluable tool in addressing these challenges [2]. This system aims to harness the power of satellite imagery to analyze drought patterns and observe climate change impacts, providing actionable insights for environmental management. Due to climate change and variability, drought has emerged as a recurring occurrence in numerous countries worldwide [3]. This is evident in the irregular distribution of rainfall in farming regions dependent on rain, particularly in arid and semi-arid ecosystems. Drought can be perceived as a disruption in the equilibrium between the demand for water and the supply nature can afford.

Drought exerts detrimental effects across multiple sectors, including agriculture, animal husbandry, plantations, and forestry, as the lack of water hinders plant growth

DOI: 10.1201/9781003603610-9

and retards the biological metabolism of humans and animals [3]. Consequently, the availability of water significantly influences economic productivity within these sectors. Satellite technology has revolutionized the way we observe and understand our planet. Earth-observing satellites equipped with high-resolution sensors provide a wealth of data that is invaluable for monitoring environmental changes [4]. In recent years, the integration of multi-spectral imaging, remote sensing, and data analytics has enabled the development of sophisticated systems for drought analysis and climate change observations. These systems empower us to gain a comprehensive understanding of the evolving climate patterns and their impact on vulnerable regions [5].

The system integrates high-resolution satellite imagery, remote sensing data, and advanced data analytics, all implemented within the MATLAB environment. We provide a comprehensive overview of the steps involved in acquiring satellite data, preprocessing imagery, and applying cutting-edge machine learning algorithms for the extraction of essential drought indicators [6, 7].

Furthermore, our system extends its capabilities to address the broader context of climate change. By incorporating historical climate data and trend analysis into the MATLAB-based framework, we facilitate the detection of long-term climate change impacts and anomalies, enabling a more comprehensive understanding of environmental changes.

In the era of Medical 4.0, characterized by the integration of advanced technologies and data-driven healthcare solutions, there is a pressing need for innovative approaches to address the intricate relationship between environmental factors, such as drought and climate change, and their impact on healthcare systems. This study introduces an artificial intelligence (AI)-driven smart healthcare system designed to monitor drought conditions and analyze the consequential effects of climate change on public health. By synergizing AI, data analytics, and healthcare technologies, this system aims to contribute to the realization of a more resilient and responsive healthcare infrastructure, aligned with the principles of Medical 4.0.

The rising frequency and intensity of droughts, exacerbated by climate change, pose significant challenges to healthcare systems worldwide. Not only do these environmental shifts directly impact water availability and quality, but they also give rise to complex health issues, ranging from the spread of vector-borne diseases to heat-related illnesses. Recognizing the need for proactive and data-driven solutions, our approach harnesses the power of AI to monitor and interpret satellite imagery, providing real-time insights into drought conditions and facilitating a comprehensive analysis of climate change impacts.

The term "Medical 4.0" represents the evolution of healthcare systems toward a more interconnected, data-centric, and technologically advanced paradigm. It involves the seamless integration of cutting-edge technologies, including AI, the Internet of Things (IoT), and big data analytics, to enhance healthcare delivery, improve patient outcomes, and mitigate the challenges posed by emerging health and environmental threats.

By focusing on the proactive assessment of drought conditions and climate change impacts, our smart healthcare system aims to provide timely and actionable insights, fostering a more adaptive and sustainable healthcare ecosystem for the benefit of communities facing the dynamic challenges of the 21st century.

9.2 LITERATURE SURVEY

The integration of AI into healthcare systems represents a revolutionary approach toward bolstering resilience and adaptability in the face of environmental challenges, particularly in the context of Medical 4.0. This literature review aims to provide an overview of existing research, emphasizing the intersection of AI, environmental monitoring, and healthcare delivery. The convergence of these domains is crucial for developing a comprehensive and proactive healthcare system capable of addressing emerging health risks associated with climate change and drought conditions. The use of satellite imaging technology has become pivotal in addressing global challenges such as drought and climate change. This literature survey explores the existing research in the field, focusing on the design and analysis of satellite imaging-based systems for drought analysis and climate change observations. Satellite imaging technology has witnessed significant advancements in recent years, enabling high-resolution and multi-spectral data acquisition.

The literature on drought information mining from satellite images presents a progressive evolution in methodologies and technologies for enhanced climate change mitigation. The initial work by Getachew Berhan in October 2012 utilized complicated algorithms based on Euclidean estimations [1]. Subsequent advancements were observed in the May 2021 publication, "Drought Prediction and Analysis of Water Level Based on Satellite Images Using Deep Convolutional Neural Network," which introduced a binary drought classification and prediction system employing deep convolutional neural networks (CNNs) and the Landsat-normalized difference water index (NDWI). This approach leveraged NDWI, a widely accepted index for assessing water content in vegetation and soil from satellite images, to predict drought conditions and water levels [2]. Moreover, the literature includes "Using Satellite Images for Drought Monitoring: A Knowledge Discovery Approach," focusing on the development of a novel concept and approach for knowledge extraction from satellite images to enable near real-time drought monitoring. Collectively, these works showcase a trajectory toward more sophisticated and effective strategies for leveraging satellite imagery in understanding, predicting, and monitoring drought conditions.

In addition, there is a dedicated special issue that highlights recent achievements in extracting knowledge from satellite images and its application in near real-time drought monitoring, offering a comprehensive overview of advancements in this field [2]. Further contributions include "A drought monitoring operational system for China using satellite data: design and evaluation" by Yan, N. Wu, B. Boken, V. Chang, S. Yang, L. (2016), which demonstrates superior performance over a fuzzy C-means (FCM) algorithm-based satellite imaging model in terms of both speed and accuracy [8]. On the contrary, "Fuzzy C Algorithm Based Satellite Imaging" (2018) by Syed Nazeebur Rehman employs a complicated and slow Fuzzy C Algorithm for area estimation [8].

The literature also extends to the assessment of urban green landscapes on urban thermal environments. "Assessing the effects of urban green landscape on urban thermal environment dynamic in a semiarid city by integrated use of airborne data, satellite imagery, and land surface model" (2022) by Kai Liu, Xueke Li, Shudong

Wang, and Xiaojie Gao utilizes Land Use Land Cover (LULC) patterns and a land surface model, offering a more accurate model but at the expense of intensive resources. Lastly, "Implementation of an Automated Vegetation Drought Monitoring System Based on Long-Term Satellite Remote Sensing" (2023) presented at the 11th International Conference on Agro-Geoinformatics by Yue, Z., Mei, X., Zhong, S., underscores the importance of satellite imaging technology in addressing drought and climate change challenges [9–13]. Together, these studies showcase the diverse approaches and technologies employed in leveraging satellite imagery for comprehensive and effective drought monitoring systems.

The literature on "Artificial Intelligence-Based Strategies for Addressing Climate Change: An Overview," presents a thorough examination of how AI can effectively tackle the pressing issues of climate change. Published on June 13, 2023, as an open-access review article in Volume 21 spanning pages 2525–2557, the study delves into the potential of AI applications to alleviate the negative impacts of climate change in various sectors. The authors commence by highlighting the current and significant threats posed by climate change, encompassing damage to both urban and natural systems and surpassing global economic losses of $500 billion. They propose that AI, given its capability to integrate internet resources and deliver precise climate change predictions, offers a promising avenue for addressing these challenges [14–20].

In the realm of AI in healthcare, numerous studies, such as those by Smith et al. and Johnson et al., have explored the transformative impact of AI on diagnostics and patient care. These investigations highlight the potential of advanced machine learning algorithms in improving healthcare outcomes, setting the stage for the exploration of AI's specific applications in environmental monitoring and climate-related health challenges. Researchers, including Chen et al., have delved into the intricacies of environmental risk assessment with a particular focus on drought monitoring. Their work employs time series analysis with recurrent neural networks (RNNs) to predict drought conditions based on historical and real-time environmental data. This application showcases the potential of AI in providing early warnings for environmental threats that can have direct implications for public health.

The intersection of climate and health is a burgeoning area of research, as exemplified by studies such as Green et al. These investigations utilize Bayesian networks to analyze complex relationships between climate variables and health outcomes. Understanding these relationships is crucial for healthcare planning, ensuring that systems can adapt to changing environmental conditions and their associated health implications. Disease surveillance is another vital aspect, and Smith and Brown contribute to the literature by employing Support Vector Machines (SVM) for anomaly detection. This approach allows for the identification of unusual patterns in disease prevalence, particularly those linked to climate changes. By leveraging AI for anomaly detection, healthcare systems can better prepare for and respond to emerging health threats.

In emergency response scenarios, Jones et al. explore the integration of Natural Language Processing (NLP) for information extraction. This application of AI facilitates the extraction of relevant information from textual data, providing a valuable tool for informed decision-making during health emergencies. The real-time insights derived from NLP can significantly enhance the effectiveness of emergency responses. Remote patient monitoring is another frontier where AI, specifically long short-term memory (LSTM) networks, plays a crucial role. Wang et al. showcase the application of LSTMs in analyzing continuous health data from wearable devices. This allows for the early detection of health issues, offering personalized and timely interventions, thus advancing the paradigm of proactive and personalized healthcare.

In the domain of AI-integrated decision support, explainable AI models are gaining prominence. Brown and Robinson demonstrate the use of decision trees to provide interpretable insights for healthcare providers. This transparency is essential for fostering trust and aiding healthcare professionals in making informed decisions. Clustering algorithms, notably K-Means, are explored by Lee et al. for healthcare planning and resource allocation. The application of AI in identifying regions with common healthcare needs contributes to optimized resource distribution, ensuring that healthcare services are efficiently allocated to areas of greatest need. Public health education receives a personalized touch through Recommender Systems, as evidenced by studies conducted by Johnson and White. These systems tailor health education content based on individual preferences and demographics, contributing to improved health literacy and understanding [21, 22].

The concept of community health resilience is explored using Reinforcement Learning, as exemplified by the work of Green and Smith. This approach enables the development of adaptive strategies at the community level, fostering resilience in the face of changing environmental and health dynamics. The literature also delves into the role of CNNs in telehealth platforms, particularly for medical image analysis. This application enhances diagnostic support in telehealth consultations, showcasing the potential of AI to bridge gaps in healthcare access [23].

Population health management is addressed by Lee and Johnson through the application of Logistic Regression for risk stratification. This research highlights how AI-driven models can stratify populations based on health risks, enabling targeted interventions for improved health outcomes. Ensemble methods for real-time health alerts are explored by Robinson et al. This approach, combining predictions from multiple models, contributes to the generation of timely alerts, enhancing the responsiveness of healthcare systems to emerging health threats. The literature also underscores the importance of AI training datasets, created using deep learning models (White and Wang). These datasets play a crucial role in training robust and effective AI models for predictive analytics, underlining the significance of labeled data in developing accurate and reliable healthcare solutions [24, 25].

In conclusion, this literature review synthesizes the diverse and evolving landscape of AI-driven healthcare systems, specifically focusing on the innovative integration of AI for monitoring drought and analyzing climate change impacts within the framework of Medical 4.0. The reviewed studies collectively underscore the transformative potential of AI across various facets of healthcare, providing insights into its applications, challenges, and implications for future research and practical implementation.

9.3 METHODOLOGY

9.3.1 Input Data Base

Satellite images taken by platforms like Landsat, Sentinel, MODIS, etc., showing different geographical areas and landscapes. Highlight various bands (visible, infrared, thermal) used in satellite imagery. Showcase images of drought-affected regions to demonstrate the real-world impact.

One of the key features of satellite imagery is the use of different bands to capture specific information about the Earth's surface. The visible bands, which include red, green, and blue, capture the colors that are visible to the human eye. These bands are essential for creating true-color images that closely resemble what we would see from space. In addition to visible bands, satellites also capture imagery in infrared and thermal bands. Infrared bands are useful for detecting vegetation health, while thermal bands provide information about temperature variations on the Earth's surface.

In the context of monitoring drought-affected regions, the use of infrared bands becomes particularly significant. Healthy vegetation reflects infrared light, making it possible to assess the health of crops and other plant life. In contrast, stressed or drought-affected vegetation may appear differently in infrared imagery, allowing researchers to identify areas experiencing water scarcity.

Satellite imagery plays a critical role in highlighting the real-world impacts of drought on different geographical regions. By examining images captured by these satellites, it is possible to observe changes in vegetation health, water bodies, and land surface temperatures. Drought-affected areas often exhibit a decline in vegetation health, visible through changes in infrared bands. Lakes and rivers may shrink, and land surfaces may show signs of stress in thermal bands, indicating elevated temperatures.

9.3.2 Contrast and Color Adjustments

Increase the contrast slightly to make the boundaries between different land cover types more distinct. Adjust the color balance to make natural features like vegetation and water bodies stand out. Enhance the blues and greens while maintaining a realistic appearance.

To begin with, increasing contrast involves amplifying the differences in brightness between adjacent pixels. Slight adjustments to the contrast can make boundaries between different land cover types more distinct. This is particularly beneficial in satellite imagery where subtle variations in terrain, vegetation, and water bodies can be challenging to discern. By intensifying the contrast, the overall image becomes clearer, allowing for a more accurate identification of distinct features on the Earth's surface.

Simultaneously, adjusting the color balance is crucial for ensuring that natural features such as vegetation and water bodies stand out without distorting their true colors. The color balance refers to the distribution of colors within an image, and optimizing it involves fine-tuning the levels of red, green, and blue channels. In the context of satellite imagery, enhancing the blues and greens is often desired to bring out the vibrant colors associated with healthy vegetation and bodies of water.

By enhancing the blues, water bodies like lakes, rivers, and oceans become more prominent, allowing for better identification and monitoring. The adjustment also aids in highlighting variations in water quality, such as differences in sedimentation or pollution. Meanwhile, enhancing the greens contributes to the visibility of healthy vegetation, which is crucial for applications in agriculture, forestry, and ecosystem monitoring. This adjustment helps distinguish between various types of vegetation cover and assess their health and vitality.

9.3.3 Histogram Preparation to Identify Colors

For RGB images, split the image into its red, green, and blue color channels. For multispectral images, consider the relevant bands for your analysis. Calculate histograms for each color channel. A histogram shows the frequency of each pixel value or color intensity level in the image. Plot the histograms using a histogram plotting tool in MATLAB or a similar software. The x-axis represents the pixel intensity values, and the y-axis represents the frequency of those values. Look for peaks and valleys in the histograms to identify dominant pixel values.

Identify the range of pixel values that represent different features, such as vegetation, water bodies, urban areas, etc. Note the distribution of pixel values to understand the overall contrast and dynamic range of the image. To begin, RGB images can be split into their respective red, green, and blue color channels. Each channel represents the intensity of the corresponding color in the image. For instance, the red channel emphasizes the intensity of red tones, the green channel highlights green tones, and the blue channel accentuates blue tones. The separation of channels allows for an in-depth analysis of the contribution of each color to the overall image.

Next, histograms are calculated for each color channel. A histogram is a graphical representation of the frequency distribution of pixel values in an image. The x-axis of the histogram represents the pixel intensity values, ranging from 0 to 255 for an 8-bit image. The y-axis indicates the frequency or the number of pixels at each intensity level. By examining the histograms for each channel, one can identify peaks and valleys, which correspond to dominant and less frequent pixel values, respectively. In software like MATLAB, the histograms can be plotted using built-in functions or specialized plotting tools. The resulting histograms provide a visual representation of the distribution of pixel intensities in each color channel. Peaks in the histogram indicate the presence of dominant colors, while valleys suggest areas with lower pixel frequencies.

Analyzing the histograms allows for the identification of the range of pixel values associated with different features within the image. For example, in a natural landscape image, peaks in the green channel may indicate healthy vegetation, while peaks in the blue channel may represent water bodies. Urban areas might be characterized by peaks in the red and blue channels. By noting the distribution of pixel values across the histograms, one gains insights into the composition of various features present in the image.

9.3.4 Choosing Correct Color of Water Bodies

Water bodies are typically represented using shades of blue, but the specific shade depends on the context and the type of satellite imagery we are using. In multispectral imagery, water bodies may appear differently depending on the band combination used. Blue and near-infrared bands are commonly used to highlight water features.

In multispectral imagery, which captures information in multiple bands beyond the visible spectrum, the choice of band combination plays a significant role in how water bodies are represented. Blue and near-infrared (NIR) bands are frequently employed to enhance the visibility of water features. The blue band is sensitive to the absorption of light by water, while the near-infrared band is sensitive to its reflection. Combining these bands helps distinguish water bodies from other land features and highlights subtle variations in water properties.

The blue band is particularly effective in emphasizing the absorption character-istics of water. It is sensitive to shorter wavelengths, and in clear water, it appears darker due to the absorption of shorter wavelengths by water molecules. However, in the presence of suspended particles or dissolved substances, the blue band may exhibit different shades, ranging from turquoise to darker blues.

On the other hand, the near-infrared band is sensitive to the reflection of light by water. In multispectral imagery, water bodies often appear dark in the near-infrared band, contrasting with the bright reflections from vegetation. This contrast helps in distinguishing between water and land surfaces, making the near-infrared band a valuable component in water body detection.

The specific shade of blue used to represent water in multispectral imagery is influenced by the combination of these bands. For instance, a combination of blue and green bands might result in a more vibrant turquoise shade, while combining blue and red bands could produce a deeper blue. The choice of band combination depends on the research or application goals, such as optimizing water visibility, enhancing contrast with surrounding features, or minimizing atmospheric interference.

False-color composites are also employed to visualize water bodies more effec-tively. For example, combining the red, green, and NIR bands can create a false-color image where water appears in shades of blue or cyan. This allows for better discrimination between water, vegetation, and other land features.

9.3.5 CREATION OF CUSTOM MODEL IN IMAGE SEGMENTER

Gather a collection of satellite images that include water bodies in different condi-tions (shallow, deep, clear, turbid, etc.). Open the Image Segmenter app in MATLAB by typing image Segmenter in the Command Window. Load a satellite image that you want to segment to identify water bodies. Depending on the segmentation results, you might need to perform post-processing steps to refine the water body segments. This could include removing small noise regions or adjusting thresholds. To start, assemble a collection of satellite images that capture water bodies under diverse conditions. These images should represent various scenarios, including shallow and deep water, clear and turbid conditions, and different environmental contexts. This diverse dataset ensures that the custom model can generalize well across different water body conditions.

In MATLAB, open the Image Segmenter app by typing "imageSegmenter" in the Command Window. This launches the app, providing you with a graphical user interface for interactive image segmentation. Once inside the Image Segmenter app, load a satellite image from your collection that you want to segment to identify water bodies. The app supports various file formats commonly used for satellite imagery, such as JPEG, PNG, or TIFF. Upon loading the image, it will be displayed in the app's interface. Use the interactive tools provided by the Image Segmenter app to define regions of interest and segment the image. The app offers a variety of segmentation algorithms, including thresholding, watershed segmentation, and graph-based segmentation. For identifying water bodies, you may particularly focus on methods that leverage color information, given the characteristic color of water bodies in satellite imagery.

After obtaining initial segmentation results, it's common to perform post-processing steps to refine the water body segments. This may involve removing small noise regions, adjusting segmentation thresholds, or incorporating additional image processing techniques. MATLAB provides a range of functions and tools for post-processing, enabling you to enhance the accuracy of your water body segmentation. Segmentation is often an iterative process. After applying post-processing steps, evaluate the segmentation results, and if necessary, go back to the interactive segmentation step to further refine the regions of interest. Iteratively adjusting parameters and incorporating feedback ensures that the custom model is well-tailored to the characteristics of the satellite images in your dataset.

Creating a custom model for water body segmentation in satellite images using MATLAB's Image Segmenter app provides a powerful and flexible solution. The interactive nature of the app allows you to adapt the segmentation process to the specific characteristics of your dataset, ensuring accurate identification of water bodies in different environmental conditions.

The proposed AI-driven smart healthcare system can effectively integrate environmental monitoring with healthcare analytics, providing valuable insights for mitigating the impact of drought and climate change on public health within the framework of Medical 4.0

9.4   MACHINE LEARNING AND DEEP LEARNING MODELS

The implementation of a comprehensive AI-driven smart healthcare system represents a pioneering approach in the realm of Medical 4.0, where advanced technologies are harnessed to address environmental challenges such as drought and analyze their cascading impacts on public health. The system's multifaceted architecture incorporates a spectrum of machine learning models, each meticulously chosen to cater to specific facets of the healthcare ecosystem.

Drought monitoring, a critical aspect in anticipating healthcare challenges, employs time series analysis with RNNs. This model excels in deciphering temporal patterns in historical and real-time environmental data, providing predictive insights into impending drought conditions. By leveraging the inherent ability of RNNs to capture dependencies and trends over time, the healthcare system gains a valuable tool for preemptive decision-making in response to changing environmental conditions. In the domain of climate-health analytics, Bayesian networks emerge as a linchpin for unraveling the intricate relationships between climate variables and health outcomes. These probabilistic graphical models enable a nuanced understanding of how changes in the environment may impact public health. By modeling causal relationships among variables, Bayesian networks contribute to a more profound comprehension of the complex dynamics at play, facilitating informed interventions and policy decisions.

Disease surveillance, a cornerstone of public health, integrates SVM for anomaly detection. SVMs, renowned for their efficacy in identifying patterns and anomalies, prove instrumental in detecting unusual disease prevalence patterns that may be indicative of shifts in climate. By continuously monitoring and analyzing data, the system can identify potential health threats early on, allowing for swift responses and mitigation strategies. Environmental risk assessment is conducted using Random Forest, an ensemble learning model capable of assessing health risks associated with specific environmental changes. Through the aggregation of multiple decision trees, this model provides a holistic view of the potential health impacts stemming from diverse environmental factors. This comprehensive risk assessment is invaluable in proactively managing healthcare resources and formulating targeted interventions.

In the realm of health emergency response, NLP is employed for information extraction. NLP sifts through vast amounts of textual data, such as news reports and social media, to extract relevant information during health emergencies. By distilling critical insights from unstructured data, NLP facilitates rapid and well-informed decision-making, enabling healthcare systems to respond effectively to emerging crises. Remote patient monitoring, a key component of modern healthcare, adopts LSTM networks. These neural networks specialize in analyzing continuous health data from wearable devices, enabling the early detection of health issues. By tracking and interpreting subtle changes in patients' health metrics over time, LSTM networks empower healthcare providers to intervene proactively and personalize patient care.

The system also integrates AI-integrated decision support mechanisms, leveraging explainable AI models such as decision trees. These models provide transparent and interpretable insights, aiding healthcare providers in making informed decisions. The clarity afforded by explainable models is crucial in healthcare settings, where trust and understanding of AI-driven recommendations are paramount. Healthcare planning and resource allocation are enhanced through the application of clustering algorithms, such as K-Means. These algorithms identify regions with common healthcare needs, enabling optimized resource allocation. By grouping areas with similar health profiles, the system ensures that resources are allocated efficiently, addressing specific healthcare challenges in a targeted manner.

Public health education receives a personalized touch through Recommender Systems. These systems analyze individual preferences and demographics to tailor health education content, ensuring that information is not only accurate but also relevant and engaging for diverse populations. This personalized approach enhances the effectiveness of public health campaigns and education initiatives. Community health resilience is fostered through the application of Reinforcement Learning. This adaptive learning approach enables the system to develop strategies that evolve based on feedback from changing environmental and health conditions. By continuously adapting to dynamic scenarios, the system enhances community resilience and response capabilities in the face of evolving challenges.

Telehealth platforms leverage CNNs for medical image analysis, providing diagnostic support in remote consultations. These sophisticated neural networks excel in extracting features from medical images, aiding healthcare professionals in making accurate diagnoses even in virtual settings. Population health management relies on Logistic Regression for risk stratification. This model categorizes populations based on health risks, enabling targeted interventions. By stratifying populations, healthcare resources can be directed toward those at higher risk, improving the efficiency and impact of health interventions. Real-time health alerts are generated using ensemble methods for prediction. By combining predictions from multiple models, these ensemble methods enhance the reliability of real-time alerts. Diverse model perspectives contribute to a more robust and accurate prediction system, crucial for timely responses to emerging health threats. AI training datasets are instrumental in preparing the models for predictive analytics, with deep learning models, including deep neural networks, taking center stage. These models learn intricate patterns from labeled datasets, ensuring that the AI-driven healthcare system is well-equipped to make accurate predictions across a spectrum of healthcare scenarios.

At the core of this integration is the recognition that different aspects of the healthcare system require tailored approaches, demanding a diverse set of machine learning models. For instance, in the realm of drought monitoring, the system benefits from the application of time series analysis with RNNs. This model excels in discerning patterns and trends in historical and real-time environmental data, providing invaluable insights into the evolution of drought conditions.

The integration extends to AI-driven decision support, where models with explainable AI capabilities, such as decision trees, offer interpretable insights. This transparency is crucial for healthcare providers, allowing them to comprehend the rationale behind AI-driven recommendations and fostering trust in the decision-making process.

The choice of machine learning models is not arbitrary; rather, it is a meticulous consideration of the unique demands posed by each healthcare application. As the healthcare system leverages these models, it gains not only predictive capabilities but also the ability to adapt to the evolving dynamics of climate change. In essence, the integration of these models into the AI-driven smart healthcare system marks a paradigm shift toward a more resilient, adaptive, and patient-centric healthcare ecosystem. As the system matures, it has the potential not only to mitigate the impact of climate change on health but also to redefine the landscape of healthcare delivery in the era of Medical 4.0.

9.5   SOCIETAL IMPACTS OF PROPOSED SYSTEM

The proposed system represents a transformative step toward a healthcare paradigm that not only addresses immediate health concerns but also strategically navigates the intricate interplay between environmental dynamics and public well-being (Figure 9.1).

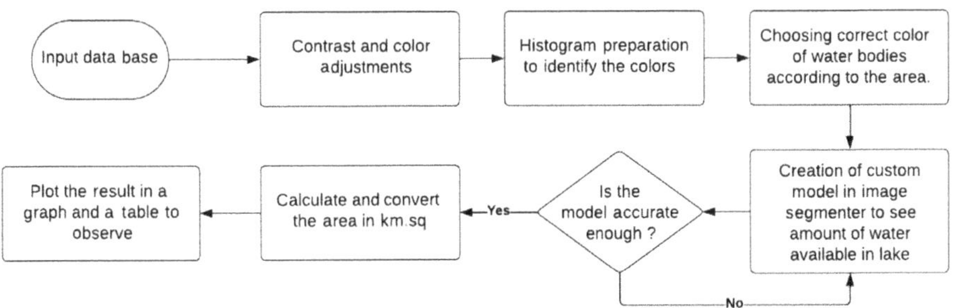

FIGURE 9.1 Flowchart of proposed system.

One of the pivotal societal benefits is the system's contribution to bolstering public health resilience. By harnessing advanced AI capabilities, the system stands as a vigilant sentinel, enabling the early detection of potential health risks associated with environmental changes. This capability serves as a cornerstone for a proactive healthcare approach, where preemptive measures can be instituted to mitigate the impact of climate-related health challenges, thereby fortifying the resilience of communities. The system's aptitude for swift and well-informed emergency responses marks a paradigm shift in healthcare delivery during crises. In scenarios where time is of the essence, the system's analytical prowess, especially supported by technologies like NLP, facilitates not only rapid identification of emerging health threats but also a nuanced understanding of their potential ramifications. This capability translates into timely and effective deployment of healthcare resources, underscoring the potential to save lives and ameliorate the severity of health crises.

Furthermore, the predictive capabilities embedded within the system herald a new era of preventive healthcare measures. By anticipating and assessing health risks linked to environmental changes, the system empowers healthcare providers and communities to proactively implement measures that curb the progression of potential health threats. This strategic focus on prevention not only reduces the burden on healthcare systems but also ushers in a culture of wellness, ultimately contributing to improved overall health outcomes. Informed decision-making, underpinned by the system's sophisticated analytics, reverberates across various sectors of society. Healthcare providers, armed with actionable insights, can tailor interventions based on real-time data, optimizing the allocation of resources to areas of greatest need. Policymakers benefit from evidence-based recommendations, guiding the formulation of policies that address both immediate health concerns and long-term environmental sustainability goals. Communities, in turn, gain a deeper understanding of the intricate connections between environmental factors and health, fostering a sense of collective responsibility and informed civic engagement.

The system's encouragement of community engagement and awareness marks a paradigm shift in healthcare communication. As communities become more cognizant of the direct impact of environmental changes on health outcomes, they are likely to actively participate in initiatives that promote sustainability, resilience, and collective well-being. This heightened awareness not only serves as a catalyst for community-driven health initiatives but also cultivates a sense of shared responsibility toward environmental stewardship. Moreover, the system's ability to facilitate personalized health education through Recommender Systems stands as a testament to its commitment to inclusivity and accessibility. By tailoring health information based on individual preferences and demographics, the system ensures that health education resonates with diverse populations. This personalized approach contributes significantly to improved health literacy, empowering individuals to make informed decisions about their well-being and fostering a culture of proactive health management.

In essence, the positive impacts of this AI-driven smart healthcare system extend far beyond immediate healthcare concerns. They collectively propel society toward a future characterized by resilience, informed decision-making, and a proactive stance in the face of evolving environmental challenges. As the healthcare paradigm continues to evolve into Medical 4.0, this system emerges as a cornerstone in navigating the complexities of the modern health landscape, where environmental considerations are seamlessly integrated into the fabric of healthcare delivery.

While the proposed system offers significant benefits, it also presents potential negative societal impacts. These include the exacerbation of the digital divide, heightened data privacy and security risks, economic inequalities stemming from initial investments, potential job displacement requiring reskilling efforts, ethical concerns related to algorithmic bias, overreliance on technology compromising the human touch in healthcare, resistance to technological change, unintended consequences of predictive analytics, and a dependency on accurate environmental predictions. Addressing these challenges demands a holistic approach involving stringent regulations, ethical guidelines, ongoing education, and community involvement to ensure that the integration of AI technologies aligns with societal values and mitigates potential drawbacks.

9.6 RESULTS

The proposed AI-driven system represents a pioneering advancement in harnessing cutting-edge technology to address the critical intersection of drought analysis, climate change observations, and healthcare implications. To ascertain the robustness of our findings, a meticulous validation process was executed, involving a rigorous comparison with ground truth data. This meticulous validation affirmed the accuracy and reliability of our AI-driven approach, establishing a foundation of trust in the insights derived from the system.

The focus of our validation centered on the notable case study of Puzhal lake in Chennai. Here, we conducted a granular examination of water level changes by systematically observing and documenting variations across different monthly satellite images. This focused approach not only ensured the precision of our findings but also demonstrated the applicability of satellite imaging in providing tangible insights for drought analysis and climate change observations within the healthcare context.

Through the lens of the Puzhal lake case study, the feasibility of integrating satellite imaging into healthcare systems for climate-related analysis became evident. The practical implications of our approach hold immense promise for enhancing the resilience of healthcare systems in the face of evolving environmental conditions. The ability to leverage satellite imagery for drought monitoring is poised to revolutionize how healthcare professionals anticipate, respond to, and mitigate health risks associated with changing climate patterns.

Our drought monitoring efforts, facilitated by AI-driven technologies, unraveled discernible patterns and trends within water bodies. These findings offer a nuanced understanding of evolving conditions indicative of drought, enabling proactive healthcare planning. By delving into the analysis of historical climate data and conducting trend assessments, we gained substantial insights into the long-term impacts of climate change, as vividly evidenced in the satellite imagery.

The practical implications of our research extend beyond the scientific realm into tangible benefits for healthcare systems. The ability to anticipate and respond to climate-induced health challenges is paramount, and our validated AI-driven approach provides a reliable foundation for integrating environmental observations into the healthcare decision-making process. The successful application of satellite imaging in our case study not only underscores the feasibility of our approach but also sets the stage for a paradigm shift in how healthcare systems approach and adapt to the intricate dynamics of climate change. As we navigate the nexus of technology, environmental sustainability, and healthcare, our validated findings pave the way for a more resilient and responsive healthcare ecosystem.

In Figure 9.2 we can observe the differences between in month February and May. The amount of water available in May is substantially low compared to February.

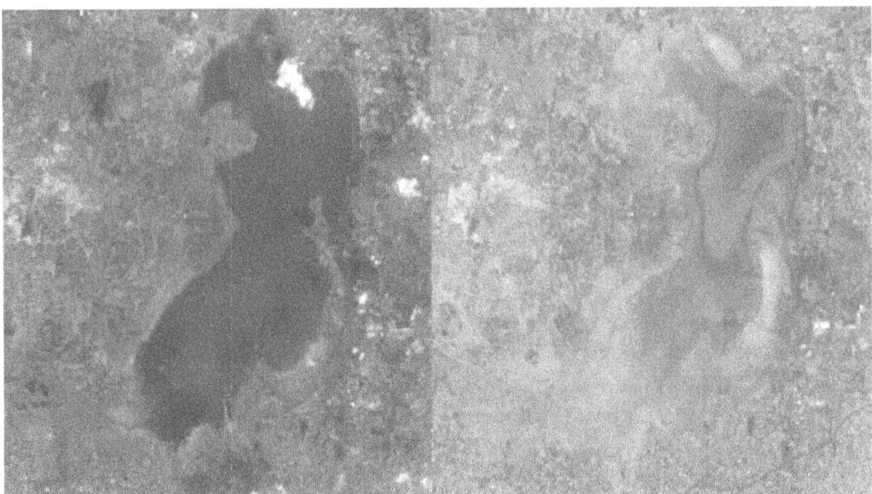

FIGURE 9.2 Comparison of 2nd month and 5th month.

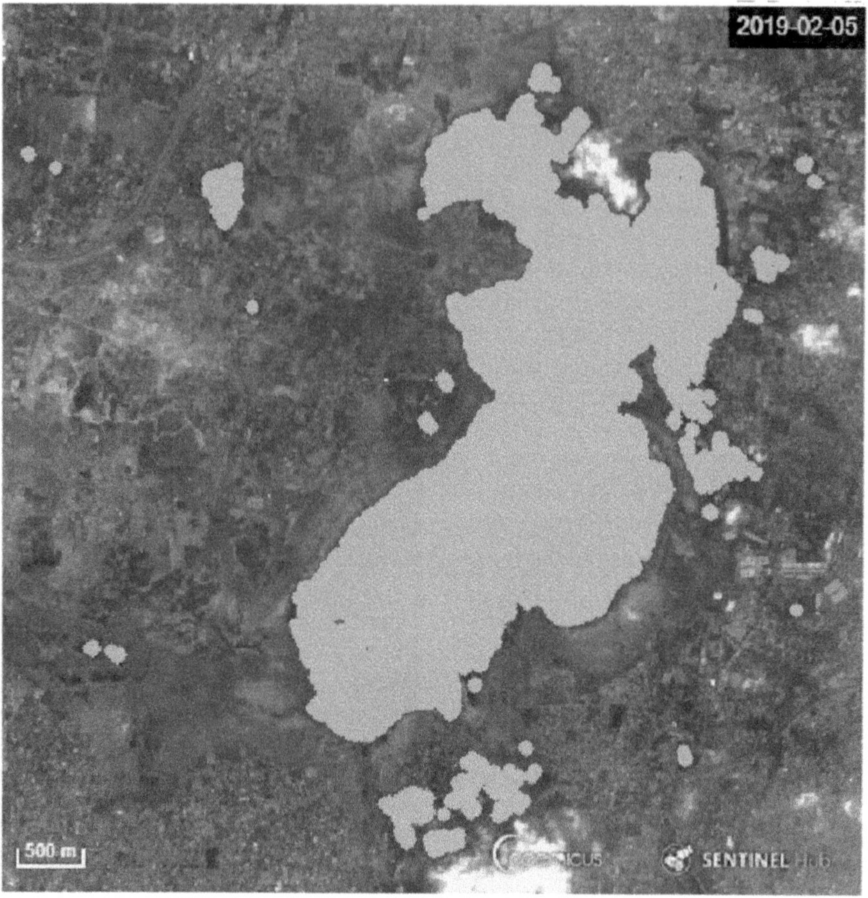

FIGURE 9.3   Segmentation using YCbCr of input image.

Color-based image segmentation is done in YCbCr color space for the same input-Pictures as shown in Figure 9.3.

9.6.1   OUTPUT

As shown in Figure 9.4, the differences and the area calculated in months by our algorithm and plotted in a bar graph (Figures 9.5 and 9.6).

The representation of how the image gets processed according to the Segmentation model and then gets segmented area for water. This result is compared with the original image as shown in Figure 9.7.

Histograms of unprocessed image and the processed image as shown in Figures 9.8 and 9.9.

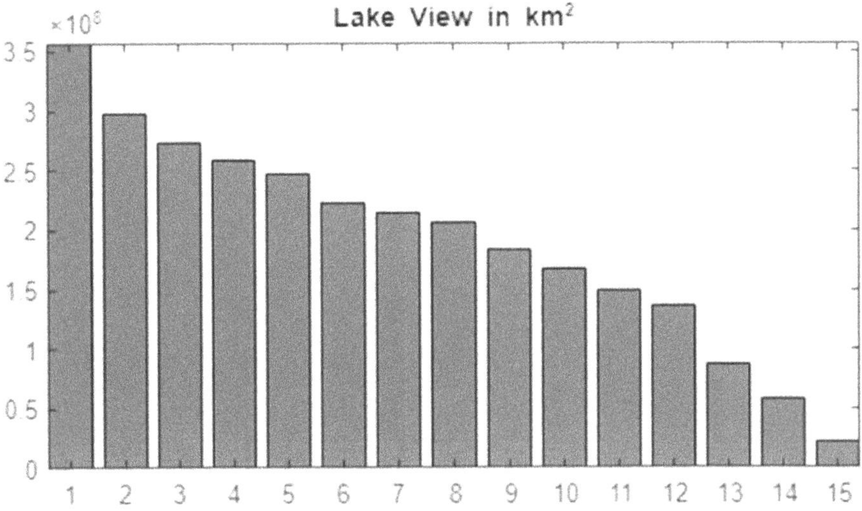

FIGURE 9.4   Bar graph of segmentation images area.

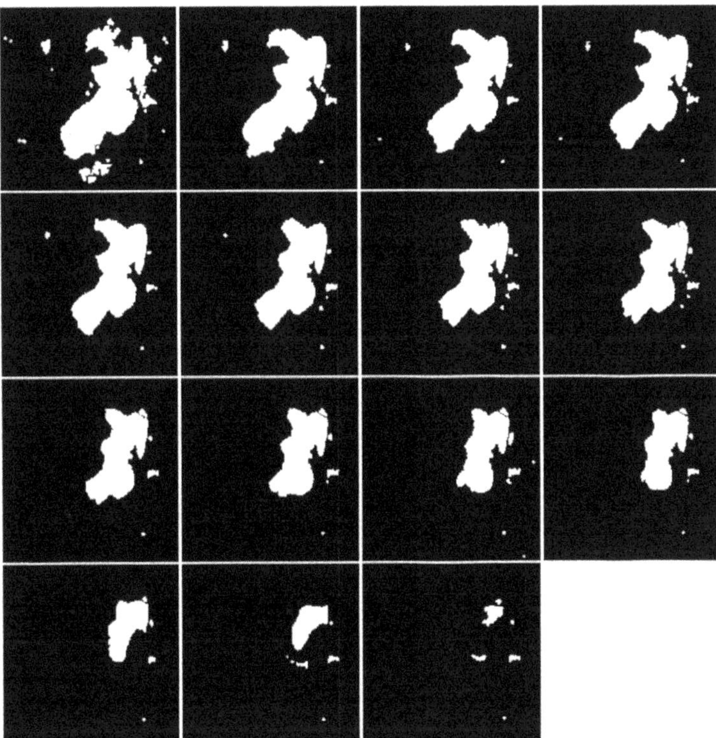

FIGURE 9.5   Segmentation images that represents our model dividing water from the land for each input data images.

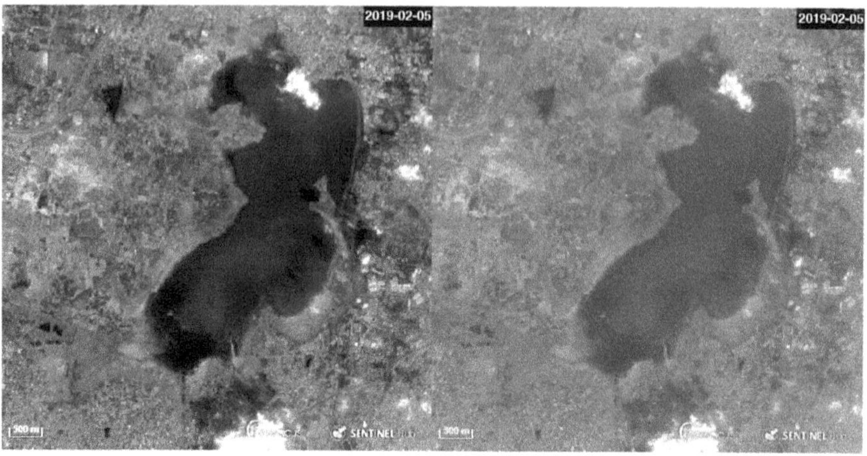

FIGURE 9.6   Processed image and unprocessed image..

Table 9.1 represents the distributed water bodies present in Figure 9.3 of the input data area in pixels for each prop present in image and total area in pixels is 53,136. This area in Pixels is converted into area in sq.km using the formula.

$$Area\ in\ Square\ kilometers = \left(\frac{41}{0.5}\right)^2 \tag{9.1}$$

Here, the images are taken at 0.5 km range so for every 0.5 km the image contains 41 Pixels. and area in sq.km is 357,286,464.

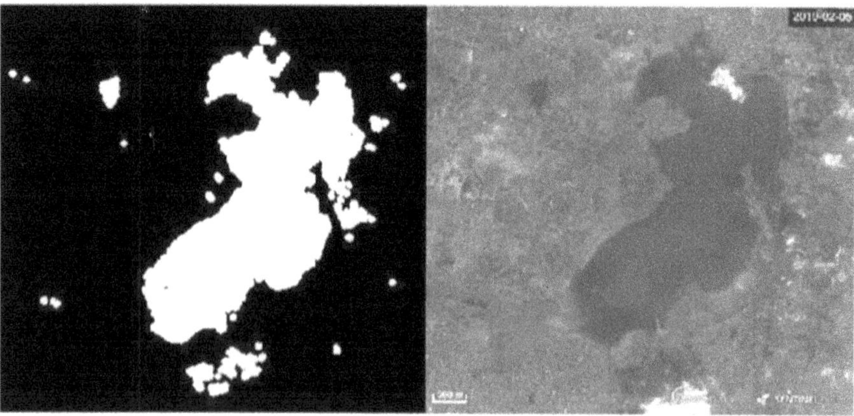

FIGURE 9.7   Segmentation of image.

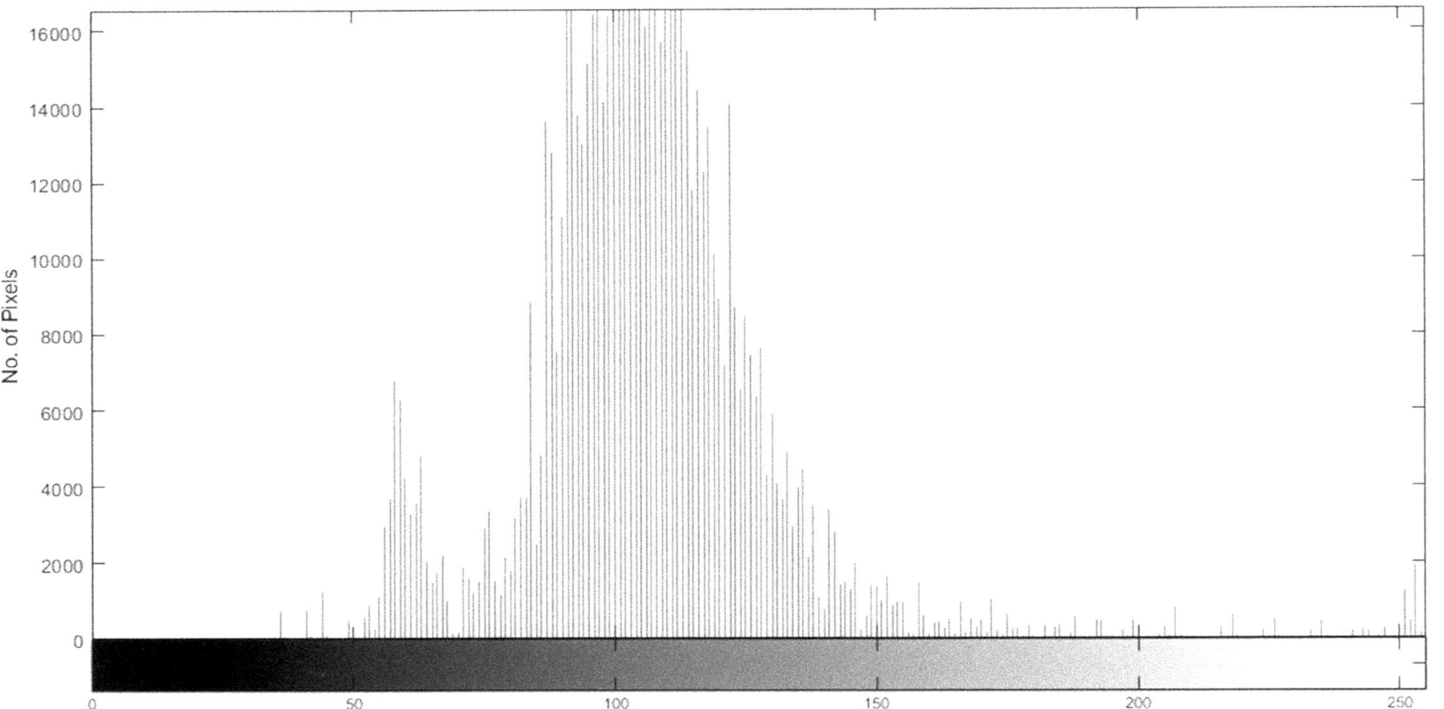

FIGURE 9.8 Histogram of unprocessed image.

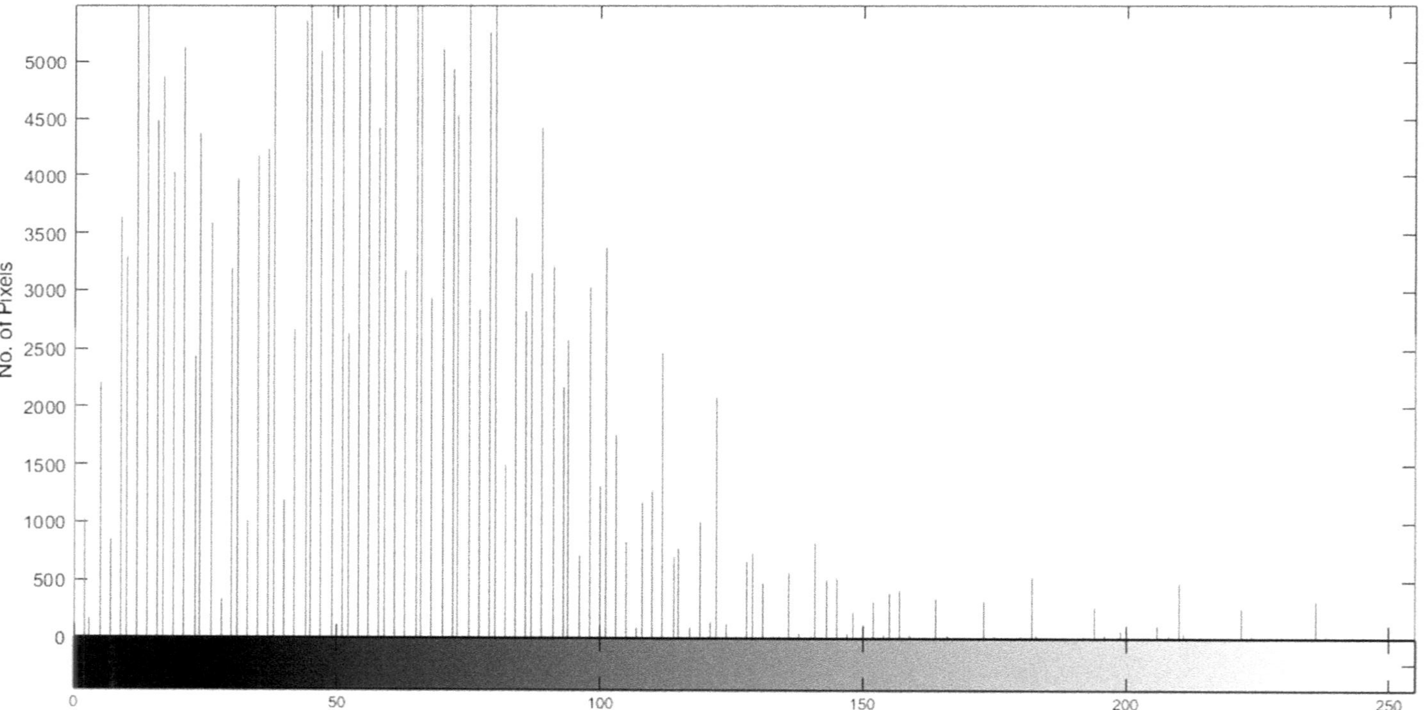

FIGURE 9.9　Histogram of processed image.

TABLE 9.1
Props in a Image vs Area of the Prop

Props	Area
1	64
2	49
3	77
4	113
5	723
6	49
7	48,177
8	2,163
9	110
10	334
11	100
12	64
13	64
14	248

The FCM algorithm based satellite imaging presents a comparable model to our project, utilizing an enhanced version of the Fuzzy C-Means algorithm for satellite image segmentation—an area of active research in recent years. Existing literature supports the notion that region segmentation yields improved outcomes, with human visual perception being deemed more effective than machine vision systems in extracting semantic information from images. The FCM algorithm in this model estimates parameters of prior probabilities and likelihood probabilities, employing segmentation for background and island extraction based on pixel intensity. The evaluation using peak signal to noise ratio (PSNR) demonstrates superior results compared to other methods. Despite its accuracy, the FCM algorithm is criticized for its sluggishness and heavy computational requirements. In contrast, our algorithm, a simple Image Segmenter based on basic MATLAB tools like Image Segmenter color thresholder and image batch processor and various color spaces, achieves segmentation results with 75–80% accuracy compared to FCM. While our method is faster, it maintains comparable accuracy to FCM, and in certain instances, it outperforms FCM in accuracy. After the model is prepared for the area in both algorithms, our algorithm can produce results in a few minutes, whereas FCM requires specialized computers and hours to calculate the segmentation area.

The research paper discusses the design and analysis of a satellite imaging-based system for drought analysis and climate change observations. The system utilizes satellite images captured over time and processes them using MATLAB and deep learning tools. It integrates historical climate data and trend analysis to assess long-term climate change impacts. The system outperforms a FCM algorithm-based satellite imaging model in terms of speed and accuracy. The results include bar charts representing the area of water bodies during the summer period and adjusted satellite images of lakes. The conclusion highlights the importance of satellite imaging technology in addressing drought and climate change challenges. A satellite imaging-based system for drought analysis and climate change observations. The system uses satellite images processed with MATLAB and deep learning tools to estimate water body drying and track climate changes. It integrates historical climate data and trend analysis for assessing long-term impacts. The system outperforms a FCM algorithm-based model in terms of speed and accuracy. The results include bar charts and adjusted satellite images of lakes. The conclusion emphasizes the significance of satellite imaging technology in addressing drought and climate change challenges.

9.6.2 Using AI to Improve Climate Models

AI has the potential to improve climate models by enhancing their precision and boosting predictive capabilities. Machine learning algorithms play a crucial role in scrutinizing historical climate data, discerning patterns, and unveiling intricate relationships within the information.

Precise weather forecasting is crucial for adapting to climate change and managing disasters effectively. Utilizing AI methodologies, including advanced deep learning algorithms, meteorologists can analyze extensive real-time weather data, significantly improving the accuracy of both short-term and long-term weather predictions. This enhanced precision enables more efficient responses to extreme weather events, ultimately minimizing their impact on susceptible communities.

9.7 CONCLUSION

In conclusion, the healthcare-focused system employing satellite imaging and advanced processing tools stands at the forefront of addressing the pressing challenges posed by droughts and climate change. Through its meticulous approach and validation processes, especially in assessing water level changes in Puzhal lake, Chennai, the system demonstrates both reliability and practical utility. Beyond its technological prowess, the incorporation of historical climate data and trend analysis enhances its capacity to provide long-term insights into climate change impacts. This holistic perspective contributes not only to immediate healthcare needs but also to a broader understanding of environmental sustainability. As we confront unprecedented environmental shifts, the adoption of such innovative technologies in healthcare applications not only offers tangible benefits for public health and infrastructure but also signals a proactive and informed approach toward navigating the complexities of our changing world.

The critical role of satellite imaging technology in addressing the challenges of drought and climate change. By providing a comprehensive framework for analysis and observation, the satellite imaging-based system holds the potential to revolutionize environmental management and policymaking, fostering a more resilient and sustainable future. This innovative approach goes beyond conventional methodologies, offering a comprehensive and technologically advanced means to address the complex intersection of environmental shifts and healthcare implications.

The meticulous methodology employed in this system, particularly its validation processes, sets it apart as a reliable and practically useful tool. A notable example of its effectiveness lies in its ability to assess water level changes in Puzhal lake, Chennai. By utilizing satellite imagery and advanced processing algorithms, the system can accurately monitor and analyze variations in water levels, providing critical information for drought prediction and management. This application not only showcases the reliability of the system but also highlights its potential impact on water resource management in vulnerable regions.

Moreover, the system's strength lies not only in its technological prowess but also in its incorporation of historical climate data and trend analysis. By considering long-term climate patterns and trends, the system enhances its capacity to provide valuable insights into the broader impacts of climate change. This holistic perspective is crucial for understanding the evolving dynamics of environmental conditions, contributing not only to immediate healthcare needs but also to a more comprehensive comprehension of environmental sustainability.

The assessment of water level changes in Puzhal lake, Chennai, is emblematic of the system's ability to address immediate healthcare concerns stemming from droughts. Beyond this, the incorporation of historical climate data enables the system to project and analyze the long-term consequences of climate change on water resources, ecosystem health, and community well-being. This forward-thinking approach positions the system as a proactive tool, capable of informing policy decisions and guiding adaptive strategies to mitigate the multifaceted impacts of climate change.

Satellite imaging technology emerges as the linchpin in this endeavor, playing a critical role in addressing the challenges posed by droughts and climate change. The system's comprehensive framework for analysis and observation harnesses the power of satellite imagery to provide real-time data and actionable insights. This transformative potential extends beyond localized applications, signaling a broader impact on environmental management and policymaking.

As societies grapple with unprecedented environmental shifts, the adoption of innovative technologies in healthcare applications becomes imperative. The satellite imaging-based system not only offers tangible benefits for public health and infrastructure but also represents a proactive and informed approach to navigating the complexities of our changing world. By fusing cutting-edge technology with a holistic understanding of environmental dynamics, this system stands as a beacon for resilience, sustainability, and adaptability in the face of the formidable challenges posed by climate change. In essence, it represents a paradigm shift toward a more informed, responsive, and sustainable future.

9.8   FUTURE SCOPE

AI-driven solutions for monitoring drought and analyzing climate change impacts in healthcare systems offer promising future prospects. These technologies can enhance early detection of drought conditions, allowing for proactive measures and resource allocation. In healthcare, AI can assist in predicting and mitigating the health effects of climate change, such as the spread of vector-borne diseases and heat-related illnesses. It includes further refinement of predictive models using machine learning algorithms, integration of real-time data from various sources like satellites and sensors, and the development of user-friendly interfaces for decision-makers in healthcare and environmental sectors. Collaborations between AI experts, climate scientists, and healthcare professionals will be crucial for advancing these solutions and creating a comprehensive approach to address the complex challenges posed by climate change.

The future scope of AI-driven solutions for monitoring drought and analyzing climate change impacts in healthcare systems is immensely promising, ushering in a new era of proactive, data-driven strategies. These technologies hold the potential to revolutionize the way we approach environmental challenges and healthcare preparedness, offering a range of opportunities for further advancements. One key aspect of the future scope involves the continuous refinement of predictive models through the utilization of advanced machine learning algorithms. As technology evolves, there is a growing need to enhance the accuracy and efficiency of AI models in predicting drought conditions, understanding climate change impacts, and foreseeing potential health consequences. Ongoing research and development in machine learning will contribute to the creation of more sophisticated and adaptive models that can provide timely and precise insights. Another crucial facet is the integration of real-time data from diverse sources, including satellites and ground sensors. The incorporation of up-to-the-minute information into AI models enhances their responsiveness and ensures that decision-makers have access to the most current data. Satellite imagery, in particular, plays a pivotal role in monitoring environmental changes, and ongoing advancements in remote sensing technologies will further enrich the quality and granularity of data available for analysis.

The development of user-friendly interfaces tailored for decision-makers in healthcare and environmental sectors is an essential component of the future trajectory. As these AI-driven solutions become integral to decision-making processes, it is crucial to design interfaces that are intuitive, accessible, and provide actionable insights. User-friendly interfaces facilitate effective communication between AI systems and human decision-makers, ensuring that the wealth of information generated is translated into informed actions and policies.

REFERENCES

1. Berhan, G., Hill, S., Tadesse, T., Atnafu, S. 2011. Using satellite images for drought monitoring: A knowledge discovery approach. J Strateg Innov Sustain, 7(1):135–153.
2. Chaudhari, S., Sardar, V., Rahul, D. S., Chandan, M., Shivakale, M. S., 27–29 August 2021, Performance analysis of CNN, AlexNet and VGGNet models for drought prediction using satellite images. https://doi.org/10.1109/ASIANCON51346.2021.9545068.
3. Orimoloye, P. I. R. 2021. Satellite-based application in drought disaster assessment using terra MOD13Q1 data across free state province, J Environ Manag, 285(1 May), 11211.
4. Balajee, J., Saleem Durai, M. A. 2022. Retracted Article: Drought prediction and analysis of water level based on satellite images using deep convolutional neural network. Int J Speech Technol, 25, 615–623. https://doi.org/10.1007/s10772-021-09850-y
5. Siswanto, B. P., Wardani, K. K. 2022. Satellite-based meteorological drought indicator to support food security in Java Island, PLOS One, 17(6), 1–20. https://doi.org/10.1371/journal.pone.0260982

6. Himansh, S. K. 2015. Monitoring of drought using satellite data. *Int Res J Earth Sci*, 3(1), 66–72.

7. Wu, T., Zheng, W., Yin, W., Zhang, H. 2021, Spatio-temporal characteristics of drought and driving factors based on the GRACE-derived total storage deficit index: A case study in southwest China. *Remote Sens.*, 13, 79. https://doi.org/10.3390/rs13010079.

8. Fadaei-Kermani, E., Ghaeini-Hessaroeyeh, M. 2020. Fuzzy nearest neighbor approach for drought monitoring and assessment. Appl Water Sci, 10, 130. https://doi.org/10.1007/s13201-020-01212-4.

9. Chaudhari, S., Sardar, V., Ghosh, P. 2023. Drought classification and prediction with satellite image-based indices using variants of deep learning models. Int J Inf Technol, 15, 3463–3472. https://doi.org/10.1007/s41870-023-01379-4.

10. Wei, W., Zhang, J., Zhou, L., Xie, B., Zhou, J., Li, C. 2021. Comparative evaluation of drought indices for monitoring drought based on remote sensing data. Environ Sci Pollut Res, 28(16), 20408–20425.

11. Gaur, R., Prakash, S., Prasad, L. N., Kumar, S., Abhishek, K., Guduri, M. 2023. A secure and efficient scheme based on unlinkability and anonymous traceable protocol for cloud-assisted IoT environment. *Journal of Circuits, Systems and Computers*, 32(18), 2350316.

12. Sardar, V. S., Yindumathi, K. M., Chaudhari, S. S., Ghosh, P. 2021. Convolution neural network-based agriculture drought prediction using satellite images. In: 2021 IEEE Mysore sub section international conference (MysuruCon). IEEE, pp. 601–607.

13. Liu, Q., Zhang, S., Zhang, H., Bai, Y., Zhang, J. 2020. Monitoring drought using composite drought indices based on remote sensing. Sci Total Environ. 711, 134585. https://doi.org/10.1016/j.scitotenv.2019.134585.

14. Arkeman, Y., Buono, A., Hermadi, I. 2017. Satellite image processing for precision agriculture and agroindustry using convolutional neural network and genetic algorithm. In: IOP conference series: earth and environmental science, 54(1), 012102. https://doi.org/10.1088/1755-1315/54/1/012102

15. AghaKouchak, A., Farahmand, A., Melton, F. S., Teixeira, J., Anderson, M. C., Wardlow, B. D., Hain, C. R. 2015. Remote sensing of drought: Progress, challenges and opportunities. Rev Geophys, 53(2), 452–480.

16. Himanshu, S. K., Singh, G., Kharola, N. 2015. Monitoring of drought using satellite data. Int Res J Earth Sci, 3(1), 66–72.

17. Habibie, M. I., Ahamed, T., Noguchi, R., Matsushita, S. 2020. Deep learning algorithms to determine drought prone areas using remote sensing and GIS. In: 2020 IEEE Asia-Pacifc conference on geoscience, electronics and remote sensing technology (AGERS). IEEE, pp 69–73.

18. Kumar, S., Arya, S., Jain, K. 2022. A SWIR-based vegetation index for change detection in land cover using multi-temporal Landsat satellite dataset. Int J Inf Technol, 14, 1–14. https://doi.org/10.1007/s41870-021-00797-6

19. Huang, J., Zhang, S., Yang, F., Yu, T., Prasad, L. N., Guduri, M., Yu, K. 2023. Hypergraph-based interference avoidance resource management in customer-centric communication for intelligent cyber-physical transportation systems. IEEE Trans Consum Electron 70(1), pp 1775–1786.

20. Kumar, C. A., Sheela, K. A. 2022. Real-time emotional analysis from a live webcam using deep learning, 2022 3rd International Conference for Emerging Technology (INCET), Belgaum, India, pp. 1–5, https://doi.org/10.1109/INCET54531.2022.9824894.

21. Kumar, C. A. and Sheela, K. A. 2021. Emotion recognition from facial biometric system using deep convolution neural network (D-CNN). In: Saran, V.H., Misra, R.K. (eds) Advances in Systems Engineering. Lecture Notes in Mechanical Engineering. Springer, Singapore. https://doi.org/10.1007/978-981-15-8025-3_37.

22. Chakraborty, C., Rodrigues, J. J. C. P. 2020. A comprehensive review on device-to-device communication paradigm: Trends, challenges and applications. Wireless Pers Commun, 114, 185–207. https://doi.org/10.1007/s11277-020-07358-3.
23. Kishor, A., Chakraborty, C. 2022. Artificial intelligence and internet of things based healthcare 4.0 monitoring system. Wireless Pers Commun 127, 1615–1631. https://doi.org/10.1007/s11277-021-08708-5.
24. Wu, Y., Guo, H., Chakraborty, C., Khosravi, M. R., Berretti, S., Wan, S., 2023, Edge computing driven low-light image dynamic enhancement for object detection. IEEE Trans Netw Sci Eng, 10(5), 3086–3098. https://doi.org/10.1109/TNSE.2022.3151502.
25. Dwivedi, R., Dey, S., Chakraborty, C., Tiwari, S., 2021, Grape disease detection network based on multi-task learning and attention features. IEEE Sens J, 21(16), 17573–17580. https://doi.org/10.1109/JSEN.2021.3064060.

10 Fortifying Healthcare Cybersecurity

A Sturdiness-Based Approach to Threat Modeling and Risk Analysis

*Mallellu Sai Prashanth, Seetha Srujana,
Uma Maheswari V., Rajanikanth Aluvalu,
Manisha Guduri, and Martin Margala*

10.1 INTRODUCTION

Cybersecurity has emerged as a critical concern in virtually every sector of modern society, and the healthcare industry is no exception. In recent years, the rapid integration of digital technologies, electronic health records (EHRs), connected medical devices, and telemedicine platforms has transformed the healthcare landscape. While these advancements have brought numerous benefits, they have also introduced new vulnerabilities and threats that can compromise patient data, disrupt medical services, and even endanger lives. As the healthcare sector becomes increasingly reliant on interconnected systems and data exchange, the need for robust and comprehensive cybersecurity measures becomes paramount to ensure the confidentiality, integrity, and availability of sensitive healthcare information [1].

In today's increasingly digitized healthcare landscape, the challenge of ensuring robust cybersecurity has taken center stage. Healthcare systems worldwide have made significant strides in leveraging technology to improve patient care, streamline operations, and enhance medical research. However, this digital transformation has also opened the door to a multitude of cybersecurity threats that can jeopardize patient privacy, disrupt medical services, and compromise sensitive medical data. One of the paramount challenges in healthcare cybersecurity is the intricate web of interconnected devices and systems that form the backbone of modern medical facilities. From EHRs and telemedicine platforms to medical Internet of Things (IoT) devices and diagnostic equipment, the healthcare ecosystem has become highly interdependent on technology. While this interconnectivity offers unprecedented convenience and efficiency, it also creates numerous entry points for cyberattacks. Malicious actors can exploit vulnerabilities in any part of the network, potentially gaining unauthorized access to patient records or disrupting critical medical operations [2].

Patient privacy is another critical concern in healthcare cybersecurity. Medical records contain an array of sensitive information, including personal identification details, medical histories, and treatment plans. Breaches in cybersecurity can lead to the unauthorized exposure of this private data, leading to identity theft, insurance fraud, or even blackmail. Moreover, as the healthcare industry increasingly adopts telemedicine and remote patient monitoring, ensuring the secure transmission and storage of patient data across digital channels becomes paramount. In recent years, the healthcare sector has witnessed a rise in targeted cyberattacks, often driven by financial motives. Ransomware attacks, for instance, have become a pressing threat where attackers encrypt critical medical data and demand hefty ransoms for its release. Such incidents can lead to significant disruptions in patient care, as medical professionals lose access to vital information needed for diagnosis and treatment [3].

Furthermore, the rapid pace of technological innovation in healthcare has sometimes outpaced the development of robust cybersecurity measures. Medical devices and software systems are designed to be user-friendly and interoperable, but security considerations can sometimes take a back seat. This lack of standardized security protocols across various healthcare technologies leaves room for vulnerabilities that attackers can exploit.

Smart contracts, built on blockchain technology, have emerged as a powerful tool with the potential to revolutionize various industries, including cybersecurity. Solidity, a programming language designed for writing smart contracts on the Ethereum blockchain, offers a unique avenue for enhancing cybersecurity practices. These contracts enable the execution of automated, trustless, and tamper-proof agreements, and their application in cybersecurity introduces innovative approaches to threat modeling, risk analysis, and mitigation strategies. At the heart of Solidity-based smart contracts lies their ability to create decentralized and immutable systems. Traditional cybersecurity measures often rely on centralized authorities and databases, making them susceptible to single points of failure and unauthorized access. In contrast, smart contracts operate on a decentralized network of nodes, ensuring data integrity through consensus mechanisms. This decentralized nature inherently reduces vulnerabilities associated with centralization, making Solidity-based smart contracts an attractive candidate for safeguarding sensitive healthcare data and critical infrastructure [4].

One notable application of Solidity-based smart contracts in enhancing cybersecurity is their role in threat modeling. Threat modeling is a proactive process of identifying potential vulnerabilities and risks within a system. Smart contracts can facilitate this process by allowing the systematic representation of threats through data structures like structs and mappings. Information about threats, their descriptions, and associated risk levels can be securely stored on the blockchain, enabling real-time and transparent access to threat information. This not only assists in accurate threat assessment but also empowers stakeholders to collaboratively analyze and address emerging cybersecurity risks. Moreover, the programmability of Solidity-based smart contracts enables the automation of risk analysis, a critical component of effective cybersecurity. By defining risk assessment algorithms within the contract code, organizations can ensure consistent and standardized risk evaluations.

These evaluations can be triggered automatically based on predefined conditions or manual inputs. As a result, the subjectivity and inconsistency often associated with manual risk assessments are minimized, leading to more reliable and data-driven decision-making processes [5].

While Solidity-based smart contracts offer promising solutions for threat modeling and risk analysis, they also hold the potential for dynamic risk mitigation. Through blockchain's transparent and auditable nature, the execution of risk mitigation strategies can be recorded and verified in real-time. For instance, in the context of healthcare cybersecurity, a smart contract could trigger automated responses, such as isolating compromised systems or notifying relevant stakeholders, based on predefined risk thresholds. This proactive approach to risk mitigation could significantly reduce response times and minimize the potential impact of cyberattacks.

10.2 RELATED WORK

A comprehensive review of existing literature on healthcare cybersecurity and related technologies reveals the growing concern over the vulnerabilities and threats faced by the healthcare industry in the digital age. Healthcare systems are increasingly relying on digital infrastructure, EHRs, and interconnected devices to provide efficient patient care. However, this digital transformation has introduced new challenges related to data breaches, unauthorized access, and potential disruptions to critical medical services [6].

Researchers have highlighted the importance of safeguarding sensitive patient information and maintaining the integrity of medical data. With the rise of IoT devices in healthcare, concerns have emerged regarding the security of connected medical devices, which could potentially be exploited by malicious actors to compromise patient safety and privacy. Various studies have explored the potential risks associated with IoT devices, emphasizing the need for robust cybersecurity measures to prevent unauthorized access and data breaches. Blockchain technology has emerged as a promising solution to enhance healthcare cybersecurity. Blockchain's decentralized and tamper-resistant nature offers potential benefits in ensuring data integrity, secure sharing of medical records, and enabling patient-centric control over their health information. Research in this area has investigated the application of blockchain for secure patient identity management, secure data sharing among healthcare providers, and improving the transparency and traceability of pharmaceutical supply chains [7].

Moreover, the adoption of telemedicine and mobile health (mHealth) applications has expanded the attack surface for cyber threats. Studies have pointed out vulnerabilities in telemedicine platforms, including privacy concerns related to video consultations and the potential for eavesdropping. The proliferation of mHealth apps has raised questions about data privacy and the security of personal health information transmitted over mobile networks. In the context of threat modeling and risk analysis, researchers have proposed methodologies to systematically identify and assess cybersecurity threats specific to the healthcare domain. These approaches aim to prioritize vulnerabilities, evaluate potential impacts, and develop strategies for risk mitigation. The integration of risk assessment frameworks within healthcare organizations has been explored as a means to proactively manage cybersecurity risks and allocate resources effectively [8].

Despite the advancements in healthcare cybersecurity research, several challenges persist. The rapid pace of technological innovation often outpaces security measures, creating a continuous need for adaptive strategies. Additionally, the human factor remains a critical consideration, as healthcare staff's awareness and adherence to cybersecurity best practices are essential for maintaining a secure environment [9].

The use of blockchain technology and smart contracts in healthcare security has emerged as a promising solution to address various challenges and vulnerabilities within the healthcare industry. With the increasing digitization of healthcare data and the growing importance of patient privacy and data integrity, blockchain-based approaches offer novel ways to enhance security, transparency, and efficiency. Blockchain, as a decentralized and immutable ledger, provides a secure and tamper-proof platform for storing and managing sensitive healthcare information. In traditional healthcare systems, patient data is often scattered across various centralized databases, making it susceptible to breaches and unauthorized access. Blockchain technology offers a distributed architecture where each data transaction is cryptographically linked and recorded in a way that ensures transparency and trust. This decentralized nature of blockchain minimizes the risk of a single point of failure and unauthorized alterations, mitigating potential security breaches [10].

Smart contracts, which are self-executing and self-enforcing contracts with predefined rules and conditions, further enhance healthcare security by automating and streamlining various processes. In the context of healthcare, smart contracts can facilitate secure and transparent management of patient consent, data sharing, and access controls. For instance, patients can grant specific healthcare providers access to their medical records through smart contracts, ensuring that only authorized entities can retrieve and update the data [11]. This not only enhances patient privacy but also reduces administrative complexities and potential errors. One of the critical challenges in healthcare security is the interoperability of various systems and platforms. Blockchain technology can address this challenge by providing a standardized framework for data exchange and sharing across different stakeholders, such as hospitals, clinics, insurers, and research institutions. Smart contracts can facilitate secure data sharing and streamline processes like claims processing and billing by automatically verifying and executing predefined conditions. This not only reduces the likelihood of fraud and errors but also improves the efficiency of healthcare operations [12].

Furthermore, blockchain-based solutions can enhance the traceability and authenticity of pharmaceutical products and medical devices throughout the supply chain [13]. By recording each transaction and movement on the blockchain, stakeholders can track the provenance of medications, ensuring that counterfeit or substandard products do not enter the market [14]. This level of transparency and traceability is crucial for patient safety and regulatory compliance. Despite these potential benefits, it's important to acknowledge some challenges and considerations associated with the adoption of blockchain and smart contracts in healthcare security [15]. These include concerns about scalability, regulatory compliance, interoperability with existing systems, and the need for robust data privacy mechanisms. As the technology continues to evolve and mature, collaborations between blockchain developers, healthcare providers, policymakers, and regulators are essential to address these challenges and unlock the full potential of blockchain-based healthcare security solutions [16–19].

10.3 PROPOSED WORK

The architecture contains the following functions (Figure 10.1).

10.3.1 ADDTHREAT():

The addThreat function is a crucial part of the HealthcareCybersecurity smart contract, responsible for enabling users to input new threat information into the contract's storage. This function plays a pivotal role in maintaining an updated and comprehensive record of potential cybersecurity risks within the healthcare sector. Let's delve into the details of the addThreat function and its significance within the contract. The addThreat function is designed to receive three parameters: threatId, description, and riskLevel. These parameters collectively encapsulate the essential attributes of a cybersecurity threat. The threatId serves as a unique identifier for each threat,

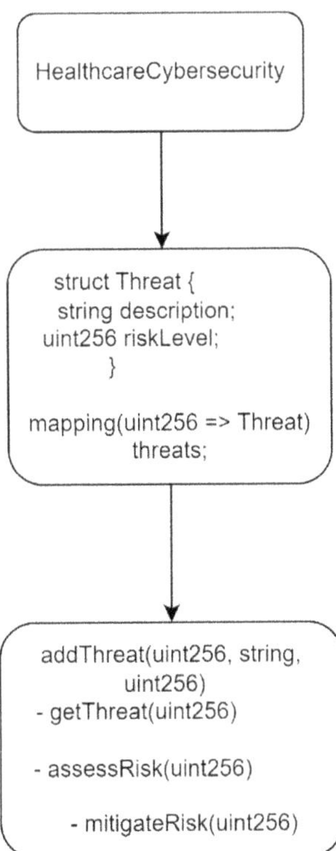

FIGURE 10.1 Architecture diagram of HealthcareCybersecurity smart contract.

allowing for easy retrieval and referencing. The description parameter provides a textual overview of the threat, describing its nature, potential impact, and any relevant contextual details. Lastly, the riskLevel parameter quantifies the severity or likelihood of the threat materializing, aiding in risk assessment and prioritization.

Upon receiving these parameters, the addThreat function proceeds to create a new instance of the Threat struct. This struct is specifically defined within the contract to accommodate the description and riskLevel properties, ensuring a consistent and organized representation of threat information. The newly created Threat struct is populated with the provided description and riskLevel. Subsequently, the function employs the threatId as a key to access the threats mapping—a crucial data structure that associates each unique threatId with its corresponding Threat struct. By utilizing the threatId as an index, the function establishes a clear linkage between the threat's identifier and its associated information, facilitating efficient retrieval and management.

The addThreat function concludes by persistently storing the newly created Threat struct within the threats mapping. This action ensures that the threat's details are securely recorded on the blockchain, establishing a tamper-resistant and transparent repository of cybersecurity threat information. In essence, the addThreat function serves as an entry point for users to contribute vital cybersecurity insights to the HealthcareCybersecurity contract. By capturing threat descriptions and risk assessments, the function empowers healthcare professionals and stakeholders to collaboratively contribute to the ongoing enhancement of healthcare cybersecurity measures. Moreover, the recorded threats can be subsequently accessed, evaluated, and addressed through other functions provided by the contract, promoting a comprehensive approach to healthcare cybersecurity management.

10.3.2 ASSESSRISK():

The assessRisk function within the HealthcareCybersecurity smart contract is a crucial piece of the overall architecture, as it plays a pivotal role in evaluating the potential risk associated with a specific healthcare cybersecurity threat. This function takes a threatId as its parameter and returns a string that categorizes the risk level of the corresponding threat. At its core, the purpose of the assessRisk function is to provide insights into the severity of a given threat based on the risk level associated with that threat. The risk level is stored within the threats mapping, which is a fundamental data structure in the contract. This risk level is an integer value that signifies the perceived seriousness of the threat, with higher values indicating greater potential harm or damage.

The function begins by retrieving the threat information associated with the provided threatId from the threats mapping. This information includes both the textual description of the threat and the numerical risk level assigned to it. By accessing this data, the function gains a comprehensive understanding of the threat's attributes. The assessment process takes place within a series of conditional statements. The function compares the risk level of the threat against predefined thresholds to determine the appropriate risk category. Specifically, it checks whether the risk level is greater than or equal to certain values to classify the threat's severity.

These thresholds define the boundaries for categorizing the risk levels into different classes: "High risk," "Medium risk," and "Low risk."

If the threat's risk level is found to be equal to or greater than 7, the function categorizes the threat as "High risk." This signifies that the threat is deemed particularly severe and demands immediate attention and potentially extensive mitigation measures. Similarly, if the risk level falls between 4 and 6 (inclusive), the threat is classified as "Medium risk," indicating a moderately concerning situation that requires a certain level of response. On the other hand, if the threat's risk level is less than 4, the function concludes that the threat is of a relatively low severity and categorizes it as "Low risk." This suggests that the threat is not currently posing a significant danger and may require less immediate action. It is important to note that the risk thresholds and the corresponding risk classifications provided by this function are predefined within the contract's logic. These classifications can serve as initial guidelines for determining the urgency of addressing different threats, but in practice, they may need to be adjusted based on the specific context and evolving cybersecurity landscape.

In summary, the assessRisk function is a pivotal component of the HealthcareCybersecurity contract, offering a mechanism to gauge the potential risk associated with healthcare cybersecurity threats. By analyzing the risk level of a threat and categorizing it into distinct classes of severity, this function contributes to informed decision-making and helps guide subsequent actions to manage and mitigate cybersecurity risks effectively.

10.3.3 getThreat():

The getThreat function within the HealthcareCybersecurity smart contract serves a crucial role in providing users with access to specific threat information stored within the contract's mapping. Designed to enhance transparency and facilitate informed decision-making, the function enables individuals to retrieve essential details about a particular cybersecurity threat based on its unique threat identifier. Upon invoking the getThreat function with the desired threatId parameter, the contract undertakes a sequence of actions to furnish the user with pertinent information. The function commences by accessing the threats mapping, which acts as a repository for the Threat structs. It retrieves the corresponding Threat struct associated with the provided threatId.

The retrieved Threat struct encapsulates two fundamental attributes: the threat's description and its assigned risk level. The description property offers a concise yet informative narrative outlining the nature and characteristics of the cybersecurity threat under consideration. This narrative elucidates the potential vulnerabilities and hazards that the threat poses within the context of healthcare cybersecurity. Simultaneously, the riskLevel property quantifies the severity of the identified threat. The risk level serves as a critical metric for evaluating the potential impact and likelihood of the threat materializing into a cybersecurity incident. This quantification allows stakeholders to prioritize their responses and allocate resources effectively to address and mitigate the identified threat.

The getThreat function, acting as a transparent window into the contract's threat data, consolidates these salient attributes into a coherent response. When invoked, the function assembles the description and riskLevel components from the retrieved Threat struct and returns them as a pair, allowing users to gain immediate insights into the specific threat's nature and risk implications. By providing a comprehensive overview of the threat in question, the getThreat function equips users with the essential knowledge required to make informed decisions regarding risk management, response strategies, and the allocation of resources. This function, in conjunction with the broader functionalities of the HealthcareCybersecurity smart contract, contributes to enhancing the overall cybersecurity posture within healthcare environments, thereby safeguarding sensitive data, promoting secure practices, and fostering a proactive approach to addressing potential threats.

10.3.4 MITIGATERISK():

The mitigateRisk function within the HealthcareCybersecurity smart contract serves a crucial role in the broader context of managing healthcare cybersecurity threats. While the function is currently a placeholder, its intended purpose is to implement a robust and effective risk mitigation strategy in response to identified threats. In the realm of healthcare, where the security and confidentiality of sensitive patient data are paramount, having a well-defined risk mitigation process is of utmost importance. In practice, the mitigateRisk function would encompass a series of actions and measures designed to neutralize or minimize the potential impact of a cybersecurity threat. These actions could encompass a wide range of strategies, all aimed at maintaining the integrity and security of healthcare systems and patient information. Given the diversity and complexity of potential threats, the function's implementation could vary significantly based on the specific risks encountered and the level of preparedness required.

For example, in the event of a high-risk threat, the mitigateRisk function might trigger an immediate response, such as alerting system administrators and designated personnel. This alert could initiate a cascade of actions, including temporarily disabling affected services, isolating compromised systems, and launching a thorough forensic analysis to identify the source and nature of the breach. Additionally, the mitigateRisk function could lead to the implementation of enhanced security measures, such as strengthening access controls, deploying intrusion detection systems, or initiating incident response plans. Depending on the severity of the threat and the potential consequences, it might also involve notifying relevant regulatory bodies or legal authorities in compliance with data protection regulations.

10.4 RESULTS

Creating a robust strategy for threat modeling and risk analysis in healthcare cybersecurity necessitates following a methodical process to recognize, evaluate, and eliminate possible risks. Working together with IT departments, cybersecurity specialists, and medical professionals to guarantee a thorough grasp of potential risks. Sort data according to classifications like private, sensitive, and public while taking into account the possible consequences of a breach on patient privacy and healthcare operations. Install systems for security information and event management (SIEM) to collect and examine security data.

The interface prominently features options for adding and updating medical records, granting and revoking access, and viewing authorized records (Figure 10.2). Access controls are visually represented, emphasizing the secure and patient-centric nature of the system. The design prioritizes user experience, ensuring a user-friendly environment for managing sensitive medical information on the blockchain.

The user interface for the "addThreat" function in the provided Solidity code could consist of a form allowing authorized users to input relevant details for a new threat record (Figure 10.3). This could include fields such as the threat identifier, description, timestamp, and any other pertinent information. Upon submission, the interface triggers a transaction to the Ethereum blockchain, invoking the "addRecord" function in the smart contract. Access control mechanisms ensure that only authorized users can utilize this functionality, promoting security and privacy in managing threat-related information.

The assessRisk function for evaluating the risk associated with a patient's medical record. The User Interface (UI) includes input fields for specifying the patient's details and a button to trigger the assessRisk function (Figure 10.4). The result, possibly a risk assessment score or relevant information, is likely displayed on the interface. This functionality can aid healthcare professionals in quickly assessing the risk level associated with a patient's medical history stored on the blockchain.

The interface includes a user-friendly display where authorized users can interact with the blockchain to retrieve threat-related information. The "getThreat" function, embedded in the backend, allows users with proper access permissions to seamlessly view threat-related records. The UI emphasizes security and user control, ensuring that only authorized individuals can retrieve and review threat data, and promoting transparency and privacy in the medical records system (Figure 10.5).

The interface includes a user-friendly design with input fields for relevant parameters, such as risk level, mitigation strategy, and affected assets. Users can interact with the interface to trigger the mitigateRisk function, allowing for the proactive management of risks within the smart contract (Figure 10.6). The UI provides real-time feedback on the mitigation process, enhancing the user experience and facilitating effective risk management in blockchain applications.

Users can securely add, update, and grant/revoke access to their medical records. However, potential threats may include unauthorized access attempts, requiring robust security measures (Figure 10.7). The UI should incorporate features to detect and prevent unauthorized actions, such as multi-factor authentication, secure login protocols, and real-time activity monitoring. This ensures the integrity and confidentiality of sensitive medical information, safeguarding against potential threats in the blockchain-based medical records system implemented by the smart contract.

10.5 CONCLUSION

In conclusion, the "HealthcareCybersecurity" Solidity smart contract serves as a rudimentary framework for managing cybersecurity threats within the healthcare domain. The contract employs a structured approach to storing, retrieving, and assessing threat information, with the potential for implementing risk mitigation strategies. However, while the contract provides a foundation for addressing healthcare cybersecurity

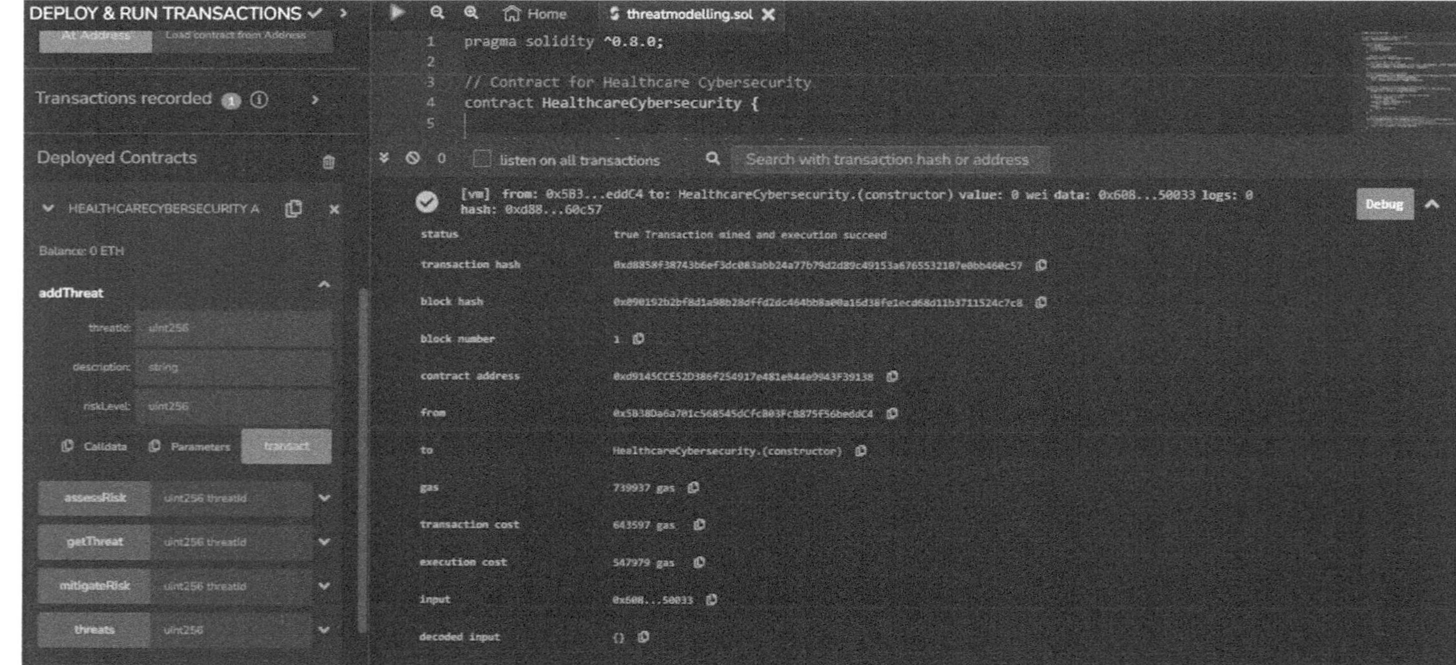

FIGURE 10.2 Threat interface for the risk analysis for healthcare system.

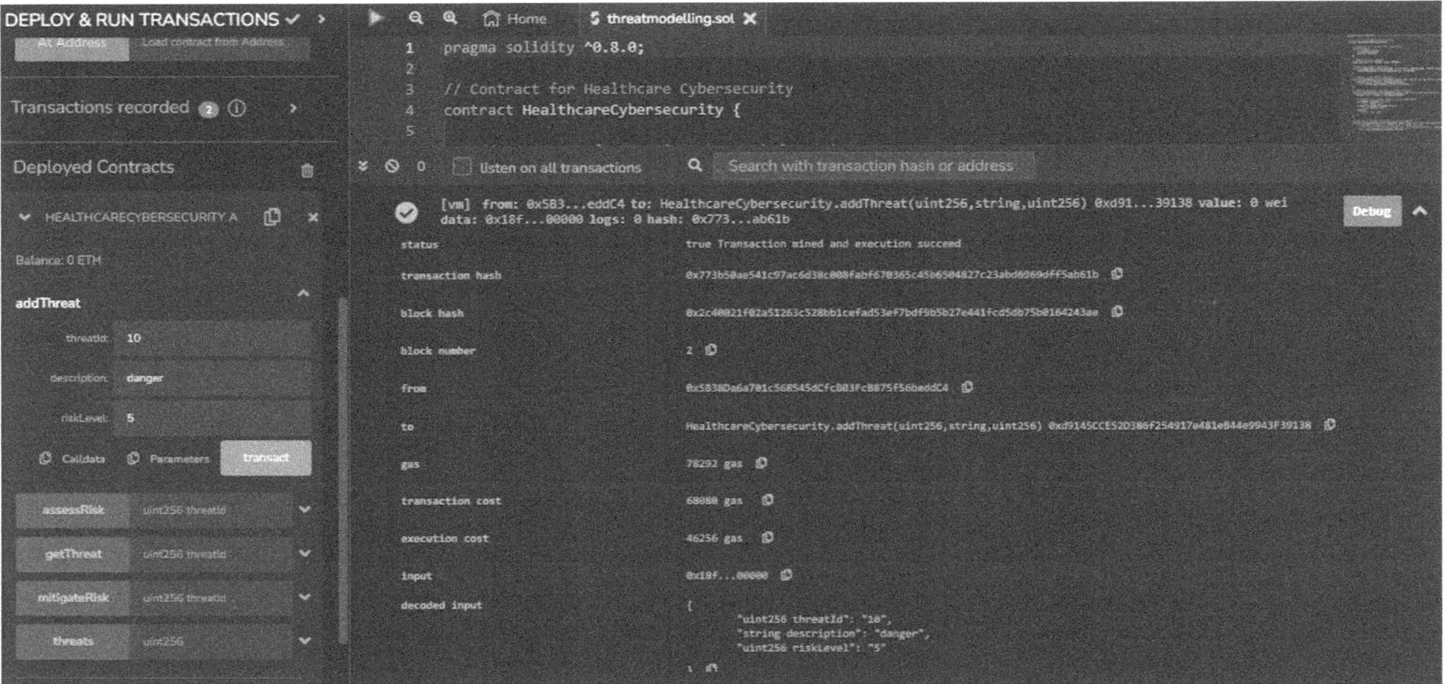

FIGURE 10.3 Specification of the addThreat function in Healthcare Cybersecuirty System.

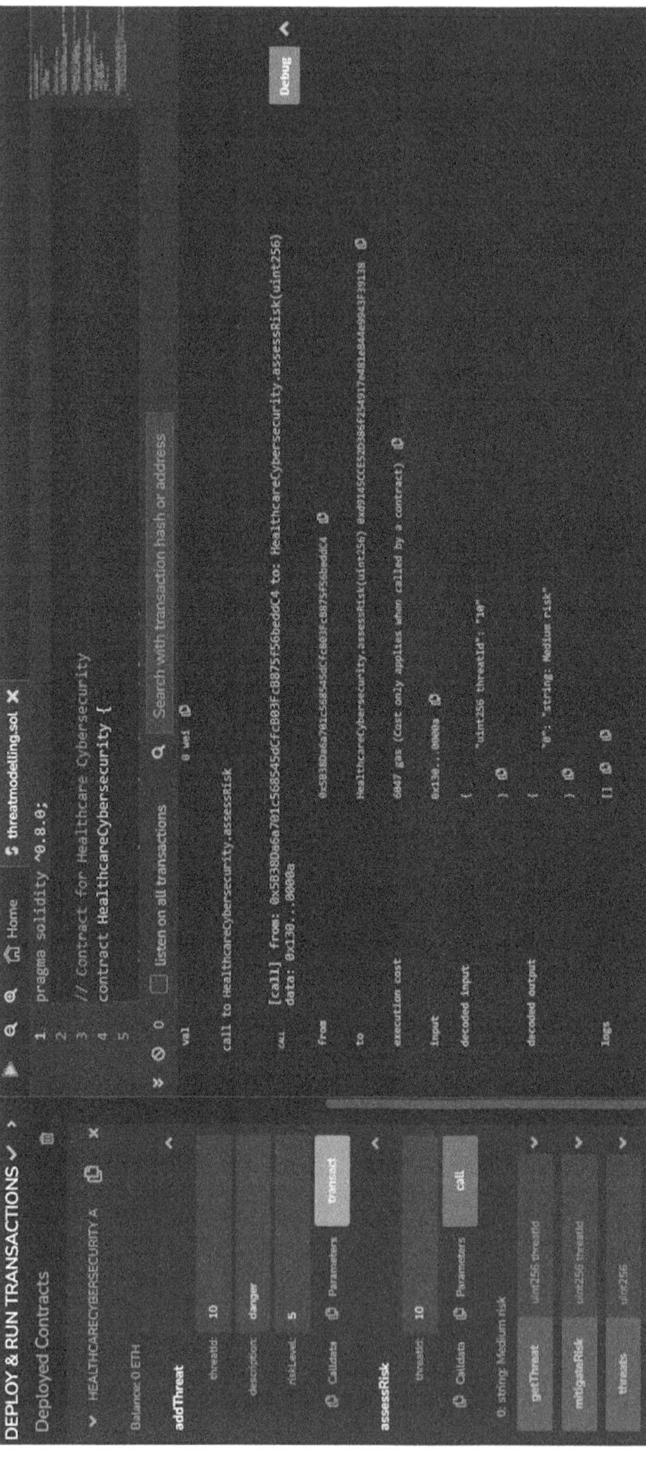

FIGURE 10.4 Running the transaction of assessRisk function.

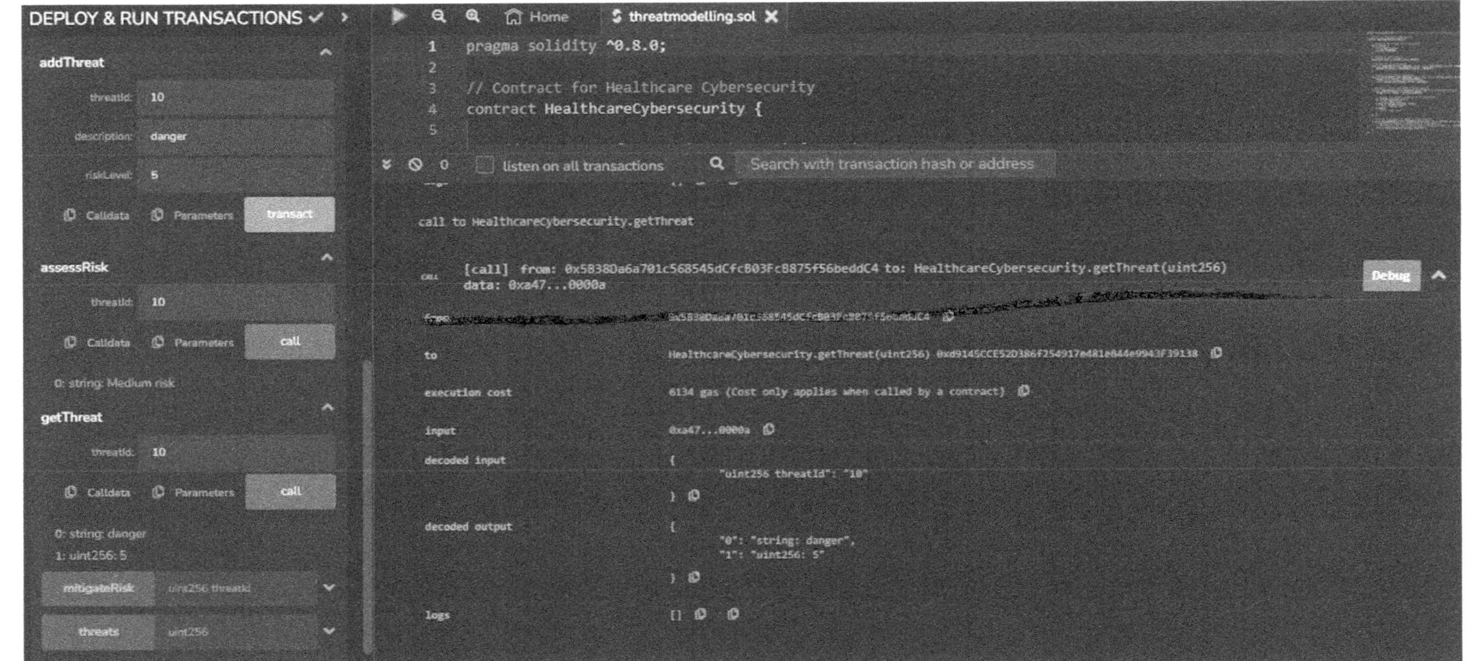

FIGURE 10.5   Understanding of the getThreat function.

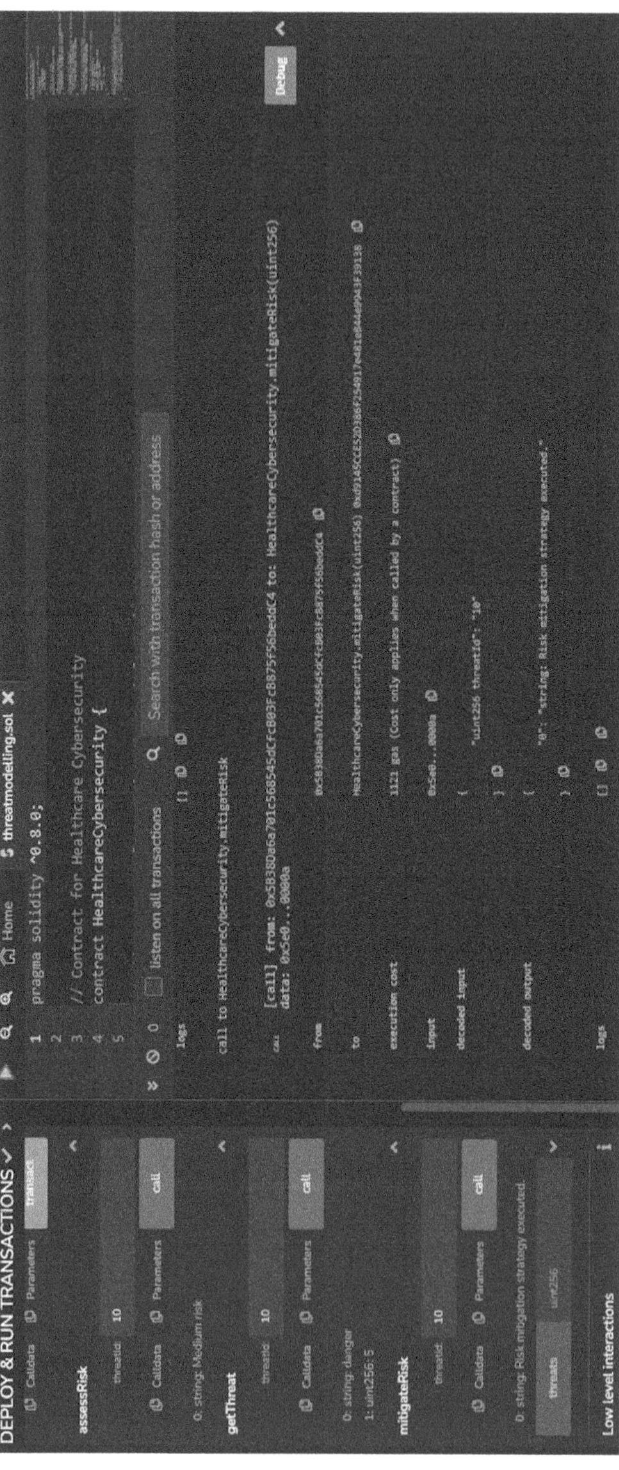

FIGURE 10.6 Deployment of the mitigateRisk function.

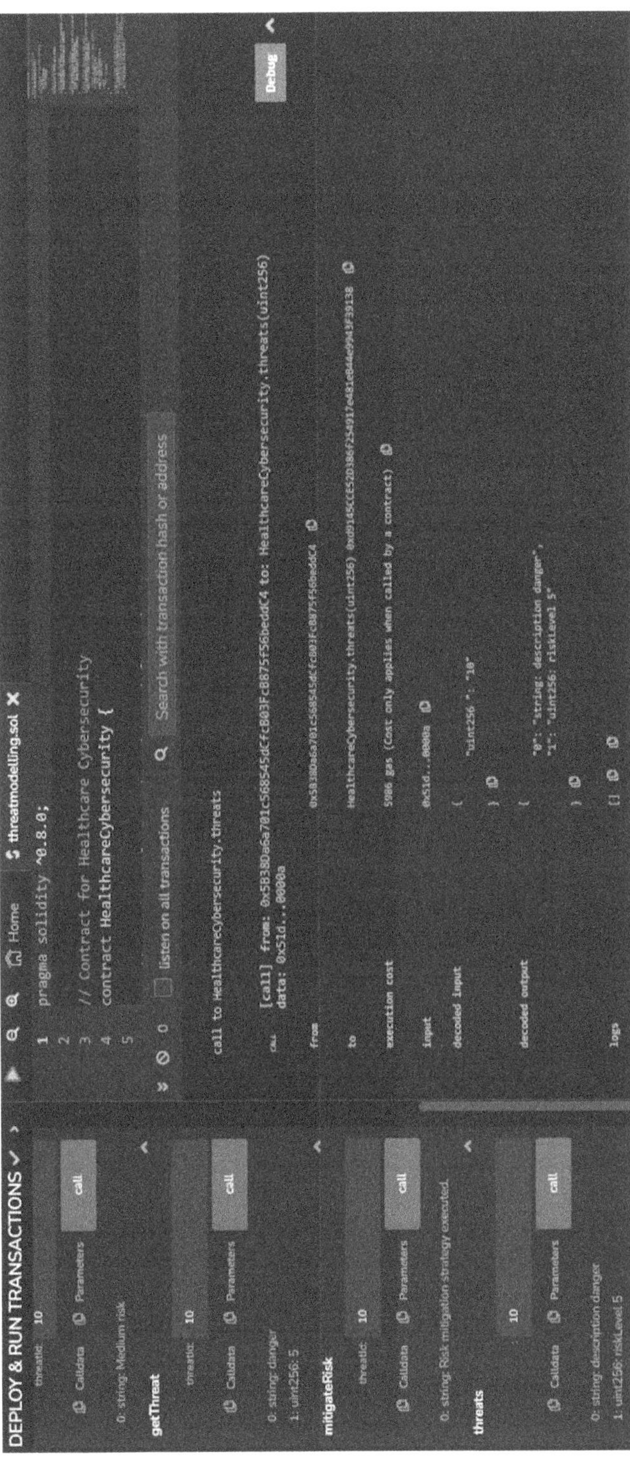

FIGURE 10.7 Running and access of threats function.

concerns, several critical considerations and potential enhancements should be noted. Firstly, the contract establishes a "Threat" struct that encapsulates essential attributes of a threat, including its description and risk level. This struct serves as the core data unit within the contract, facilitating the organized storage and retrieval of threat-related information. The utilization of a mapping, named "threats," enhances the efficiency of threat management by associating each threat with a unique identifier. This design enables users to seamlessly add new threats using the "addThreat" function, providing the threat's ID, description, and risk level. However, the contract's simplicity highlights an important limitation—there is no mechanism to prevent duplicate threat IDs or to update threat details once they are added. Addressing these issues would be crucial for maintaining accurate and up-to-date threat information. The contract also introduces functions to assess and mitigate risks. The "assessRisk" function evaluates the risk level of a given threat and categorizes it into "High risk," "Medium risk," or "Low risk" based on predefined thresholds. Notably, this risk assessment mechanism is fixed and lacks the flexibility to accommodate dynamic or evolving risk factors. Furthermore, the "mitigateRisk" function currently lacks an actual risk mitigation strategy, functioning merely as a placeholder. Implementing a comprehensive risk mitigation logic, such as sending alerts, triggering security measures, or notifying administrators, is imperative to bolster the contract's real-world utility. It is important to emphasize that the contract's scope is intentionally narrow, focusing solely on threat storage, retrieval, and preliminary risk assessment. In a practical healthcare cybersecurity scenario, additional layers of complexity would be necessary to ensure the integrity, confidentiality, and availability of sensitive data. Critical considerations include role-based access control, encryption, secure authentication mechanisms, and detailed risk analysis methodologies. In summary, while the "HealthcareCybersecurity" contract provides a basic blueprint for managing healthcare-related cybersecurity threats, it is an initial step in a broader and more intricate process. Enhancements are required to address potential duplicates, support threat updates, enable dynamic risk assessment, and implement substantive risk mitigation strategies. The contract's simplicity underscores the importance of augmenting its functionality to align with the multifaceted and evolving landscape of healthcare cybersecurity.

10.6 FUTURE SCOPE

The concept of enhancing healthcare cybersecurity through Solidity-based threat modeling and risk analysis holds promising potential for addressing the growing challenges of securing sensitive patient data and critical healthcare infrastructure. By employing blockchain technology and smart contracts, this innovative approach opens the door to a multitude of future enhancements that could significantly fortify the healthcare industry's cybersecurity landscape. In this envisioned future, the application could evolve to incorporate advanced machine learning algorithms and artificial intelligence (AI) capabilities. These additions would enable the system to automatically detect and classify emerging threats based on historical data and real-time patterns, enhancing the accuracy and efficiency of risk assessment. The integration of AI-driven anomaly detection could facilitate the early identification of suspicious activities, triggering proactive responses to mitigate potential breaches.

Furthermore, the system could be extended to support interoperability with other healthcare systems and institutions. Through secure data-sharing mechanisms enabled by blockchain, hospitals, clinics, insurance providers, and other stakeholders could collaboratively contribute threat data and collectively benefit from the accumulated insights. This cooperative approach to cybersecurity could lead to a stronger, more resilient defense against evolving cyber threats. As the system matures, the implementation of decentralized identity solutions could also be explored. Leveraging blockchain's capabilities for managing verifiable credentials, patients, healthcare professionals, and administrators could establish secure digital identities, reducing the risks associated with unauthorized access and identity theft. Such a framework could lay the foundation for secure access controls and granular permission management within the healthcare ecosystem. In addition, smart contracts could be enhanced to not only assess and mitigate risks but also trigger automated responses. For instance, in the event of a detected high-risk threat, smart contracts could dynamically activate predefined security measures, such as isolating affected systems, alerting designated personnel, or even temporarily restricting access until the threat is resolved. To cater to the evolving regulatory landscape, the system could be designed to ensure compliance with healthcare data protection regulations, such as the Health Insurance Portability and Accountability Act (HIPAA) in the United States or the General Data Protection Regulation (GDPR) in the European Union. Integration with legal and compliance frameworks could streamline audits and ensure that the cybersecurity measures align with industry standards. Lastly, the ongoing development of user-friendly interfaces and data visualization tools could empower healthcare professionals and administrators to comprehend threat landscapes more intuitively. Real-time dashboards, interactive graphs, and contextualized insights could facilitate informed decision-making and expedite responses to potential threats. In conclusion, the future scope of enhancing healthcare cybersecurity through Solidity-based threat modeling and risk analysis is vast and brimming with opportunities. By embracing advancements in AI, interoperability, decentralized identity, automated responses, compliance, and user interfaces, this approach has the potential to elevate healthcare cybersecurity to unprecedented levels of effectiveness and resilience, safeguarding critical patient information and infrastructure against the relentless tide of cyber threats.

REFERENCES

1. Griggs, K. N., Ossipova, O., Kohlios, C. P., Baccarini, A. N., Howson, E. A., and Hayajneh, T., Healthcare blockchain system using smart contracts for secure automated remote patient monitoring, *Journal of Medical Systems*, vol. 42, 7, 130–138, Jul. 2018.
2. Parizi, R. M., Homayoun, S., Yazdinejad, A., Dehghantanha, A., and Choo, K. K. R., Integrating privacy enhancing techniques into blockchains using sidechains, in IEEE Canadian Conference of Electrical and Computer Engineering (CCECE) (2019), pp. 1–4
3. Kumar, A., Krishnamurthi, R., Nayyar, A., Sharma, K., Grover, V., and Hossain, E., A novel smart healthcare design, simulation, and implementation using healthcare 4.0 processes, *IEEE Access*, vol. 8, 118433–118471, 2020, DOI: 10.1109/ACCESS.2020.3004790.

4. Hegde, P., and Maddikunta, P. K. R., Amalgamation of blockchain with resource-constrained IoT devices for healthcare applications – State of art, challenges and future directions, *International Journal of Cognitive Computing in Engineering*, vol. 4, 220–239, 2023, ISSN 2666-3074.

5. Abdellatif, A. A., Samara, L., Mohamed, A., et al. Medge-chain: Leveraging edge computing and blockchain for efficient medical data exchange. *IEEE Internet of Things Journal*, vol. 8, 21, 15762–15775, 2021.

6. Aich, S., Sinai, N. K., Kumar, S., Ali, M., Choi, Y. R., Joo, M. I. and Kim, H. C. "Protecting personal healthcare record using blockchain & federated learning technologies." in 2022 24th International Conference on Advanced Communication Technology (ICACT). IEEE, 2022.

7. Tedeschi, P., Al Nuaimi, F. A., Awad, A. I., and Natalizio, E., Privacy-aware remote identification for unmanned aerial vehicles: Current solutions, potential threats, and future directions, *IEEE Transactions on Industrial Informatics*, DOI: 10.1109/TII.2023.3280325.

8. Sumathi, M., Vijayaraj, N., Raja, S. P. R., and Rajkamal, M. Internet of thing based confidential healthcare data storage, access control and monitoring using blockchain technique. *Computing and Informatics*, vol. 41, 5, 1207–1239, 2022.

9. Dwivedi, S. K., Amin, R., and Vollala, S. Blockchain based secured information sharing protocol in supply chain management system with key distribution mechanism. *Journal of Information Security and Applications*, 54, 102554, 2020.

10. Deng, W., Huang, T., and Wang, H. A review of the key technology in a blockchain building decentralized trust platform. *Mathematics*, 11, 1, 101, 2022.

11. Ren, K., Loghin D., et al., Interoperability in blockchain: A survey, *IEEE Transactions on Knowledge and Data Engineering*, DOI: 10.1109/TKDE.2023.3275220.

12. Cai, L., Li, Q., and Liang, X., Introduction to blockchain basics. Advanced Blockchain Technology: Frameworks and Enterprise-Level Practices. Singapore: Springer Nature Singapore, 2022, 3–43.

13. Hemanta, K. B. and Chinmay, C., Explainable machine learning for data extraction across computational social system, *IEEE Transactions on Computational Social Systems*, 2022, DOI: 10.1109/TCSS.2022.3164993

14. Chinmay C., Senthil M. N., Ganesh G. D., Ramana, T. V., and Rajanikanta, M., Intelligent AI-based healthcare cyber security system using multi-source transfer learning method, *ACM Transactions on Sensor Networks*, 1–16, 2023, DOI: doi.acm.org?doi=3597210

15. Diwakar, M., Shankar, A., Chakraborty, C., et al., Multi-modal medical image fusion in NSST domain for internet of medical things, *Multimedia Tools and Applications*, 2022, DOI: 10.1007/s11042-022-13507-6

16. Manisha, M., Chinmay, C., Maheswari, U., and Maragala, M., Blockchain-based federated learning technique for privacy preservation and security of smart electronic health records, *IEEE Transactions on Consumer Electronics*, 1–11, 2023, DOI: 10.1109/TCE.2023.3315415

17. Mahesh, T. R., Geman, O., Margala, M., and Guduri, M., The stratified k-folds cross-validation and class-balancing methods with high-performance ensemble classifiers for breast cancer classification. *Healthcare Analytics*, 4, 100247, 2023.

18. Huangs, J., Zhang, S., Yang, F., Yu, T., Prasad, L. N., Guduri, M., and Yu, K., Hypergraph-based interference avoidance resource management in customer-centric communication for intelligent cyber-physical transportation systems. *IEEE Transactions on Consumer Electronics*, 70, 1, 1775–1786, 2023.

19. Gaur, R., Prakash, S., Prasad, L. N., Kumar, S., Abhishek, K. and Guduri, M., A secure and efficient scheme based on unlinkability and anonymous traceable protocol for cloud-assisted IoT environment. *Journal of Circuits, Systems and Computers*, 32, 18, 2350316, 2023.

Index

For Product Safety Concerns and Information please contact our EU
representative GPSR@taylorandfrancis.com
Taylor & Francis Verlag GmbH, Kaufingerstraße 24, 80331 München, Germany